Cash's Textbook of Neurology
for Physiotherapists

Cash's Textbook of Neurology for Physiotherapists

edited by
PATRICIA A. DOWNIE FCSP

with a Foreword by
Dame Cicely Saunders DBE, FRCP
Chairman, St Christopher's Hospice, London

fourth edition

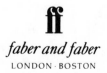

faber and faber
LONDON · BOSTON

First published in 1974
by Faber and Faber Limited
Reprinted 1975, 1976
Second edition 1977
Reprinted 1979
Third edition 1982
Fourth edition 1986

Printed in Great Britain by
Butler and Tanner Ltd
Frome and London

British Library Cataloguing in Publication Data

Cash's textbook of neurology for physiotherapists.
—4th ed.
1. Nervous system—Diseases
I. Downie, Patricia A.
616.8   RC346

ISBN 0-571-13728-8

Contents

Contributors

Mrs H. W. Atkinson MCSP, HT, DipTP
Head of School and Principal Lecturer
Coventry (Lanchester) Polytechnic School of Physiotherapy
Priory Street, Coventry CV1 5FB

R. Birch Esq FRCS
Consultant Orthopaedic Surgeon, St Mary's Hospital *and*
The Royal National Orthopaedic Hospital
London

Miss R. Cartwright MCSP
Superintendent Physiotherapist, Chailey Heritage Hospital
North Chailey, Lewes, Sussex BN8 4EF

Professor C. A. Corr PhD
Professor in the School of Humanities
Southern Illinois University at Edwardsville
Edwardsville, Illinois 62026

Mrs D. M. Corr RN, BSN
Assistant Professor in the Nursing Faculty
St Louis Community College at Forest Park
St Louis, Missouri 63110

Miss P. M. Davies MCSP, DipPhysEd
Instructor, The Postgraduate Study Centre
Medical Department, Bad Ragaz, Switzerland

Miss A. Evans MCSP, ONC
Senior Physiotherapist, Midland Spinal Injuries Unit
Robert Jones and Agnes Hunt Orthopaedic Hospital
Oswestry, Shropshire SY10 7AG

Mrs S. Franklyn MCSP
Senior Physiotherapist
c/o The Parkinson's Disease Society
36 Portland Place, London WC1N 3DG

Dr F. W. Frazer MCSP, BA(Hons), PhD
District Physiotherapist, South Birmingham Health Authority
Selly Oak Hospital, Birmingham B29 6 JD

Dr R. B. Godwin-Austen MD, FRCP
Consultant Neurologist
Nottingham University Hospitals *and*
Derby Hospitals

Mrs B. Goff MCSP, ONC, DipTP
Formerly: Teacher, Oswestry and North Staffordshire
School of Physiotherapy
Robert Jones and Agnes Hunt Orthopaedic Hospital
Oswestry, Shropshire SY10 7AG

C. Grant Esq FRCS
Senior Registrar, Department of Orthopaedics
St Mary's Hospital, London

D. A. Hill Esq BSc, MCSP, DipTP
Head of Department of Occupational Therapy and Physiotherapy
University of Ulster at Jordanstown
Newtownabbey, Co Antrim BT37 0QB

Dr G. P. Hosking MB, MRCP, DCH
Consultant Paediatric Neurologist
The Ryegate Centre and The Children's Hospital
Sheffield S10 5DD

Dr G. L. Kidd MSc, PhD
Senior Lecturer in Physiology, Director, BMR Research Unit
Department of Physiology, University of Liverpool

Miss J. M. Lee BA, MCSP, DipTP
Course Leader, (Physiotherapy) Department of Health and
Community Studies
Teesside Polytechnic, Middlesborough TS1 3BA

Dr P. D. Lewis DSc, MD, MRCP, FRCPath
Reader in Histopathology *and* Honorary Consultant Neurologist
The Royal Postgraduate Medical School *and*
Hammersmith Hospital London W12 0HS

Dr G. T. McCarthy MB, FRCP, DCH
Consultant Neuropaediatrician
Chailey Heritage Hospital *and*
The Royal Alexandra Hospital for Sick Children, Brighton

T. McSweeney Esq MC(NUI), MCH(ORTH), FRCS, FACS
Consultant Orthopaedic Surgeon
Robert Jones and Agnes Hunt Orthopaedic Hospital
Oswestry, Shropshire SY10 7AG

Mrs O. R. Nettles MCSP, ONC
25 Goffs Park Road, Crawley
Sussex RH11 8AX

Mrs B. O'Gorman MCSP
Superintendent Physiotherapist, St Christopher's Hospice
London SE26 6DZ

Dr D. J. Oliver BSc, MB, BS, MRCGP
Medical Director, The Wisdom Hospice
St Williams Way, Rochester
Kent ME1 2NU
(Previously Senior Registrar, St Christopher's Hospice)

Miss M. I. Salter MBE, MCSP
Formerly: Superintendent Physiotherapist, JSMRU
RAF Chessington KT9 2PY

Dame Cicely Saunders DBE, FRCP
Chairman, St Christopher's Hospice,
London SE26 6DZ

Miss C. Shumway BSc(Mass), RPT, MCSP, PGDip
Superintendent Physiotherapist
Cheyne Centre for Spastic Children
Cheyne Walk, London SW3 5LX

Dr J. M. Sutherland MD(Glas), FRCP(Edin), FRACP
Honorary Consultant Neurologist, Royal Brisbane Hospital
Honorary Reader in Neurology, University of Queensland
Honorary Neurologist, Toowoomba General Hospital

Miss J. M. Todd BSc, MCSP
Superintendent Physiotherapist The Wolfson Medical Rehabilitation Centre
Atkinson Morley's Hospital
London SW20 0NQ

Dr J. P. H. Wade BA, MD, MRCP
Senior Registrar, The National Hospital for Nervous Diseases
Queen Square, London WC1N 3BG

Foreword

by Dame Cicely Saunders DBE, FRCP

The aim of treatment and care for some patients with a neurological disease can be the restoration of full function and health. Here the physiotherapist is a vital member of a team with clear and optimistic goals. But for many who find themselves in the situations discussed in this textbook the aim will rather be to 'strengthen the things that remain', and to share with the patient in coming to terms with loss. Hardest of all for the team as well as for the patient will be the progressive deterioration of some diseases, the constant setting of short-term goals and the acceptance that even they become unrealistic. All have somehow to find the ability to adapt and develop in this situation also.

It is not only the patient who has to come to terms with what is happening but the whole family who have to face a new way of life. The entire therapeutic team may be called on in their different ways to give them the support they will need, whether it be in hospital, special unit or the patient's own home.

If physiotherapists are to play their full part in such a team they have to be secure in their own role, with confidence in their particular knowledge and skills. This textbook will be an essential resource for constant referral.

The knowledge available here will be a major help as all try to recognise and encourage both the strengths and the possibilities of the whole family, and the essential independence that can persist and grow even in the midst of dependence, whether it be, hopefully, a temporary need, or instead a whole new way of life.

Cicely Saunders

Chairman, St Christopher's Hospice
London SE26 6DZ

Editor's Preface

Sir Thomas Browne MD, a seventeenth-century writer, offered literary advice in a treatise entitled *To a Friend Intending a Difficult Work*:

> Think and think again on the work you intend; consider how strong your shoulders be; You must be a good swimmer, a Delian even, yet in this stormy sea swim not without a buoy;
> . . .
> Variety of wits, discord of studies, parties, heresies, divide the fates of the noblest productions; and you may fail to please them all, unless you are wise beyond Wisdom. . . .

An editor of a multi-author book is faced with problems not least of which is the control of the authors! In their exuberance to impart knowledge they heed not the guidelines: maximum lengths are exceeded - Oh! I didn't think you meant it (3000 words overlong); deadlines are passed - Oh! No one keeps to a deadline (now you know why books are delayed!). I could go on, but I find comfort in Sir Thomas Browne that even in those distant days the same problems arose. For this new edition I am grateful to all the contributors who co-operated to enable what is a radically revised edition to be assembled.

Disorders of the neurological system provide physiotherapists with a large percentage of their work. Neurophysiological advances have enabled the rationale of many of the techniques used to be better understood, and physiotherapists are now able to *select* from the *different* approaches those *particular* patterns which are most appropriate to the *individual* patient. This is re-iterated throughout the various treatment chapters.

At the same time therapists are reminded that while 'cure' is satisfying, 'caring always', even when the patient is visibly deteriorating as in motor neurone disease, can be even more richly satisfying. Charles and Donna Corr eloquently expand this theme, reminding us that 'we try to cure them [patients] because we care for them'. Indeed Lois Dyer (1982) has said that 'the traditional heavy emphasis on cure should change to that of care and support'. This notion of support is also reflected throughout the book and particularly that support which is needed to be given to relatives.

This radical revision has enabled me to invite new contributors thus bringing new slants on old themes – *plus ça change, plus c'est la même chose*. I have already expressed my grateful thanks to *all* the contributors, new and old. I am particularly grateful to Professor Charles Corr and his wife for the opening Chapter on *Developing a Philosophy of Caring* – they have experience in the hospice movement in the USA and are regular visitors to England, Dr Gillian McCarthy has wide experience of the interdisciplinary management of children with neurological disorders, and I thank her not only for her own chapters but also for generous advice. I was asked to include some advanced neurophysiology, and Dr Geoffrey Kidd accepted my invitation to write a chapter – he chose *The Myotatic Reflex* because he felt it was fundamental to a physiotherapist's understanding of so much of her work. His reputation as a lecturer at physiotherapy meetings is well-known, and I am sure that all readers will, like me, be appreciative of his willingness to provide a chapter to this book. As always, I say thank you to Mrs Audrey Besterman who has provided yet more illustrations – they do so enhance the text allowing the technicalities to be more readily absorbed by the reader. The Chinese were so right when they said 'One picture is better than a thousand words'. Friends United Press, Richmond, Indiana have kindly given permission for the inclusion of the verse on page 31.

Dame Cicely Saunders allowed herself to be persuaded to write a Foreword – she has always been a staunch supporter of physiotherapists and at present is President of the London branch of the Chartered Society of Physiotherapy. I have known her for many years and it gives me much pleasure to have her among the contributors to this book.

I end as I began with Sir Thomas Browne – whether I am 'wise beyond Wisdom' only the reader can decide but let me quote further:

> While you slave at this book, I would not have you think you are boiling asparagus. Rub out, restore, return to the anvil ... Pledging your time and labour to pure truth, yet watch that you study not your own small fame, while you claim to serve truth ...

P.A.D., 1985

REFERENCES

Browne, Sir Thomas. To a Friend Intending a Difficult Work. In Keynes, G. (ed.) (1964). *The Works of Sir Thomas Browne*, pp. 153–5 vol. 3. Faber and Faber, London.

Dyer, L. (1982). Professional development. *Physiotherapy*, **68**, 390–3.

Chapter 1

Developing a Philosophy for Caring

by C. A. CORR PhD *and* D. M. CORR RN, BSN

It is vitally important for care-givers to master the skills of their profession and to remain current with advances in scientific knowledge that bear upon the application of those skills. It is equally important for care-givers to attend to the obligations and values which are upheld by their profession, to the contexts within which they work, and to their own needs, both as practitioners and as human beings. The new edition of this book is a fine resource principally for the former sort of continuing education. This chapter is an effort to contribute especially to the latter work, the self-reflection on principles, goals, needs, and their practical interaction. In particular, this chapter will outline elements that might be considered appropriate to the development of a working philosophy for caring, one that takes into account interpersonal relationships in care-giving, potential sources of stress, and ways of minimising or managing dis-stress in caring.

AN APPROACH TO CARING

Any approach to caring will be defined by the obligations which it respects and by the values which it embodies. These are, respectively, the criteria whereby it discriminates 'right' from 'wrong', on the one hand, and 'good' from 'bad' on the other hand. Our obligations are expressed in the principles or means according to which our actions are guided; our values are the ultimate goals or ends which we seek to foster. Let us consider each of these in turn as they apply to our present purposes, first in themselves and then in terms of the concept of 'rehabilitation'. As we do this, we will propose some obligations and values which we support, but we recognise that our primary responsibility here is to stimulate individual reflection rather than to advance our own convictions.

Obligations and principles

An old medical adage urges any health care system or practitioner 'to cure sometimes, to comfort often, to care always'. Those whose professional work has to do with health care will be familiar with, and may often take part in, possibilities for cure. For many care-givers, effecting a cure represents an especially satisfying outcome for their efforts. We suspect, however, that cure is achieved only in a relatively small portion of cases. Certainly, many presenting conditions are not curable or are beyond the stage when they might have been susceptible to cure. In such circumstances, our obligations as health care professionals do not go away, they simply shift their character. To cure is usually one of the best ways to express comfort and care, but when the former is not possible the latter remain incumbent upon us.

We say this because curing is, or should be, essentially a species of comforting and caring. We do not care for people only in order to be able to cure them; we try to cure them because we care for them. Further, as the hospice movement has shown so well, comfort and care are not second-best alternatives to be left to less qualified professionals or amateurs (Saunders, 1976). In hospice, as in the whole of the health care system, health care practitioners should find their proper identities precisely as concerned givers of care. When Dyer (1982) says that 'the traditional heavy emphasis on cure should change to that of care and support', we believe this is because she recognises that the latter encompass the former, but not necessarily vice versa.

There are many ways in which ethical issues arise for professionals in the health care system (Sim, 1983). For example, care-givers are frequently reminded that the precept 'do no harm' (*primum non nocere*) is a more fundamental moral and professional obligation than the injunction to 'do good' (Jonsen, 1978). We do wish to do good to (or for) our patients, but it is even more important that we do not do harm (whether physically or in any other significant respect) to those we serve, whether through abandonment and a failure to act or through an ill-conceived, over zealous, or ill-timed intervention. Thus, it is better not to intervene at all than to make a bad situation worse through our ineptitude, just as it is better to do something useful (however minimal that may be) than to permit a bad situation to deteriorate to one that it is even less satisfactory. Both the doing of good and the avoidance of harm are embraced in the familiar Christian injunction to 'do unto others as you would have them do unto you'. And both are part – though only a part – of what it means to respect 'the patient as person', a familiar slogan in recent years and one that brings us to the value underpinnings of these putative obligations.

Values and goals

Respecting the patient as person calls upon us to regard patients as unique individuals and to see them in the totality of their being, with physical, psychological, social, and spiritual dimensions alike. But why should we value patients as persons? What is it about them that health care serves as its basic goal? We believe the personhood of patients is to be valued because it is as persons that we are all fellow human beings, fellow members of the human community. Further, it is as a person that each of us possesses the capacity to be an agent of creativity, to bring into existence moral, spiritual, social, and aesthetic value.

To use another language, human beings are to be respected, even in their weakness, vulnerability, limitation, and dependence, because human life is sacred. This is a way of saying that such life has intrinsic value, that it is not merely a utilitarian means to an end. At the same time, one can also say that human life is not an absolute or ultimate value. The sacrifice of human life for legitimate reasons, e.g. in martyrdom, on behalf of the lives of others, or in self-defence, is typically given religious credence in the light of what are taken to be higher or more ultimate values.

We neeed not pursue this discussion to draw the moral for health care practitioners. The end that they serve is not life itself, but health or well-being. Their task is to assist those they serve to achieve what has been called 'integrity' or a sense of wholeness. The meaning of this concept is paradoxical in some respects. For example, integrity is sometimes served by the surgical removal of a diseased organ. At other times, it is found in physical and psychological adjustment to a handicap or in learning to use an adaptive device to compensate for limitations in functional ability. In most instances, the full meaning of health or well-being goes beyond the mere absence of disease. In other cases, it can be compatible even with a chronic or terminal illness. In all circumstances, it is quality of life that we are finally discussing. This is not to dismiss quantity of life, which is normally the proximate goal that we seek. But it is to say that there is a more ultimate value in the qualitative order that can and should sometimes take precedence over mere prolongation of living (and of dying).

Rehabilitation

The word 'rehabilitation' is a familiar term in the vocabulary of professional care-givers and one that is particularly well known to physiotherapists. Etymologically, it means to restore to, or, to re-establish a previous privilege, rank, character, reputation, or condition. The root word here is 'habilitate', a term derived from the Latin that might be rendered as 'to capacitate', 'to qualify for', or 'to be endowed with ability'. More generally, this refers to the action of *enabling*, as in the modern German usage where 'habilitation' designates the process and its concluding dissertation (*Habilitationsschrift*) whereby one qualifies to teach at the university level.

In the universe of health care, it would appear that for some the term 'rehabilitation' carries as its primary meaning much the same connotation as cure. That is, it signifies the restoration to full functioning at a previous level or one that is taken as normative for the individual's age, sex, etc. This is a wholly desirable goal, one with which we have no quarrel when it is feasible and appropriate. But it should be evident that this 'strong' meaning of rehabilitation is beyond reasonable expectation for many individuals in our society. Many of these individuals can regain some degree of functioning, though not the full scope or efficiency which they formerly enjoyed. Some can achieve an equivalent, though not identical, level of functioning through some process of adaptation or correction. Others have simply lost the particular ability, and will need external compensation or support to the degree that it is an important one in their lives.

The point here is that the goal to be achieved is the root source from which all else follows. It is therefore of great importance to define and to articulate goals carefully, both for professional work in general and in the context of a particular case. What we identify as our goals will determine what we recognise as our obligations, and will govern our concrete decisions both as to actions which we choose to undertake and as to those which we choose to omit.

IMPLEMENTING THIS APPROACH

The work of care-givers takes place in interactions with fellow human beings. Three of the most important of these in implementing any approach to caring are interactions: with patients; with their families; and with colleagues, the care-giving team, the health care system, and society itself.

Interactions with patients

In consequence of the values suggested above, our primary concern in interactions with patients is to foster their individual autonomy. We take this to refer to the self-control and quality of living which every individual prizes. In the service of this end, two things are required: (1) we must meet people where they are; and (2) we must respect the 'little deaths' throughout life which they have already experienced or are currently experiencing (Purtilo, 1976). Meeting people where they are means that human beings are not just patients; they are multidimensional beings with individual needs. The practical meaning of 'quality of living' must be defined by each concrete individual, not by his or her care-givers. Further, each person who comes into our care will already have had a varied history of experiences with loss and grieving. These, too, affect present and projected quality in living.

Care-givers would do well, then, to begin by practising active listening, the condition for which is our willingness to make a gift of our presence both as caring human beings and as skilled professionals. Only in this way can care-givers come to know what the individual prizes as values or meanings in his or her own life. The process of recapitulating and reframing the significance of one's life from a new perspective has been called 'life review' in the elderly (Butler, 1963). But this is not exclusively a process of ageing since its main function is the establishment or re-establishment of meaning and value.

To fail to attend to very personal articulations of this sort is almost surely to blunder and to intrude upon the privacy and dignity of a competent person. This occurs, for example, when care-givers intervene where they are not wanted or when they fail to offer services that would be desired if their purpose and availability was appreciated. By contrast, we assist people to tell their own stories (Brady, 1979) when we offer not only our skills but also our humanity. That is why Downie (1983) has argued that often our most important response to a patient may be one of simply sitting down and listening to his or her concerns.

It is in this light, for example, that physiotherapy for the terminally ill has its place (Shanks, 1982), both as a service on behalf of quality in living and as a basis for important human interchanges. Even a passive exercise as simple as opposition maintains physical contact, bridges the gap of isolation and loneliness, and demonstrates that caring continues even when active treatment is no longer feasible.

Interactions with families

Most patients are not isolated entities, but integral parts of social units. This is seen perhaps most clearly in the case of young children who are embedded in family contexts and for whom parents are essential decision makers. The moral is that care for an individual will be inadequate if it does not simultaneously address the legitimate needs and productive resources of the human networks in which most human beings are engaged. Care-givers must not come between the members of such networks or take sides with families against their patients. Rather, the roles which challenge them are to serve as advocates for patients and as providers of support for both patients and families. This is an effort to re-create a mini-community to address the new needs of disease and disability. It calls for mobilising and guiding the individuals involved in a common effort. Once again, active listening is essential to discern weakness, vulnerability, and strength. Just as we ought not to limit our concern solely to a particular organ or biochemical system, in a similar way we cannot neglect family and other social dimensions of persons if we hope to maintain confidence and achieve optimal quality in living for those we serve. Of course, when there are conflicting interests, the primary responsibility of the care-giver is always to the patient first and foremost.

Interactions with colleagues, team, system, and society

The immediate end that we seek to achieve in conjunction with colleagues, the care-giving team, and the health care system on behalf of patients and families is co-ordination and continuity of care. This is not always easy when vulnerable and dependent people are involved, and when co-operation is required from many providers within a complex bureaucratic system. A suitable beginning can be found in a problem-solving technique that jointly determines plans, goals, and approaches. Further teamwork involves the sharing of skills, knowledge, and experiences. Such sharing is not lightly undertaken when assets have been acquired only after great expenditure of time and energy, or when professional and disciplinary boundaries loom large. But it means the difference between the all-too-familiar, fragmented heterogeneity of multidisciplinary services, on the one hand, and the smooth integration of mutual respect in the organic unity of a truly interdisciplinary team. Teamwork of the latter sort is essential because it draws on a broader range of resources than any one care-giver could hope to offer, because it recognises that different care-givers are appropriate to different patients or at different times, and because it provides latitude for the patient to choose moments and individuals for self-disclosure.

Within a context of this sort both individual care-givers and the interdisciplinary team can be forceful advocates for patient and family needs. They will be able to contribute to the education of the larger society, just as they take care not to exploit the larger community unfairly or to misuse its resources. A balanced perspective which recognises and respects a shared set of obligations and values makes possible a common effort towards the creation of a better and more caring community at all levels (and even within overtly hierarchical systems).

STRESS AND SUPPORT IN CARING

Some degree of stress is likely to be found in every profession and in most aspects of human life. Stress cannot be completely eradicated while we remain alive. Indeed, in some measure stress may be essential for truly creative living. The issue is not whether there will be stress in our lives, but what it will be like, whether we will recognise it, and how we will cope with it. Will stress be stimulating or overwhelming, will we channel it into productive directions or will we simply give in to its pressures and find ourselves paralysed or exhausted?

The term 'burnout' seems to refer to situations in which stress can neither be endured nor turned to any productive purpose. It implies a burden that once may have been challenging or manageable but which has now become unbearable or unmanageable. Edelwich and Brodsky (1980) have described four stages of disillusionment in the process of burnout - enthusiasm, stagnation, frustration, and (finally) apathy – and attention has recently been given to implications for physiotherapists and other professional care-givers (Wolfe, 1981; Schuster et al, 1984; Squires and Livesley, 1984). But burnout is not restricted to the health care system. It is a well-publicised syndrome these days among groups as diverse as air traffic controllers and grammar school teachers. Dysfunctional stress will most likely be revealed in emotional, behavioural, physical, social, and/or spiritual manifestations.

Care-givers may have particular reason to be legitimately concerned about dysfunctional stress. They frequently come into contact with disability, loss, and dependence, they may work in contexts that too often engender a sense of frustration, and often they are idealistic and have a high personal need to serve. Let us consider some typical sources and types of stress, as well as constructive ways to mitigate or manage its implications.

Stress: sources and types

Stress arises out of three principal sources: the strengths or weaknesses of our own intrapersonal resources; interpersonal or social relationships; and systemic contexts or professional roles.

Intrapersonal stress: This arises from within me when *I* am unable to cope with the demands of everyday living in a satisfying manner. *I* might lack sufficient patience, energy, a sense of humour, imagination, flexibility, stamina, or many other individual qualities. As a result, *I* may not cope well even in situations where others might find little or no difficulty. This should not be unexpected. As individuals, none of us do equally well in all aspects of living. Maturation is essentially a process of coming to appreciate our personal strengths and weaknesses. In this process, we may learn to change ourselves or to compensate for some deficiencies. Some skills need to be developed in us all, others apply mainly to specific individuals or situations, and some can be neglected or set aside.

Interpersonal stress: This has to do with relationships between people and is usually evidenced either in a sense of isolation or in a need to be overly dependent. Primarily, this sort of stress has to do with our ability to get along with other human beings in ways that are satisfactory for all concerned. Stress is generated when we cannot achieve an appropriate balance between the private and the public dimensions of our lives. Everyday activities and ordinary social intercourse become onerous and difficult because we find ourselves all too frequently clashing with or being rebuffed by the people around us. Some degree of interpersonal stress is perhaps inevitable and only to be expected in the complex and fast-paced societies of today. But extraordinary levels of inner tension and of anti-social behaviour suggest contemporary failings that are more than just private in nature.

Contextual or vocational stress: This is more than just interpersonal, since it relates primarily to a specific context within the society or to a particular social role. The nature of the work itself, expectations as to its proper outcome, the availability of suitable rewards or satisfactions, and the general atmosphere of the institutional environment or work situation all have to do with the presence or absence of vocational stress. That is, what we bring to a particular professional activity, how it is valued (or not valued) by society, and what it consists of in itself will all have a bearing on whether or not it becomes a source of stress in our lives. In many vocations that depend upon teamwork, stress arises from conflicting views of obligations, poorly shared or inadequately articulated values, and perceived impotence and frustration.

Stress: prevention, support, and management

Dealing effectively with stress is essentially a matter of anticipation and prevention, social or professional support, and individual management. The point is not just to protect ourselves, since that can be done in a dysfunctional way as when professional demeanour is employed as a defence against emotional involvement with patients and families (Quint, 1967). Rather, the aim is a healthy resolution, one which incorporates adaptation and balance at the personal, social, and vocational levels (Lattanzi, 1983, 1985).

Stress is best addressed ahead of time in the careful selection of staff for particular professions or roles. Much can be achieved with sound people; little can be expected of those operating at a significant deficit in relevant capacities. Following selection, staff need careful education and training – both at the outset and in a continuing programme – that prepare them for their responsibilities, encourage them to function effectively within the team or system, and enable them to manage work-related stress. Constructive supervision models values and establishes the tone of the overall environment. In addition, support from colleagues and within the team is invaluable in sustaining high quality care. Each of these contributes to the growth and development of a care-giver, while minimising difficulties and limitations.

At the same time, care-givers must take part in their own sustenance and support. They can do this by striving to maintain a balanced life of pleasurable and satisfying activities, by securing time alone for reflection, clarification, and self-integration, by developing outlets for sharing and emotional expression, by fostering personal or group-related rituals in which experiences can be overtly acknowledged, and by nurturing an overarching personal philosophy or life view. In other words, the values and the lived meanings within the personal lives of care-givers are the inevitable foundation upon which social and professional activities will be conducted. Specifically with regard to work itself, those considering a career in health care would do well to learn about the profession that interests them, to undertake a training period, an apprenticeship, or a limited trial experience, and to consider the contexts in which they will work before making life-long or relatively permanent commitments.

A CONCLUDING REMARK

A professional vocation is not just a job, but a calling. That of care-giver is a noble vocation in which one is called to provide aid to others with respect to their health and well-being. Training for such a vocation is essential, but it is not sufficient. On its own, that would only result in the task-orientation of a mechanic. For professional care-givers, technical knowledge and skill are essential, but a degree of reflection, self-awareness, deliberation, and human availability are also required. In this way, what care-givers have to offer and what they might do are viewed not merely in themselves but in perspective. That is, actions and interpretations of obligations are governed by conscious values. As important as technical knowledge and skills undoubtedly are, perhaps the ultimate test of a professional lies in the appreciation of instances when those skills are not appropriate, when simple human presence is sufficient, or when giving way to another would better serve the needs of the patient in question.

Thurman (1976) has written the following about times of sorrow, but it applies equally to other trials and tribulations throughout life:

I share with you the agony of your grief,
  The anguish of your heart finds echo in my own.
  I know I cannot enter all you feel
  Nor bear with you the burden of your pain;
I can but offer what my love does give:
  The strength of caring,
  The warmth of one who seeks to understand
  The silent storm-swept barrenness of so great a loss.
This I do in quiet ways,
  That on your lonely path
  You may not walk alone.

The responsibility of professional care-givers is to walk alongside those they serve in skilful and perceptive ways for a relatively short and limited time in order to assist others to bear their burdens more effectively. The reward for so doing is the privilege of entering into the life of another and the satisfaction of helping to make that life better in some way or degree. None of this can be achieved without a continuing effort towards developing a personal philosophy for caring.

REFERENCES

Brady, E. M. (1979). Telling the story: ethics and dying. *Hospital Progress*, **60**, 57-62.

Butler, R. N. (1963). The life review: An interpretation of reminiscence in the aged. *Psychiatry*, **26**, 65-76.

Downie, P. A. (1983). The place of physiotherapy in hospice care. In *Hospice Care: Principles and Practice*, pp. 148-59, (jt. eds. Corr, C.A. and Corr, D. M.). Faber and Faber, London.

Dyer, L. E. (1982). Professional development. *Physiotherapy*, **68**, 390-3.

Edelwich, J. and Brodsky, A. (1980). *Burnout: Stages of Disillusionment in the Health Professions*. Human Sciences Press, London.

Jonsen, A. R. (1978). Do no harm. *Annals of Internal Medicine*, **88**, 827-32.

Lattanzi, M. E. (1983). Professional stress: adaptation, coping, and meaning. In *Death and Grief in the Family*, pp. 95-106, (jt. eds. Hanson, J. C. and Frantz, T. T.). Aspen Systems Corporation, Rockville MD.

Lattanzi, M. E. (1985). An approach to caring: caregiver concerns. In *Hospice Approaches to Pediatric Care*, pp. 261-77, (jt. eds. Corr, C. A. and Corr, D. M.). Springer Publishing Co, New York.

Purtilo, R. B. (1976). Similarities in patient response to chronic and terminal illness. *Physical Therapy*, **56**, 279-84.

Quint, J. C. (1967). *The Nurse and the Dying Patient*. Macmillan, New York.

Saunders, C. M. (1976). The challenge of terminal care. In *Scientific Foundations of Oncology*, pp. 672-3, (jt. eds. Symington, T. and Carter, R. L.). William Heinemann Medical Books Limited, London.

Schuster, N. D., Nelson, D. L. and Quisling, C. (1984). Burnout among physical therapists. *Physical Therapy*, **64,** 299-303.

Shanks, R. (1982). Physiotherapy in palliative care. *Physiotherapy*, **68,** 405-7.

Sim, J. (1983). Ethical considerations in physiotherapy. *Physiotherapy*, **69,** 119-20.

Squires, A. and Livesley, B. (1984). Beware of burnout. *Physiotherapy*, **70,** 235-8.

Thurman, H. (1976). *Meditations of the Heart*. Friends United Press, Richmond, USA.

Wolfe, G. A. (1981). Burnout of therapists: inevitable or preventable? *Physical Therapy*, **61,** 1046-50.

BIBLIOGRAPHY

Cherniss, C. (1980). *Professional Burnout in Human Service Organizations*. Praeger, New York.

Cherniss, C. (1980). *Staff Burnout: Job Stress in the Human Services*. Sage Publications, London.

Corr, C. A. and Corr, D. M. (jt. eds.) (1983). *Hospice Care: Principles and Practice*. Faber and Faber, London; Springer Publishing Co, New York.

Downie, P. A. (1978). *Cancer Rehabilitation: An Introduction for Physiotherapists and the Allied Professions*. Faber and Faber, London.

Downie, R. S. and Telfer, E. (1969). *Respect for Persons*. George Allen and Unwin, London.

Downie, R. S. and Telfer, E. (1980). *Caring and Curing; A Philosophy of Medicine and Social Work*. Methuen, London.

Purtilo, R. B. (1975). *Essays for Professional Helpers: Some Psychosocial and Ethical Considerations*. Charles B. Slack, Thorofare, New Jersey.

Purtilo, R. B. (1978). *Health Professional/Patient Interactions*, 2nd edition. W. B. Saunders Company, London.

Purtilo, R. B. and Cassel, C. K. (1981). *Ethical Dimensions in the Health Professions*. W. B. Saunders Company, London.

Ramsey, P. (1970). *The Patient as Person*. Yale University Press, London.

Saunders, C. M. (ed.) (1978). *The Management of Terminal Disease*. Edward Arnold, London.

Selye, H. (1976). *The Stress of Life*, revised edition. McGraw-Hill, London.

Chapter 2

Clinical Diagnosis of Neurological Conditions

by P. D. LEWIS D Sc, MD, MRCP, FRCPath

As in other branches of medicine, the art of the neurologist consists of making a diagnosis from the patient's own account of his illness and from a physical examination, aided by appropriate radiographic or laboratory tests. Once the diagnosis has been reached, suitable treatment can be given and the outlook predicted. What distinguishes neurology from its sister specialties is the degree of attention to detail in taking the medical history and in examining the patient. This quest for detail, so mysterious to the non-neurologist, is linked to a wealth of knowledge of nervous anatomy, physiology and pathology, accumulated over more than a century, the application of which at the bedside often enables a precise diagnosis to be made. The meticulous enquiry into the patient's symptoms and search for physical signs was once the approach of all specialist physicians. However, as some diseased organs became easily and accurately studied by diagnostic tests (like chest radiographs), clinical methods in these fields of medicine became somewhat less important. Until quite recently, abnormalities of structure in the living brain could only be visualised by specialised radiological methods, sometimes carrying risks and sometimes needing anaesthesia. Now that computerised tomography (CT-scanning) has become generally available, the brain can be x-rayed as readily as the chest, resulting in a trend toward simpler clinical neurological assessment.

TAKING A NEUROLOGICAL CASE-HISTORY

For the neurologist, a complete and accurate history is essential. Very often a precise diagnosis can be made from the history, and examination is simply confirmatory; the converse, a physical examination which provides signs not predictable from the history, tends to come as a surprise. The description of the tempo of the illness – acute or chronic, coming on slowly or abruptly, steadily progressive or remitting, often suggests the type of pathological process. Vascular problems are usually of acute onset, tumour symptoms tend steadily to progress, demyelinating disease may remit. The characterisation of symptoms is then attempted, the neurologist assisting the patient with suitable questions. Headaches, 'dizziness' and 'fainting' are three of the most frequent problems dealt with in neurological clinics. It is the task of the neurologist to decide if the patient's headaches result from a brain tumour or simply (and as usually is the case) from muscular tension or from migraine. Dizziness may signify disease of the balance mechanisms in the ear and brainstem. Faints may or may not mean neurological disease: epilepsy may resemble fainting attacks, and careful enquiry with specific questions is often needed to obtain a clear picture of such episodes. Other symptoms of special significance to the neurologist include disturbances of memory or concentration; loss of vision; double vision; facial pain or weakness; difficulty with speech or swallowing; weakness, wasting, pain or numbness in a limb; abnormal movements; trouble with walking; and disturbance of bladder control. Each of these symptoms, described by the patient, has a range of possible causes which need to be considered; thus it will set in train a particular process of enquiry as the neurologist attempts – on the basis of the information given by the patient – to form a clear image of the nature and localisation of the underlying neurological disorder.

THE NEUROLOGICAL EXAMINATION

To a certain extent the neurological examination begins from the moment the patient enters the consulting room. Gait, mental attitude, alertness and speech may all give important diagnostic clues. However, the formal examination of the nervous system follows completion of history-taking. Testing of the head, trunk and limbs for motor and sensory function is preceded by an evaluation of mental state and intellectual level. The patient's overall appearance and behaviour, mood, orientation, thought processes, memory and intelligence may be affected in many brain diseases, and need to be assessed. A disturbance of speech may point to a disorder of the dominant cerebral hemisphere or of motor control.

The carotid arteries are felt and listened to in the neck to check on arterial blood flow to the brain, neck movement is tested and the skull is felt (and listened to for abnormal sounds). Functions of the cranial nerves are then examined in turn. Sense of smell (olfactory nerves); visual fields, visual activity, optic fundi – using the ophthalmoscope (optic nerves); examination of the pupils (oculomotor nerves) and of eye movements (oculomotor, trochlear and abducent nerves); facial sensation, corneal sensation and reflexes, jaw movement (trigeminal nerves); facial movement (facial nerves); hearing (auditory nerves); palatal sensation and movement (glossopharyngeal and vagus nerves); movements of sternomastoid and trapezius muscles (spinal accessory nerves); and tongue movement (hypoglossal nerves) are the major cranial nerve functions assessed in a full neurological examination. Abnormalities observed in any of these will suggest the anatomical basis of the patient's complaint.

The systematic examination of the trunk and limbs includes both motor and sensory testing; the patient's symptoms should suggest which of these is carried out first, since either can be tiring. In order to decide if muscle function is normal or abnormal the doctor must first carefully look at the limbs for signs of muscle wasting, abnormality of posture (suggesting muscular imbalance), involuntary movements (which may be a sign of extrapyramidal disease) and fasciculation (often a sign of damage to motor nerve cells). He then evaluates the tone of the limb musculature (the state of tension in the muscles, which may be increased or decreased under abnormal conditions), assesses power systematically, muscle group by muscle group, looks for signs of incoordination of movement, and tests the tendon reflexes (which can reveal derangement of function at or above or below the spinal segments each represents). Once again motor testing aims to localise the neurological abnormality.

Sensation from different zones of skin is conveyed to the nervous system via different spinal nerves and spinal cord segments, while distinct forms of skin sensation (e.g. pain and touch) have separate pathways in the nervous system. Clearly, careful sensory testing can also be of great localising value. In practice the neurologist will often test pain sensation with a pin, touch with a piece of cottonwool and joint position sense by carefully moving a finger or toe. He makes much use of the vibration of a tuning fork as an overall test of sensory function.

FURTHER TESTS

Even the most skilful and experienced clinical neurologist would not expect to make an accurate diagnosis in every patient on the basis of history and examination alone. Overall, perhaps 50 per cent of clinical diagnoses will be found to be correct. Accuracy is increased by means of special tests which aim to localise the abnormality in the nervous system or to define its pathology.

Radiographs

These are invaluable for disease affecting the bones of the skull and the spine. However, they cannot show the soft tissues contained inside. For these to be seen, it is necessary either to inject into the blood vessels of the brain or cord a substance which is opaque to x-rays (arteriography, angiography) or to outline the nervous tissue by defining the fluid spaces within and outside them, using air or an opaque medium (pneumo-encephalography or ventriculography for the brain; myelography for spinal cord). The selective uptake of radioactive isotopes by diseased nervous tissue can be used to produce images of the brain (isotope scans).

The CT-scanner, mentioned earlier, has supplanted isotopic methods in those centres where it is available, and gives in many cases a definitive structural diagnosis. Its principle is the detection of minute changes of tissue density from point to point inside the head. In this way a radiographic picture of the brain itself, and not just the skull, can be assembled.

Magnetic resonance imaging (or nuclear magnetic resonance, NMR) involves similar computing techniques to CT-scanning to build up a highly informative picture of brain tissue (Figs. 2/1a and b). It is not an x-ray technique but uses a powerful magnet to produce temporary physical changes in the atoms of the brain. White matter visualisation is especially good, and multiple sclerosis can be diagnosed in NMR pictures.

Electrodiagnostic tests

These involve the amplification and recording of the electrical activity of nervous tissue and have certain diagnostic applications. Electro-encephalography is useful in the investigation of some epileptic patients, in some cases of coma and in certain forms of encephalitis.

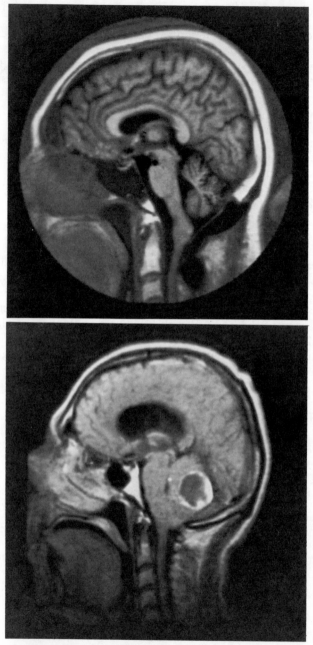

FIG. 2/1 Magnetic resonant imaging of the brain (*courtesy* Dr G. M. Bydder, NMR Unit, Hammersmith Hospital, London). (a) Normal mid-sagittal scan; (b) Sagittal scan showing a cystic cerebellar tumour

Electromyography is described on page 138 and is an essential part of the evaluation of patients with neuromuscular disease. Measurement of sensory and motor nerve conduction is equally essential in the study of lesions of the peripheral nervous system.

Cerebrospinal fluid tests

These are important in neurological diagnosis. Lumbar puncture is the usual technique for obtaining a sample. It is a necessary procedure where meningitis or subarachnoid haemorrhage is suspected, and it may give useful information in certain inflammatory diseases of brain tissue.

The tests of general medicine

These include haematological tests, blood and urine biochemistry, and may give diagnostic information. Many generalised diseases have neurological complications, and the neurologist may be the first physician to see a patient whose disease has major effects on other parts of the body. For all his special skills the neurologist is still a physician. Whether taking a medical history, examining the patient, or ordering tests it is important that he keeps sight of the broad canvas of human disease.

BIBLIOGRAPHY

Bannister, R. (ed.) (1984). *Brain's Clinical Neurology*, 6th edition. Oxford University Press, Oxford.

Bickerstaff, E. R. (1980). *Neurological Examination in Clinical Practice*, 4th edition. Blackwell Scientific Publications Limited, Oxford.

Matthews, W. B. (1975). *Practical Neurology*, 3rd edition. Blackwell Scientific Publications Limited, Oxford.

Pansky, B. and Allen, D. J. (1981). *Review of Neuroscience*. Macmillan, New York.

Patten, J. (1977). *Neurological Differential Diagnosis*. Starke, London.

Chapter 3

The Development of the Nervous System

by G. T. McCARTHY MB, FRCP, DCH
and H. W. ATKINSON MCSP, HT, DipTP

The development of the nervous system from conception to maturity is a complex and fascinating study. Our understanding of neurological development has increased enormously in the past 25 years. This has arisen in a number of ways:

1. Detailed observation of the normal baby at birth and during the first year or two of life (André-Thomas et al, 1960; Prechtl and Beintema, 1964; Saint-Anne Dargassies 1966, 1972, 1977; Prechtl, 1977; Touwen, 1976; Brazelton, 1973, 1984).
2. Detailed neurological evaluation of the premature baby (Dubowitz and Dubowitz, 1981; Dubowitz et al, 1984).
3. Elegant detailed neuropathology of the infant brain correlated with neurological signs (Wigglesworth and Pape, 1978; Hambleton and Wigglesworth, 1976).
4. The development of the more precise tool of ultrasound to observe progress in the preterm infant brain (Pape and Wigglesworth, 1979; Levene et al, 1982).

'In many ways there are greater differences between the brain of a 28-week gestation infant and that of a 36-week infant than there are between a 3-month-old baby and an adult' (Wigglesworth and Pape, 1978).

Development is a concept which implies both growth and maturation. Growth is not just an increase in size, but the development of increasingly more complex interconnections within the brain. The nervous system arises from the neural plate which folds to form the neural tube about the 3rd to 4th week after conception (O'Reilly and Gardner, 1977). The development of a series of flexures then occurs which separate into the different regions of the brain, and the cerebral hemispheres are visible as paired vesicles at the end of the 5th week.

At first the brainstem, thalamus and basal ganglia are dominant in development, the rapid growth of the cerebral cortex and cerebellum taking place in the latter part of fetal life. The blood supply alters during development, reflecting the neuronal growth and migration of cells from the sub-ependymal plate to the cerebral cortex. During the 3rd trimester the vascular bed is re-modelled as the balance of the circulation shifts from a central to a cortical and white matter orientation (Wigglesworth and Pape, 1978). As the interconnections of the cortical neurones increase in number, myelination commences.

The newborn brain may be damaged by (a) haemorrhage, (b) ischaemia, (c) metabolic insult (e.g. hypoglycaemia or hyperbili-rubinaemia), or (d) direct trauma during delivery leading to (a) or (b).

The pattern of damage can to some extent be correlated with the infant's gestational age and brain development, although the way in which it reacts to insult may vary, e.g. maintenance of the blood pressure and adequate respiration may maintain the cere-bral circulation in some infants.

At birth the human brain is very well developed; a complex and relatively larger organ than any other animal. The relative size of the brain, 12 per cent of the body mass, is also much larger than at maturity when it is 2 per cent.

Low blood pressure may lead to damage at boundary zones between different cerebral artery territories and adjacent white matter which are just being defined at term. Boundary zones in the periventricular region between vessels supplying the basal ganglia and those penetrating through white matter from the cor-tex remain important and may be a site of damage in both term and preterm infants.

The relatively greater metabolic requirements of the basal gan-glia and thalamus, brainstem nuclei, and mid-brain make these areas more vulnerable to cerebral anoxia with the resultant pat-tern of severe dyskinetic cerebral palsy.

THE NEWBORN INFANT AT TERM

The normal newborn baby is a complex individual already cap-able of interaction with its environment and those taking care of it. The attachment of the baby to its mother is a vital step in development, and the baby is able to distinguish its mother by visual recognition, by smell and by recognition of her handling within days of birth.

The relative state of arousal of the baby was first recognised as important in describing its reaction by Prechtl and Beintema (1964), and Brazelton (1973, 1984) added important further observations (Table 3/1). The levels describe how accessible the baby is to stimulation and handling.

TABLE 3/1   (After Brazelton, 1984)

State 1:	Deep sleep, no spontaneous movement, no eye movements
State 2:	Light sleep, eyes closed, rapid eye movements, low activity level, random movements and startles, irregular respirations, sucking movements
State 3:	Drowsy or semi-dozing, eyes open or closed, activity level variable, mild startles, dazed look
Start 4:	Alert with bright look, seems to focus on source of stimulation, motor activity minimal
State 5:	Eyes open, considerable motor activity, thrusting movements of extremities, few spontaneous startles. Brief fussing vocalisation
State 6:	State of crying, intense crying difficult to break through with stimulation, motor activity high

The tone of the baby should be noted: this is defined as the resistance of parts of the body to passive movements. The posture of the baby at rest reflects tone, and should be observed in prone and supine.

In the full-term newborn baby there is predominance of extensor tone in the neck and flexor tone in the limbs. When suspended in prone, the full-term infant will maintain the head on a level with the trunk, the arms and legs remaining in a flexed position (see Fig. 3/2). As the baby matures active extension of the neck occurs, associated with hip extension – developing into the Landau response (see Fig. 3/2) from 3 to 7 months.

The preterm infant has much lower tone, seen in its posture in supine when the legs are extended and in suspended prone when the head flops forward and the arms and legs hang down in extension. Interestingly, in a group of preterm infants examined at 40 weeks' postmenstrual age by Dubowitz and Dubowitz (1981) a substantial number had better head and trunk posture than term infants. Unlike the term infants the limbs were frequently extended. It is important to recognise this difference in posture in preterm infants who have developed outside the uterus and not regard it as a sign of spasticity.

The development of vision and visual responses are important in motor development as visual orientation is used in maintaining posture and balance. The newborn baby is able to focus and many will follow vertically and horizontally in an arc. Preferential gaze on the face develops quickly within a few days.

Neonatal reflexes

The neonatal reflexes are responses which can be reproduced readily after a particular stimulus. There are also a number of responses which are patterns of movement regularly seen in the newborn period but which are not elicited after every stimulus.

The neonatal reflexes must be looked at with some circumspection. They are present even in babies with severe abnormality of the brain or even absence of the cortex as in anencephaly. Abnormal reflexes, with asymmetry, or absent or persistent reflexes should be considered significant. Stereotyped responses are particularly significant (Touwen, 1976).

MORO REFLEX

The best way to elicit this reflex is by the 'head drop' method (Fig. 3/1a). The baby is held in supine supported behind the chest and head, the head is allowed to drop about 10°. The response is abduction of the shoulders and arms, extension of the elbows followed by the 'embrace'. The legs also extend and then flex.

The Moro reflex is fully developed in the term infant. It gradually disappears over the first 3-4 months of life, first in the legs, then in the arms.

Absence of the Moro response may signify severe depression of the CNS or marked hypotonia. Persistence of the Moro, particularly an excessive response, occurs in the absence of inhibition. The Moro reflex is probably a vestibular response (Prechtl, 1965), although proprioceptive responses from the cervical vertebrae have also been considered as mediators of the response.

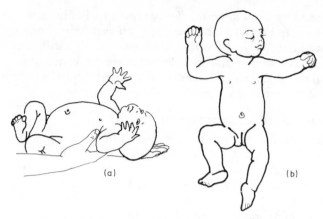

FIG. 3/1 (a) The Moro reflex. Head-drop method showing the embrace and flexion of the legs. (b) The asymmetric tonic neck response (ATNR): a normal posture seen at rest, it may be imposed by the examiner turning the head, between 2 and 4 months. A strongly imposable reflex after 6 months, or an obligatory response at any age, is evidence of significant motor handicap

PALMAR GRASP

The infant should be supine with head in the midline; an index finger is placed in the palm of each hand and the palmar surface pressed. A normal response is strong sustained flexion of the fingers for several seconds.

PLANTAR GRASP

This can be elicited by stimulating the root of the toes when active flexion will occur.

ROOTING REFLEX

With the infant supine, head in the midline, each corner of the mouth is stimulated by stroking laterally, the head turns, mouth opens and grasps, the lips may curl to the stimulated side.

SUCKING REFLEX

The index finger is placed in the baby's mouth, pad up, and the sucking action noted. A normal reaction is a sustained strong sucking action.

WALKING REFLEX

The baby is held in a standing position with the chin and head supported by one's fingers: a normal response is discernible steps with knee and hip flexion, and a step on each side. The walking response is usually lost within 4 weeks or so of birth, and supporting reactions of the legs do not reappear in the infant for several months. Passive extension of the head results in reinforcement of this reflex (Mac Keith, 1964).

ASYMMETRIC TONIC NECK RESPONSE

The asymmetric tonic neck response (ATNR) is a posture seen frequently in normal babies between 2 and 5 months. The head is turned to the side, the arm and leg on that side are extended and on the opposite side they are flexed. This is not an obligatory response except in an abnormal baby, when its persistence and reproducibility indicates pathology (Fig. 3/1b).

The disappearance of neonatal reflexes during development occurs as the nervous system matures and the neural mechanisms merge into more complex mechanisms. It is for this reason that infantile responses reappear after serious brain damage or in degenerative conditions. It is also for this reason that the reflexes persist in babies who have sustained damage to the nervous system at birth. Although plasticity in the CNS allows for remodelling of some of the damaged brain, the position of the damage is all-important in the final outcome.

Three types of neural mechanism, as defined by Touwen (1976), can be distinguished:

1. Primary or basic neural mechanisms, e.g. for visual or acoustic perception, and mechanisms for generating adequate muscle tone.
2. Mechanisms which merge into larger and more complex mechanisms or seemingly disappear completely to reappear in another form in a later stage of development, e.g. stepping movements and voluntary walking patterns.
3. Mechanisms which mature more or less independently and become linked together at a particular moment, which process results in differentiated motor patterns, e.g. the development of voluntary grasp ending with a pincer grasp, and the development of independent sitting, standing and walking.

Babies all develop differently and at their own rates. These may be slowed down by intercurrent illness, malnutrition or motor disorders. In mental handicap the development may also be disparate. Families often demonstrate similar patterns of development, e.g. rapid motor development, shuffling or late walking.

The term cephalocaudal development, while describing the

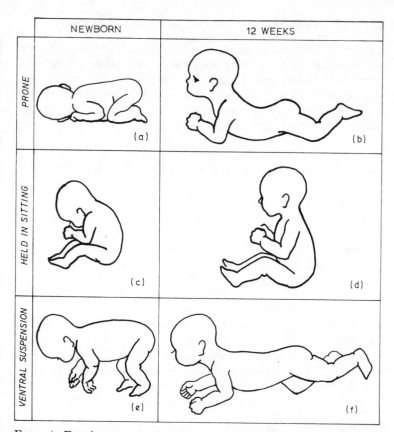

	NEWBORN	12 WEEKS
PRONE	(a)	(b)
HELD IN SITTING	(c)	(d)
VENTRAL SUSPENSION	(e)	(f)

FIG. 3/2 Development in the first 12 weeks of life. (a) The newborn infant in prone is flexed with the knees under the trunk and the arms flexed under the body; (b) By 12 weeks the arms and legs are extended. The baby is usually able to lift the shoulders and head up to look around; (c) The newborn infant held in sitting has a rounded back with the head flexed and hips and knees flexed; (d) By 12 weeks the head is maintained erect and the upper part of the back is straight, there is still a lumbar curve and the legs are still in a flexed posture; (e) Ventral suspension in the newborn usually provokes some neck extension with the head level with the body for a few seconds; (f) By 12 weeks the head is extended, the trunk straight and the hips are also extended. The *Landau reaction* is elevation of the head beyond the horizontal and arching of the spine so that it becomes concave. This degree of spinal extension is not usually reached until about 1 year. Passive flexion of the head causes loss of extensor tone – the *Landau reflex*.

Ventral suspension may demonstrate abnormal posture in the limbs and trunk and give information about a motor deficit. Marked *hypotonia* is present in future choreoathetosis or ataxia, and *hypertonia* in future spasticity

apparent acquisition of skills from head to tail, tends to obscure the important motor activity which is present in the whole baby from birth, and indeed in utero, e.g. the legs are actively moving and the hips flexing when the baby is pulled from supine to sitting at birth. Increasing control of the hips, necessary for sitting, crawling and standing, is occurring from birth.

DEVELOPMENT IN THE FIRST 2 YEARS OF LIFE

In the normal baby, development is a continuous process involving vision, hearing, motor control and function, and social and emotional responses. It is not necessarily a smooth process, so that examination of a baby at intervals is required to see the pattern clearly as demonstrated by Touwen (1976) in his study of 51 normal babies.

THE SEQUENCE OF DEVELOPMENT

There are several books on the details of developmental sequences (see Bibliography, p. 58). It is important to recognise that all babies develop in their own way, and to look at their development as a whole. The sequence outlined here is an attempt to show how the different parameters link together.

First 12 weeks (Fig. 3/2)

POSTURE AND LARGE MOVEMENTS

The development of head control, in prone, sitting and supine occurs. The head is maintained upright in supported sitting, but still lags when pulled to sitting by 12 weeks. In prone, neck extension develops and the arms begin to support the body. In ventral suspension by 12 weeks the head is held well above the line of the body, hips and shoulders extend.

VISION

Visually very alert, with increasing ability to fix and follow, and by 12 weeks follows a dangling ball 6-12 inches from face horizontally and usually vertically. Particularly preoccupied by human face. Holds a rattle for a few moments when placed in the hand, but not able to regard it.

HEARING AND SPEECH

Awareness developing, responds to meaningful sounds, quiets or smiles at sound of mother's voice and vocalises when spoken to.

SOCIAL BEHAVIOUR

Developing awareness and responding to daily routine: enjoys bathing, feeding and being handled.

12–28 weeks

POSTURE AND LARGE MOVEMENTS

There is development of head control and trunk balance. The head is maintained level with the body when pulled to sitting by about 24 weeks, and there is gradual loss of the lumbar curve by about 28 weeks. At the same time the arms are extended in prone and become stronger, lifting the shoulders and trunk off the couch.

The forward and downward parachute reactions develop (Fig. 3/3), and head righting occurs when the baby is tilted from the midline, demonstrating increasing ability to balance the trunk in

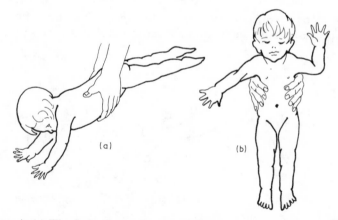

FIG. 3/3 (a) The forward parachute reaction appears at about 28 weeks. It consists of extension of the arms and hands with spreading and slight hyperextension of the fingers. It is an important reaction – asymmetry or absence of the reaction particularly denoting abnormality; (b) The downward parachute reaction also appears at around 28 weeks and consists of extension of legs and feet as the baby is lowered to the ground

space, and increasing awareness of the position of the head and body in space.

As sitting balance develops, the trunk gradually straightens. Early sitting balance is maintained by leaning forward and using the arms to prop. At first the legs tend to be flexed and slightly abducted; as trunk balance increases, the legs become straighter and rotation around the base occurs (Fig. 3/4a).

By about 24 weeks rolling over develops, usually first from prone and initiated by extension on the arms, and then from supine. The baby enjoys kicking his legs and being held in standing when he will bounce up and down (unless he is a shuffler).

VISION AND MANIPULATION

Awareness of environment increasing; moves head around to watch everything within visual fields. Uses whole hand to grasp voluntarily from about 14-16 weeks, and by 24 weeks in transferring and is able to hold an object in each hand. Beginning to watch a fallen toy within visual field but not outside it.

HEARING AND SPEECH

Vocalisation increasing, screams and laughs aloud. Responds to baby hearing test at 18 inches level with the ear.

SOCIAL BEHAVIOUR AND PLAY

Develops more complex interaction especially as hand function improves, reaches out readily for rattle and shakes it by 24 weeks.

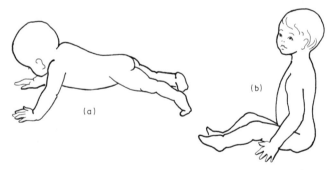

FIG. 3/4 (a) About 36 weeks, the baby, in prone, is able to take weight on fully extended arms and experiments with his feet and legs, extending them, then weight-bearing on his knees; (b) Sitting at 36 weeks. Independent sitting is usually attained around 28 to 32 weeks, but it takes several weeks before the back is straight with a lumbar lordosis and the arms are not required for support

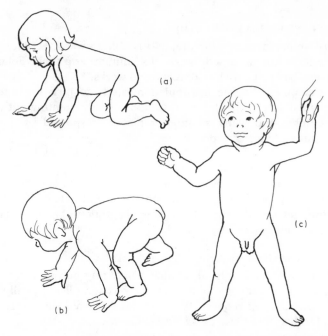

FIG. 3/5 (a) At 40 weeks, crawling; (b) At 52 weeks, 'bear walking' may precede upright walking; (c) At 52 weeks, walking with one hand held. Typical wide-based gait with a tendency to valgus feet

Takes objects to mouth, finds own hands and feet interesting. By 28 weeks beginning to be wary of strangers.

28–52 weeks

POSTURE AND LARGE MOVEMENTS

Is usually sitting without support for several minutes by 28 weeks (Fig. 3/4b). As trunk control improves and rotation around the sitting base develops, the legs become straighter and crawling is initiated by leaning forward and tucking legs under by about 36 weeks, sometimes 'Commando' crawling occurs without flexing the knees and lifting the pelvis.

Crawling – pulling to standing – cruising around furniture by side stepping occur at different rates, and 'bear-walking' may occur before walking independently (Fig. 3/5b). Usually able to walk with one hand held and may stand alone at 52 weeks (Fig. 3/5c). By 52 weeks is usually able to sit up from lying.

VISION AND FINE MANIPULATION

Visual ability develops rapidly, and is able to watch activities at 10-12 feet with sustained interest for minutes at a time. Follows the fixed-ball test $\frac{1}{8}$ inch at 10 feet by 36 weeks.

Development of fine manipulation: starts to pick up objects with radial side of hand; by 36 weeks is usually pointing with an index finger and using an inferior pincer grasp, and by 40-45 weeks uses a pincer grasp.

HEARING AND SPEECH

Becomes increasingly aware of environment; localises baby-hearing test at 3 feet level with ear and above and below. Vocalises and imitates sounds from about 36 weeks, tuneful babble – dada, conversational sounds by 52 weeks.

SOCIAL BEHAVIOUR AND PLAY

Likes to be within sight of familiar adult; play becomes increasingly complex, begins to put cubes into box and releases, will give toy to an adult on request. Will look for a toy hidden before his eyes. Drinks from a cup by 52 weeks. Chews.

Development in the second year of life - 12-24 months

POSTURE AND LARGE MOVEMENTS

The average age of independent walking is 15 months, but there is a wide variation, and children who have a different pattern of motor development – shuffling on their bottoms instead of crawling – tend to walk later. Shuffling occurs in about 15 per cent of the population, and is associated with hypotonia, especially in the trunk and legs. Physiotherapy intervention may be required to give parents advice in appropriate stimulation. When the downward parachute reaction is attempted, the baby 'sits on air', and it is difficult to get him to weight-bear through his feet.

Some children walk on their toes initially; most tend to walk on a broad base with flat feet (Fig. 3/5). By 18 months most children are walking independently, can manage to walk upstairs, but prefer to creep backwards downstairs. As balance improves, squatting to pick up a toy is possible. By 2 years he is usually able to run safely and avoid obstacles, climbs on to a large chair and can get down safely, and can walk up and down stairs holding on to the rail, two feet at a time.

As the baby develops, he is constantly practising his skills to perfect them. Touwen's (1976) study showed this clearly in a group of 51 infants who were observed at home every month until they had attained independent walking. The unfolding of development usually stimulates parents and carers to move on to the next step in their handling of the baby, but many parents need advice as they are not aware of their baby's needs. The health visitor plays an important role in interpreting development in the normal baby and observing deviations from normal.

The role of the physiotherapist has widened over the years so that she is often involved in stimulation programmes for mentally handicapped babies, including those with Down's syndrome, as well as in treatment of children with motor disorders.

The best way to gain experience is to handle as many normal babies of different ages as possible. Attendance at sessions in normal baby clinics would be ideal training to observe variations within normal development.

DISCUSSION OF DEVELOPMENTAL SEQUENCES

Mature movements are complex permutations of the basic flexion and extension synergies. Until the child can mix flexion and extension components of movement, only mass patterns can be produced. The ability to stabilise the trunk and proximal part of the limbs while allowing distal parts to move is important where skilled activity is concerned, and cerebellar activity is very important to this. Equally well, the ability to retain a fixed distal extremity while the proximal segments and trunk move over it is also essential. Much of the child's developmental progress is related to the ability to produce these two varieties of movement, not only as distinct entities, but going on at the same time.

Let us take two examples to illustrate the points mentioned above:

THE MIXTURE OF FLEXION AND EXTENSION COMPONENTS

A simple example may be seen when the sitting position is considered. This requires extension of the vertebral column, but flexion of the hips and knees. If it is impossible to extend the column unless a total extension pattern is used, then the child is unable to maintain a sitting position.

A more complex example may be seen if the lower limbs are

considered in the walking synergies. Mass movement patterns of
a more reflex variety follow certain stereotyped synergies. When
the hip and knee flex the lower limb also abducts and may laterally rotate and the foot dorsiflexes. However, to walk forward we
require to flex the hip and knee while adducting the limb. This
is followed by extending the knee while dorsiflexing the foot.
Here, alone, are some interesting synergies. The leg then prepares
to take weight, when it extends at the knee and hip and abducts
to prevent a Trendelenburg sign (drop of the pelvis on the non-
weight-bearing side) (Fig. 3/6) while the foot is dorsiflexed –
another mixture of synergies. In Figure 3/6a the abductors of the
weight-bearing limb are working to prevent the pelvis from dropping on the non-weight-bearing side. In Figure 3/6b the abductors are not working and so the pelvis has dropped into adduction
on that side, causing a compensatory lurch of the trunk. This is
called a Trendelenburg sign.

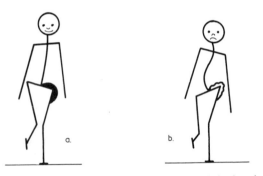

FIG. 3/6 The role of the hip abductors in weight-bearing

The push-off requires more extension of the hip, flexion of the
knee and plantar flexion of the foot. This is a very complex series
of synergies. The ability is not immediately available. The child
who has recently started walking flexes and abducts his hip. Only
later does he keep it adducted as the leg comes forward.

PROXIMAL FIXATION AND DISTAL FREEDOM AND VICE VERSA

A simple example may be seen when we consider the child in
prone lying. When he is able to take weight on one elbow while
playing with a toy with the other hand he is demonstrating distal
fixation of the supporting limb with the trunk free to move over
it, while the free limb is moving distally against the proximal
support of the steady trunk.

A more complex example of the same thing occurs with the much more mature pattern of writing. Here the supporting arm is offering distal stability to the trunk which is free to move over it. The hand which is putting pen to paper is working freely with a more proximal area of stability in the forearm. However, the forearm must also be partly free to move for each word and so movement at the shoulder has to occur. The shoulder is functioning as a stable and mobile structure at one and the same time against the stable background of the trunk which, in turn, is free to move over the other, or supporting limb. This is a very complex synergy. Little wonder that we cannot write at birth!

Many learning processes depend upon the ability to move. We require movement to be able to explore our environment, and unless this is possible our mental processes cannot develop normally. Head control is essential to movement, but is also essential for the ability to make maximum use of the sense of sight. If we cannot control our head position it is difficult to gain control over our eye activities. The eyes also need to have a stable base from which to work. Eye movements are similar to limbs. They can remain stable while the head moves, or they can move while the head stays still, or the two activities may go on at once, none of this is possible if head control is absent.

Assessment of spatial relationships depends upon movement. The relationship between hands and eyes depends upon the ability to move and explore, and the perception of depth, space, height, size and shape have all to be learned by experiences dependent upon movements of different areas of the body.

Balance activities basically start by the balance of the head upon the shoulders in prone lying. Progression is then made by balancing the shoulders over the elbows which offer a forward support in prone lying. In sitting it should be noted that the body is at first inclined forward so that head balance on the shoulders is still an extension activity and the arms are in a supporting forward position, but with extended elbows.

Later the ability to balance with the arms supporting sideways develops, and much later the arms may support by being placed behind as when sitting in a backward leaning position. This requires flexor activity in the head and neck to maintain the balance of the head on the shoulders.

Before the child is able to give a backwards support to the

sitting position he is developing rotatory ability in the trunk which is the precursor to more skilful balance activities. Maturity of balance is seen when the upper limbs can carry out skilled activities, while the legs and trunk are dealing with maintenance of equilibrium without the aid of the upper limbs.

The development of motor skills is not complete until the hands can be used in prehensile activities, and much work has been done by various authors on the development of prehension. As a summary it may be pointed out that the hand activities are inclined to develop from ulnar to radial side. The grasp and release activities of the early stages in development appear to commence with activity of the little finger and radiate out towards the thumb. Gradually the radial aspect of the hand becomes more dominant and eventually the pincer grasp between thumb and index finger develops while the ulnar side of the hand takes up a more stabilising function. Much more mature is the 'dynamic tripod' posture described by Wynn Parry in 1966 and explained by Rosenbloom and Horton (1971). Here the thumb, index and middle fingers are used as a threesome to give fine co-ordinated movements of the hand. The classic example of the use of this tripod is in writing, although it may be seen in other functional activities.

The physical, intellectual and social development of the child are so clearly linked with each other that it would take several volumes to give a complete and detailed account.

The physiotherapist makes most use of the physical aspects of development, but needs some understanding of the intellectual and social aspects to appreciate fully the whole problem.

As a brief summary it may be said that the process of integrating certain reflex mechanisms involved in movement occurs over a period of time and eventually makes controlled purposeful movement possible. The control develops in a cephalocaudal direction. It is closely linked with perception of body image, intellectual and social behaviour and, although it is not dependent upon environmental factors, these may influence the rate at which perfection develops. Motor development starts with control of the head position in prone, with the upper limbs most able to take weight in a forward or elbow support position. Later development includes rolling and supported sitting with the weight supported forwards on the hands at first, and later at the sides and even later behind. Body rotation begins to be perfected as rolling occurs and limb rotation follows trunk rotation as a rule.

Movements at first follow primitive patterns of synergy, but later the ability to combine flexion/extension patterns to give more complexity of movement develops. Ultimate maturity of movement is reached when the hands are totally free from an obligation to balance mechanisms, so that they can be freely developed as skilful tools and used in conjunction with visual and other sensory feedback mechanisms.

It should be noted that the child's development mechanisms are so arranged that he is preparing for balance in a position before he is able fully to adopt the position and certainly before he is able to use it as a base for activities of his hands. Usually the mother plays with the child so that he experiences advanced activities before he is able to perform them. In other words, he is being prepared for the activity in addition to making his own 'in-built' preparations.

Let us take an example. A child may be 7 or 8 months old before he is able to get himself into a sitting position. To sit in a balanced manner he needs to flex at the hips and extend at the trunk. He needs head control and the ability to support himself forwards on his hands. These are minimum requirements. He is prepared for this naturally by the early development of head control, the elbow and hand support prone positions, and by lying on his back playing with his feet. His mother also helps him by propping him into a sitting position so that he experiences it prior to achieving it. Help in this manner makes him experiment and he tries to balance when he is put into sitting and in fact learns to do so.

In the meantime his rolling and rotatory activities are developing. The child gradually develops the ability to get into sitting *after* he has learned to balance in that position.

THE CLINICAL VALUE OF A KNOWLEDGE OF DEVELOPMENTAL SEQUENCE

When working with handicapped children and, in particular, with the very young, it is easy to see that this information is exceedingly valuable.

When treating babies with movement defects it is important to start as early as possible and to bear in mind the normal sequence of development so that one can, as far as possible, channel the child's reactions along suitable lines and encourage step by step progress without leaving gaps which may lead to abnormality. The earlier the abnormal child is given help the more successful is the treatment likely to be. It is much more difficult to correct abnormal habits than it is to prevent them from occurring. The child's nervous system is very malleable and able to adapt very readily. Consequently it can be most easily influenced before it is fully matured. It is a great mistake to wait until the child can consciously co-operate. By this time irretrievable abnormalities will have developed. The skilled physiotherapist is able to exploit her knowledge of the nervous system to stimulate suitable responses in the child long before he is aware of co-operating.

However, many physiotherapists deal only with adults or, at least, the greater bulk of their patient load is adult. Where then does this knowledge have value? The answer is simply that injury or disease to the central nervous system frequently brings about demyelination of certain areas and may damage or destroy the nervous pathways which have been used to control certain activities. The patient frequently shows a regression of motor skills to a more primitive level. Certain of the reflex mechanisms, which have hitherto been integrated into mature movement patterns, may be partly released from cortical control and may exert an excessive influence over the patient, dominating these movement patterns into abnormality or even preventing them from occurring at all. The patient will frequently show absence or disturbance of normal equilibrium reactions, poverty of movement synergy, perception difficulties and diminution of sensory discrimination. If the physiotherapist is going to help the patient to make full use of such nervous connections as are left, she is more likely to be successful if she has a knowledge of the way in which more skilled activities develop in the first place so that she can, to some extent, simulate the conditions to facilitate redevelopment. The following example illustrates this point.

A patient with neurological symptoms can often maintain a sitting position but, on attempting to stand, he pulls himself up by placing his hands on a rigid forward support or by pulling on a helper who is standing in front of him. Frequently the head is flexed forward or, conversely, it may be thrown back so that the nose is pointing upward. In the first instance the patient is using the symmetrical tonic neck reflex pattern to aid him into standing, and in the second his legs are making use of the tonic labyrinthine effect. Neither of these is acceptable as the patterns are those of total reflex synergy, and balance in standing will never be achieved using these patterns. Such a patient has his movement excessively influenced by the tonic reflex mechanisms and requires training to modify them and to start early balance activities. He requires help in receiving weight on to his arms in a forward position. Such activities as elbow-support prone lying are suitable, progressing to hand-support forward side sitting, leading to prone kneeling and hand-support forward standing (standing but resting hands on a stool or low support in front of him). He needs to feel the sensation of weight being received forwards instead of pulling back. There are many other facets to this patient's problems which need attention, but the above example makes the point.

Many head injury cases regress to an enormous degree and intellectual and social abilities regress also. Motor training along developmental lines is accompanied, in many cases, by a brightening of intellectual activities and the beginning of social communication. The patient may never achieve behaviour patterns which are mature, but he is more likely to make balanced progress if a developmental approach is used.

REFERENCES

André-Thomas, Y. C. and Saint-Anne Dargassies, S. (1960). *The Neurological Examination of the Infant*, (eds. Mac Keith, R. C., Polani, P. E. and Clayton-Jones, E.), CDM No. 1. Spastics International Medical Publications. William Heinemann Medical Books Limited, London.

Brazelton, T. B. (1973). *Neonatal Behavioral Assessment Scale*, CDM No. 50. Spastics International Medical Publications. William Heinemann Medical Books Limited, London.

Brazelton, T. B. (1984). *Neonatal Behavioral Assessment Scale*, 2nd edition, CDM No. 88. Spastics International Medical Publications. Blackwell Scientific Publications Limited, Oxford.

Dubowitz, L. and Dubowitz, V. (1981). *The Neurological Assessment of the Pre-term and Full-term Newborn Infant*, CDM No. 79. Spastics International Medical Publications. William Heinemann Medical Books Limited, London.

Dubowitz, L., Dubowitz, V., Palmer, P. G. et al (1984). Correlation of neurologic assessment in the pre-term newborn infant with outcome at 1 year. *Journal of Paediatrics*, **105**, 3, 452-6.

Hambleton, G. and Wigglesworth, J. S. (1976). Origins of intraventricular haemorrhage in the pre-term infant. *Archives of Disease in Childhood*, **51**, 651-9.

Levene, M. I., Fawer, C. L. and Lamont, R. F. (1982). Risk factors in the development of intraventricular haemorrhage in the pre-term neonate. *Archives of Disease in Childhood*, **57**, 410-17.

Mac Keith, R. C. (1964). The primary walking response and its facilitation by passive extension of the head. *Acta Pediatrica Latin America*, **17** (Suppl. 6), 710.

O'Reilly, R. and Gardner, E. (1977). The developmental anatomy and history of the central nervous system. In *Handbook of Clinical Neurology*, Vol 30, pp. 15-40, (eds. Vinken, P. J. and De Buyn, G. W.). Elsevier North Holland, Amsterdam.

Pape, K. E. and Wigglesworth, J. S. (1979). *Haemorrhage, Ischaemia and the Perinatal Brain*, CDM No. 69/70. Spastics International Medical Publications. William Heinemann Medical Books Limited, London.

Prechtl, H. (1965). Problems of behavioral studies in the newborn infant. In *Advances in the Study of Behavior*, Vol 1, p. 75, (eds. Lehrman, D. S., Hinde, R. A. and Shaw, E.). Academic Press, New York.

Prechtl, H. (1977). *The Neurological Examination of the Full-term Newborn Infant*, 2nd edition, CDM No. 63. Spastics International Medical Publications. William Heinemann Medical Books Limited, London.

Prechtl, H. and Beintema, D. J. (1964). *The Neurological Examination of the Full-term Newborn Infant*, CDM No. 12. Spastics International Medical Publications. William Heinemann Medical Books Limited, London.

Rosenbloom, L. and Horton, M. E. (1971). The maturation of fine prehension in young children. *Developmental Medicine and Child Neurology*, **13**, 3-8.

Saint-Anne Dargassies, S. (1966). Neurological maturation of the premature infant of 28 to 41 weeks gestational age. In *Human Development*, pp. 306-25, (ed. Falkner, F.). W.B. Saunders Co, Philadelphia.

Saint-Anne Dargassies, S. (1972). Neurodevelopmental symptoms during the first year of life. I: Essential landmarks for each key age. *Developmental Medicine and Child Neurology*, **14**, 235-46.

Saint-Anne Dargassies, S. (1977). *Neurological Development in Full-term and Premature Neonates*. Elsevier/North Holland/Excerpta Medica, Amsterdam.

Touwen, B. (1976). *Neurological Development in Infancy*, CDM No. 58. Spastics International Medical Publications. William Heinemann Medical Books Limited, London.

Wigglesworth, J. S. and Pape, K. E. (1978). An integrated model for haemorrhagic and ischaemic lesions in the newborn brain. *Early Human Development*, **2**, 179-99.

BIBLIOGRAPHY

Connolly, K. J. and Prechtl, H. (eds.) (1981). *Maturation and Development. Biological and Psychological Perspectives*, CDM No. 77/78. Spastics International Medical Publications. William Heinemann Medical Books Limited, London.

Illingworth, R. S. (1980). *The Development of the Infant and Young Child*, 7th edition, Churchill Livingstone, Edinburgh.

Sheridan, M. D. (1973). *Children's Developmental Progress from Birth to Five Years: The Stycar Sequences.* NFER Publishing Co Ltd, Windsor.

Chapter 4

Aspects of Neuro-Anatomy and Physiology

by H. W. ATKINSON MCSP, HT, DipTP

THE NERVOUS SYSTEM AS A TOOL

The nervous system is the tool used by the living creature in order to be able to react to its environment. The more complex the creature, the more complicated its nervous system and the more versatile are its reactions. The system is concerned with physical (motor, sensory and autonomic), intellectual and emotional activities and, in consequence, any disorder may involve any one or all three of these major functions.

Neurone

The nervous system is composed of an enormous number of neurones, connected together and following certain pathways, in order to make functional activity possible. The neurone is the basic unit of the nervous system and comprises the nerve cell and its processes. Each neurone has a cell body and two types of processes (Fig. 4/1), dendrites and axons.

Figure 4/2 shows how each ramus carries motor, sensory and autonomic fibres and the sympathetic ganglion communicates with those above and below it in level and also sends fibres to the visceral contents. Figure 4/3 shows that the corticospinal path represents the pyramidal system and other paths may be considered to be extrapyramidal.

The synapse

This is the term used to define the area where the process of one neurone links with another. The synapse is a point of contiguity but not of continuity. Synapses may occur between the terminal

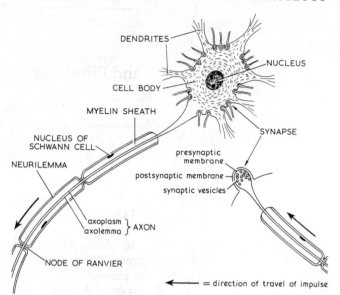

FIG. 4/1 Structure of a neurone

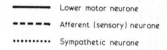

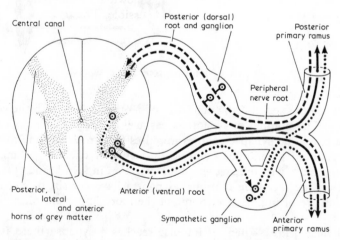

FIG. 4/2 Neurones forming a mixed spinal nerve at thoracic level

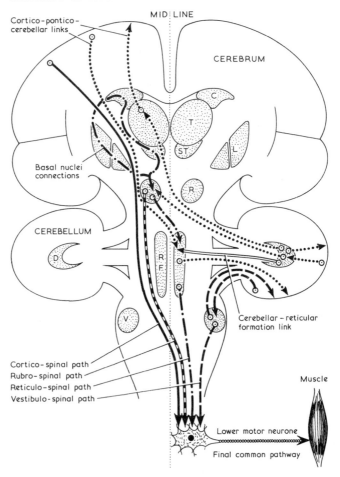

FIG. 4/3 Motor neurone connections

parts of an axon and the dendrites of another cell or with the cell body. The number of synaptic areas may be very vast in any one neurone. The synapse enables impulses from one neurone to be transmitted to another neurone by virtue of chemical changes taking place which bring about an alteration in membrane potential on the receiving neurone. Synapses have certain properties which are of importance. Some of the more important ones are:

Synaptic delay. When an impulse reaches a synapse there is a brief time lag before a response occurs in the recipient neurone.

Consequently conduction along a chain of neurones is slower than along one single neurone. Thus monosynaptic pathways conduct more rapidly than polysynaptic routes.

One-way conduction. Synapses permit conduction of impulses in one direction only, i.e. from the pre-synaptic to the post-synaptic neurone.

Vulnerability. Synapses are very sensitive to anoxia and to the effects of drugs. Polysynaptic pathways are very susceptible to anaesthesia.

Summation. The effect of impulses arriving at a synapse can be added to by other impulses. For instance the effect of impulses could be subliminal (insufficient to bring about adequate chemical change for depolarisation of the post-synaptic neurone). If, however, another spate of impulses arrives before the effect of the previous one has subsided then the two effects may complement each other and the total change be sufficient to cause depolarisation. Such a phenomenon is called summation. There are two types of summation, the type just described being dependent upon a time factor and being called temporal summation. The other type is called spatial summation. It is the result of the adding together of impulses from different neurones which converge upon the post-synaptic neurone and bring about depolarisation of its membrane.

Fatigue. The synapse is thought to be the site of fatigue in nerve conductivity.

Inhibition. Certain neurones have an inhibitory effect upon the post-synaptic neurone, possibly because they use a different chemical mediator. Thus the effect of these neurones would be to discourage depolarisation of the post-synaptic cell membrane and would be antagonistic to influences exerted by excitatory neurones. These effects can summate in the same way as the excitatory effects. Many interneurones have an inhibitory effect.

Post-tetanic potentiation. This occurs across synapses which have been subjected to prolonged and repeated activity. The threshold of stimulation of these junctions is thought to be lowered making transmission across it more easily brought about for a period of several hours. Facilitation of transmission is said to occur, and is an elementary form of learning and also forms an important part in the approach to physical treatment of patients with neurological disorders.

Supporting tissue

Neurones are delicate, highly specialised structures and require support and protection. This is afforded to them in the nervous system by specialised connective tissue called neuroglia. If neurones are damaged and destroyed their place is filled by proliferation of neuroglial material.

The axons are surrounded by a fatty sheath called myelin which has an important effect on the conduction of impulses. Because of this sheath, bundles of axons give a whitish appearance and form the white matter of the central nervous system.

When the axon and its myelin sheath leave the central nervous system they become surrounded by a membrane called the neurilemma. This is of vital importance and it should be noted that the neurilemma is absent round the fibres of the brain and spinal cord whereas it is present as soon as they leave these areas.

Nerve fibres which are surrounded by neurilemma may regenerate if they are destroyed. Hence destruction of fibres in a peripheral nerve does not necessarily mean permanent loss of function whereas destruction of the fibres in the central nervous system will mean permanent loss of function of those fibres. It should also be noted that the nerve cell is resilient to injury and has considerable recuperative powers but, if it dies, it is incapable of being replaced. Thus destruction of cell bodies means permanent loss of function.

SOME PHYSIOLOGICAL CONCEPTS

Most patients suffering from neurological disorders show movement difficulties, and it is therefore important to consider the factors which are essential for the production of normal movement and activity.

Movement in its mature and skilled form is the result of complex teamwork between a multitude of muscles and joints so that balanced movement patterns are produced which can achieve an effect for the individual. Movement and postural attitudes are so closely related that it is impossible to distinguish one from the other.

The muscles concerned in the production of movement receive their ultimate stimulation from the motoneurone pools or masses of cells housed in the anterior horns of the spinal cord or, in the case of the cranial nerves, in the motor nuclei of the brainstem. Axons from the motoneurone pools pass to the muscles and constitute the lower motor neurones or final common pathways.

Many neurones converge upon and synapse with the lower motor neurone, some coming from the extrapyramidal and pyramidal pathways, some being spinal interneurones and some coming direct from the peripheral afferent system. Whether or not impulses pass along the final common pathways depends upon two very important factors:

1. The integrity of the pathway
2. The influence exerted upon the cells of the motoneurone pool.

If the lower motoneurone pathway is not intact there is no route for the impulses to take. Fortunately each muscle is supplied by many neurones and only a severe lesion in the pathway would involve every lower motoneurone passing to any one muscle. However, this can occur and the result is a muscle which cannot be made to contract via activity in its own motor nerve supply and therefore one which is unable to participate in any teamwork towards functional activity.

Since many neurones are converging upon the cells in the motoneurone pools, including interneurones, it is possible that two types of influence may be exerted. These are *excitatory* - encouraging depolarisation - and *inhibitory* - discouraging depolarisation. The ratio between these two influences is the deciding factor as to whether the motoneurone pools are activated or not. The muscles they supply will, therefore, contract or remain inactive according to the balance of excitatory *versus* inhibitory influences being exerted upon their motoneurone pools.

When contraction occurs its intensity is dependent upon the number of muscle fibres brought into action. The number of fibres activated depends upon the number of cells in the motoneurone pool which have conveyed impulses. Thus the greater the excitatory influence on the motoneurone pool and the lower their threshold of stimulation, the greater the number of active motoneurones and the greater the resultant degree of muscle contraction.

The factors exerting an influence on the motoneurone pools

These are many and varied. Pathways which are of importance are those of the pyramidal and extrapyramidal parts of the central nervous system which convey impulses resulting in volitional, postural and equilibrium reactions. Also of importance are the lower reflex pathways which give rise to withdrawal and stretch responses which are the result of more direct influences from the afferent side of the peripheral system. The interrelationship between one and the other is very important and can be illustrated by a simple account of the stretch reflex mechanism.

Skeletal muscles may be divided into two types of fibres. The large ordinary fibres are known as extrafusal fibres and the smaller fibres, which lie parallel to the extrafusal fibres and are encapsulated, are known as intrafusal fibres. The intrafusal fibres are part of the stretch reflex mechanism of muscle and the one illustrated in Figure 4/4 has a non-contractile part and a contractile part.

The non-contractile part of the intrafusal fibres is concerned with stretch reception and is linked to the central nervous system by an afferent neurone (called an Ia fibre) which makes direct synapse with a large anterior horn cell in the motoneurone pool of the same muscle to which the intrafusal fibres belong. Stretch to the muscle and therefore to the non-contractile part of the

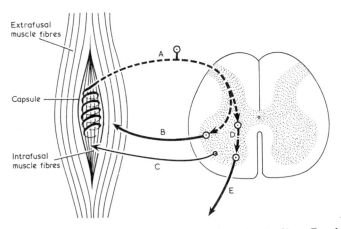

Fig. 4/4 The simple stretch reflex mechanism. A = Ia fibre; B = alpha efferent; C = fusimotor fibre (gamma efferent); D = interneurone; E = motor neurone to antagonistic muscle

intrafusal fibre has an excitatory effect on the stretch receptor, and impulses travel along the Ia fibre to the motoneurone pool where the large anterior horn cell is stimulated and conveys impulses to the extrafusal fibres causing them to contract. The large anterior horn cell is said to send an alpha efferent to the extrafusal muscle fibre. In this way the stretch on the intrafusal fibres is reduced. The afferent fibres also influence other associated motoneurones and by means of interneurones they may exert an inhibitory influence on the motoneurone pools of antagonistic muscles.

The contractile parts of the intrafusal fibres have their own nerve supply from the motoneurone pools by means of small anterior horn cells. The axons of these cells are called fusimotor fibres (gamma efferents) to distinguish them from the fibres of the large anterior horn cells. Impulses passing along these fusimotor fibres to the intrafusal muscle fibres will cause them to contract and make them exert tension upon their own non-contractile areas. Thus they are able to make the intrafusal non-contractile area more sensitive to stretch by their activity or less sensitive to stretch by their inactivity.

In other words a bias can be put upon the sensitivity of the stretch reflex mechanism depending upon the degree of activity in the intrafusal contractile tissue and the fusimotor fibres. This bias depends upon the influences being exerted upon the small anterior horn cells which are particularly linked to the extrapyramidal pathways from the central nervous system, which in turn incorporates the balance and postural mechanism. Through this system the stretch reflex mechanism in muscle can be made more sensitive or less so according to the postural needs of the moment. Thus there is interaction between excitation and inhibition and between lower reflex activity and higher control. (See Chapter 5 for a detailed description of the myotatic (stretch) reflex.)

There are at least two types of intrafusal fibres (nuclear bag and nuclear chain). There are also two types of stretch receptors, Ia and II, and there are at least two types of fusimotor fibres. This mechanism makes the muscle sensitive to both velocity and degree of stretch, enables it to adjust its resting length and to be sensitive to stretch to a varying degree whatever its resting length happens to be. Figure 4/5 illustrates the simple stretch reflex mechanism and the effect of contraction of the intrafusal fibres.

Thus it may be seen that the influence of the fibres from the extrapyramidal system can adjust muscle activity to a fine degree and since certain righting, postural and equilibrium reactions are

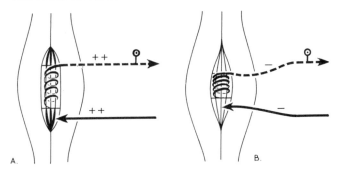

FIG. 4/5 Effect of activity of fusimotor (gamma) fibres

integrated into the extrapyramidal system it is not difficult to see that these reactions exert their influence upon the motoneurone pools via these fibres.

These postural mechanisms and reactions make possible a variety of automatic responses to various situations. The normal human being can, however, encourage or inhibit these activities at will and can carry out activities which are not entirely automatic but are dependent upon some automatic adjustments. When these background automatic adjustments are not available normal willed movement becomes inco-ordinate, posturally unsound and well nigh impossible.

DISTURBANCE OF AFFERENT INFORMATION

Loss of, or imperfection in, afferent supply may give rise to several problems. It may be the result of definite interruption of afferent pathways, giving areas of anaesthesia or paraesthesia. If the interruption lies within a peripheral nerve then the area affected will be that specifically supplied by that particular nerve. If, however, it is more centrally placed the lesion may have more diffuse effects because many fibres from different areas tend to travel together in the spinal cord.

Sensory disturbance may be due to disease processes pressing on afferent pathways giving distorted input. It may be due to faulty linkage between thalamus and cortex, which would prevent discriminative assessment of sensory information.

Disturbance in the link between spinal cord and cerebellum

would give rise to inadequate information to help the cerebellum in its postural activities.

One must also remember that visual, auditory and vestibular afferents may be affected in addition to those conveying joint sensation. These latter factors give rise to the most potent symptoms of disorientation and loss of body image.

The results of afferent disturbance vary from very slight effects to total loss of body image, disorientation and rejection of the affected area. Skin anaesthesia makes the patient vulnerable to injury since pain is absent and there is no withdrawal from harmful stimuli.

Patients with a reduction in afferent information may have difficulty with spatial perception. The relative positions, size, heights and depths of objects may be difficult for them to perceive. This, of course, is closely linked to visual impressions. Ability of hand/eye control depend to some extent upon binocular vision.

Appreciation of shapes, textures and weight is also important and depends upon eyes, hands and manipulative skills in addition to skin and kinaesthetic sensation. Loss of this variety of sensory perception magnifies the loss of body image and the patient may forget the affected area or even reject it.

Disturbance of sensory perception may, in some cases, be aggravated by lack of experience. If the patient is prevented from experiencing certain afferent stimuli because of the disability then some measure of deprivation must occur. For example, the human being normally carries the hand towards the face for a multiplicity of reasons. If the movements of the upper limb are so impoverished that this cannot occur then the link between hand and face becomes weaker and some degree of body image is lost due to lack of repetitive experience.

Conversely other disturbing things may happen. If a patient experiences an abnormal sensation often enough, he may well eventually accept this as normal and may resent any attempt to adjust or correct this. Let us take an example to illustrate: the patient's disability may make him inclined to lean his weight, when sitting, consistently on to one side. If this is allowed to continue he will accept the one-sided pressure as being natural and normal and interpret the position as being one of safety and one in which he feels secure. If attempts are then made to encourage him to take weight evenly on each side he will feel that he is leaning dangerously towards the side which has not been accustomed to receiving weight. He will not feel safe until he has regained his own 'normal' position. Thus he may reject attempts to correct his posture to a more normal one and much patience and understanding will be required to gain his co-operation.

Paraesthesia is a term used to signify disturbed and diminished sensory information. It refers to tingling and numbness of the affected area and may be the result of lesions of any part of the afferent system. However, it is most obvious in peripheral problems. Paraesthesia should not be confused with para-anaesthesia, which is a term used to denote *loss* of sensation in both lower limbs.

Dissociated anaesthesia refers to the loss of appreciation of pain and temperature while tactile information is still available. This is most often due to interruption of the lateral spinothalamic tracts within the cord and is seen in cases of syringomyelia.

Hypalgia refers to a reduction in sensitivity to pain. This occurs in certain disorders of the afferent system. Where all afferent information is reduced or lost there will obviously be hypalgia but it is most noticeable in association with dissociated anaesthesia. These two phenomena lead to damage as a result of major and minor trauma since they reduce the stimulation of protective mechanisms.

When afferent information reaches the brain it is received and interpreted. The brain processes the information so that appropriate reactions may occur. Any defect at this level makes the production of appropriate reactions difficult or impossible. The patient cannot recall, learn or relearn basic patterns of movement and may be very difficult to treat for this reason. It is important for the physiotherapist to appreciate this, since many patients are thought to be unco-operative or 'not trying', when in fact the problem is in the processing of afferent material.

ABNORMALITIES OF MOVEMENT

These may take several forms according to the area of damage.

Muscle flaccidity or paralysis (atonia)

This is the result of disturbance in the lower motor neurone. The muscle or group of muscles affected may be totally paralysed if all their available neurones are put out of action. If only some anterior horn neurones are involved the muscles will show partial paralysis and will appear to be very weak. Any muscles affected in this way would be unable to function as members of a team and consequently movement synergies requiring their participation would be abnormal and substitute patterns would be produced. If only a small muscle group is affected in this way the abnormalities are minimal, but if many groups are involved, substitution can be grotesque or even inadequate, in which case the subject is rendered relatively helpless.

Totally flaccid muscles have no lower motor neurone supply because of damage or injury to all the cells in their motoneurone pools or to all the fibres passing peripherally. Such muscles cannot be brought into action voluntarily, or as an automatic reaction or in a reflex action. They feel soft and flabby to the touch, are non-resilient, offer no protection to the structures adjacent to them and are unable to support the joints over which they pull. Because of lack of use, and therefore of blood supply, they atrophy quite rapidly losing the greater part of their muscle bulk.

Hypotonia

This term is used here to denote the reduction in preparedness for action found in the muscles when there are defects in certain areas of the extrapyramidal part of the central nervous system. In this case the excitatory influence exerted by the extrapyramidal system upon the motoneurone pools is diminished and, as a result, the muscles show a reduction in sensitivity to stretch. This may, at first sight, be confused with muscle paralysis because the muscles may appear to be totally or almost totally flail. It is, however, very different. The muscles have a normal lower motor neurone supply but the factors exerting an influence upon the motoneurone pools are seriously disturbed. There is a reduction of excitatory influence upon the small anterior horn cells which give rise to the fusimotor fibres. Because of this the fusimotor fibres are inactive and therefore activity of the intrafusal muscle fibres is diminished. Thus the muscles are less sensitive to stretch – particularly if it is applied slowly. Quick, exaggerated stretch will bring about a response via the spinal stretch reflex but the bias on the receptors is low. If the muscle is stretched by distortion of its tendon, as in the knee jerk, the response will occur but will not be quickly checked by a reciprocal response in the hamstrings because their stretch reflex mechanism will also be sluggish. The lower leg will swing backward and forward like a pendulum before it finally comes to rest again.

Hypotonia never affects muscle groups in isolation because it is not a peripheral problem. It is usually found as a general feature or, in some cases, it may be unilateral. The most common reason for hypotonia is disturbance in function of the cerebellum. It may be the result of damage or disease in the cerebellum itself or in the links between the cerebellum and the brainstem extra-pyramidal mechanisms.

The cerebellum is thought to exert its influence upon the postural reflex mechanisms by its link with the extrapyramidal system. If it fails to encourage excitation in these tonic mechanisms the fusimotor system will fail to function adequately and the stretch reflex bias will be low. This gives a background of postural instability and makes proximal fixation for distal movements unavailable. Movements therefore tend to be slow in forthcoming and when they do commence they are of an unstable, ill-controlled nature, inclined to overshoot the mark and show intention tremor. This term is used because the tremor occurs when a movement is being carried out and is not present when at rest.

Balance reactions are also disturbed and when they occur they are inclined to overcompensate. The patient may, in fact, fall because of his exaggerated balance reactions. These are occurring against a background of unstable postural tone due to diminished fusimotor activity.

Ataxia

A patient who has hypotonia inevitably shows a form of ataxia. The symptoms described under the heading 'hypotonia' are also those of ataxia. Ataxia means that movements are inco-ordinate and ill-timed, giving a deficiency of smoothness of movement. Ataxia related to hypotonia occurs partly because of the defective postural tone as a background and partly because of the phenomenon of dyssynergia.

Dyssynergia is the term used to describe the loss of fluency in a movement. The balance of activity is upset because of faulty synergy. The teamwork between muscles is lost, giving a jerky appearance to the movements, which may well be split up into a series of jerky, separated entities. Both stopping and starting of movements are difficult and overshooting occurs.

These symptoms may also be noted when hearing a patient

speak. Speech is a very mature ability, requiring intricate control of co-ordination of the appropriate muscles. Dyssynergia and accompanying problems lead to speech being broken up in the same way as was described for movement. Speech affected in this way is said to be 'scanning'.

Ataxia may also be linked with the sensory problems mentioned earlier in this chapter. It may be due to deficiency of afferent information to the cerebellum and to the cortex, making the individual unaware of his position in space. In this case the cerebellum cannot bring about the necessary postural adjustments, nor is the central nervous system receiving a feedback regarding the success of the movements. A person with this problem will show very similar symptoms to the previous form of ataxia, but he may be able to mask his problem by using his eyes and ears to excess as substitutes for his loss of skin and joint position sensation. If he is temporarily deprived of the use of his eyes – as in the dark – or of his ears – as in a noisy environment – he may be much more ataxic than when he is able to make full use of them. This is often called rombergism.

The ataxias are often accompanied by *nystagmus*, which is a form of dyssynergia in the eyes.

Occasionally ataxia may be accompanied by vestibular disturbance which gives rise to vertigo. This is a condition in which the patient's appreciation of head position is disorientated. The subject feels giddy and nauseated. These symptoms can add greatly to the problems of the ataxic patient.

Dysmetria is a term often applied to the ataxic patient. It refers to the difficulty in assessing and achieving the correct distance or range of movement. It is seen in the overshooting symptoms mentioned earlier.

Hypertonia

This denotes the opposite state of affairs to hypotonia. There are two types of hypertonia, spasticity and rigidity.

SPASTICITY

As was stated before, the fusimotor system is rendered excessively active. The sensitivity of the stretch receptors is excessively high to both slow and quick stretch stimuli. In its milder form the sensitivity to quick stretch is most noticeable, when a 'clasp-knife' phenomenon may be demonstrated. In this situation the muscles respond to quick stretch in a phasic manner when there is synchronous firing of the primary receptors, which in turn gives a synchronous contraction of extrafusal muscle in response. The primary receptors fire synchronously because their threshold has been made low due to the excessive activity of the fusimotor system. The term 'clasp-knife' phenomenon is occasionally used because the opposition of the muscle to stretch seems to build up to a climax and then to subside suddenly. The sudden reduction in opposition may be attributed to the inhibitory influence exerted by the group Ib Golgi tendon organs, when tension is applied to the musculotendinous junction. Many explanations have been offered for this phenomenon and studies are not completed.

The response to slow stretch is that of steady opposition to the stretch stimulus which, in some cases, may build up to a tremendous level whereas in other milder cases it may be very slight indeed. On the whole passive movements to joints, where the muscles are showing spasticity, are more likely to be successful if conducted slowly so as to avoid eliciting a phasic response.

This form of hypertonicity may be associated with the release of reflex activity from cortical control. If the lesion has occurred at a high level in the central nervous system then the tonic postural reflexes may be released in addition to the spinal reflexes. The released reflexes will exert a relatively uninhibited effect upon the motoneurone pools and cause patterns of increase in tone relevant to the reflexes released. For example, the released asymmetrical tonic neck reflex will cause spasticity to show in the extensor groups of the limbs on the side towards which the face is turned and in the flexors of the opposite side. The tonic labyrinthine reflex will incline the patient to show spasticity in the extensor groups if his head is in the appropriate position. The symmetrical tonic neck reflex will cause appropriate spastic patterning according to the position of the cervical spine, i.e. if the cervical spine is flexed the upper limbs will flex and the lower limbs extend.

It is rare to find one reflex mechanism released in isolation and a confusion of patterns is more likely to occur. However, knowledge of these factors enables the physiotherapist to interpret what is happening at any one time more accurately.

Spastic patterning varies from moment to moment depending upon many factors. One factor is the general position of the patient. Another is the nature of the stimulus being applied to the patient and yet another is how much effort the patient is making to obtain a voluntary movement. Strong volition often simply facilitates the excitation of the spastic patterning. This is possibly because the threshold of the appropriate motoneurone pools is already low, due to reflex release, so that the slightest volitional effort triggers them into action.

If the damage to the central nervous system is lower in level so that only the spinal reflexes are released then the spastic patterning may well be more related to flexion withdrawal. According to the stimulus applied there may be flexion or extension patterning but flexion is more likely to be predominant. Withdrawal is a response to noxious stimuli, but in this type of case it can be the response to almost any stimulus: touching of bedclothes on the affected areas, vibration, noise, sudden movement. It is well to bear this in mind since such patients must be dealt with very carefully if flexion withdrawal is not to become a permanent position for the patient.

Spasticity is never isolated to one muscle group. It is always part of a total flexion or total extension synergy. Let us take a lower limb example. If the lower limb is in extensor spasticity it will tend to adopt hip extension, adduction and medial rotation, knee extension and foot plantar flexion. Thus if one detected spasticity in the adductor groups one should expect it in all the other groups in the pattern.

It should be noted that the limb is not put into a good weight-bearing position by this patterning. The heel is unable to touch the supporting surface and the adducted limb is unable to support the pelvis adequately. Thus the patient showing this patterning is not able to experience the appropriate stimuli which will give the slow-acting postural muscles the appropriate guidance to support the limb.

For sound supporting posture we require the normal afferent stimulus of compression upon the heel of the foot. In this way the appropriate malleable postural mechanisms giving balanced co-contraction of both flexors and extensors can be encouraged. If this occurs we do not show the hyperextended knee of the mildly spastic or the complete inability to get the heel on to the ground of the severely spastic case.

The spastic patient of this type may be deprived of experiencing the very afferent stimulation which could make his postural tone more normal. This occurs in many ways to the patient with this abnormal patterning and is an important factor in his treatment. The physiotherapist must help the patient to experience afferent stimulation which he is, by his condition, denied.

Reflex release mechanisms are more often than not incomplete.

It is because this is so that many patients have interesting variations in patterning and also have some voluntary control. Obviously, the more control the patient has, the less severe is the residual problem. However, some patients require time to make use of such control as may be available and meanwhile bad habits, if unchecked, could mar the patient's eventual result.

RIGIDITY

In this type of hypertonicity the fusimotor system is also excessively active giving an increase in sensitivity to the stretch receptors in muscle. The disturbance is thought to lie at a different level from that causing spasticity since there is a considerable difference in the type of change in response to stretch.

It will be remembered that the subcortical nuclei comprising the basal ganglia are thought to help in the production of postural fixation by exerting their influence upon the stretch reflex mechanism via the reticular formation. They help to maintain adequate postural fixation while allowing the necessary malleability for voluntary movement. If they become too effective as factors in postural fixation the stretch reflex mechanism may lose its malleability due to excessive fusimotor action. Damage in the area of link between the cortex and basal ganglia may well lead to excessive postural fixation to the detriment of volitional activity. The rigidity which ensues is different from spasticity in that it does not adopt the patterns of any particular reflex mechanism because the reflexes of tonic posture are not released. The pathways in the brainstem may still be intact and consequently some control of the stretch reflex mechanism may be available. The 'clasp-knife' effect seen in spasticity is not available in rigidity because phasic stretch does not appear to be suddenly inhibited. This may be because the control centres in the brainstem exert a suppressor action upon the inhibitory mechanisms.

In rigidity the muscles respond to slow stretch by steady resistance which does not particularly build up or relax off. There is a tremor which is said to give a 'cog-wheel' effect, or the limbs may feel like lead when moved, giving rise to the term 'lead-pipe' rigidity. Explanations of this phenomenon are not complete and it must be remembered that, at present, there are many questions which remain unanswered.

Patients showing rigidity usually have lesions in the subcortical areas and show a typical posture which becomes progressively more flexed. They do not rotate in any of their movements and lack of axial rotation seriously interferes with balance reactions.

The 'rigidity' patient shows movement problems in which automatic adjustment and activities do not occur freely and therefore voluntary movement is slow and impoverished because it is unaccompanied by automatic balance reactions and because it occurs so slowly against the ever-resisting stretch mechanisms.

In spasticity movement impoverishment also occurs. Balance reactions cannot be produced against the spastic patterns and mature permutations of flexion versus extension patterns are not available, only the stereotyped reflex patterns being produced in voluntary movement.

Athetosis

When this occurs the patient shows disorder of movement because of fluctuation in the level of postural fixation. The patient adopts a succession of abnormal postures which may be quite grotesque. The condition is made more severe by excitement and emotional stress. It is thought to be due to lesions within the basal ganglia and in particular in the putamen. In this instance the basal ganglia are failing in their ability to encourage adequate postural fixation and fluctuations therefore occur.

Involuntary movements occasionally occur but the symptoms are always made worse by voluntary activity.

Choreiform activity

This is a series of involuntary movements, which occur in the face and limbs. They are quicker than those of athetosis and are also made worse by voluntary movement. Many patients show a combination of choreiform and athetoid activities. The basal ganglia are considered to be at fault in choreiform problems.

Ballismus

This is a term used to describe wild flinging movements which may occur to such an extent that they throw the patient off balance. The condition usually occurs as a result of a lesion in the subthalamic region and only affects one side. In this case it is called hemiballismus.

Dystonia

This is a term used to describe an increase in muscle tone that is antagonistic to the intended movement. The symptoms tend to prevent movement and may pull the individual into grotesque postures. It may affect one part of the body or the body as a whole. Spasmodic torticollis is thought to be a type of local dystonia. The lesion is thought to lie in the putamen.

TENDENCY TO DEVELOP DEFORMITIES

Whenever there is a tendency to adopt habitual postures of one part of the body or many parts there is a danger of adaptive shortening of some soft tissues and lengthening of others. In this way joints may become stiff and give deformities which are very difficult to correct. The least vulnerable patients are the athetoids and choreiform types since these patients are rarely still, but the spastic, rigid and flaccid types of patient may develop severe deformities if left untreated.

VULNERABILITY TO INJURY

Sensory loss leads to obvious dangers. Pain produced by damage is a protection against continuation of the damage. If pain is not felt then damage can occur with no protective reaction. Many cases of skin lesion and ulceration are due to this problem.

Many of these patients have sphincter problems and are incontinent. This renders the skin soggy and even more vulnerable. Pressure sores are a common complication. If pain is felt and the patient is unable to move away from its cause damage will also occur.

Muscle flaccidity, dyssynergia, and spasticity may all lead to ill-controlled joint positioning so that joints are put to undue strain and ligaments permanently stretched. The hyperextended knees of extensor spasticity are an example of this. The joint distortion may in some cases be great enough to cause subluxation.

Malposturing may also lead to undue pressure on nerves and blood vessels. This may give rise to secondary neuropathy, defects of venous return and oedema.

CIRCULATORY PROBLEMS

These exist in various forms in most neurological disorders.

When muscle paralysis is present the muscle pump action is

defective and venous return is reduced. This may not have a noticeable effect if only small groups are affected, but if large areas of muscle are paralysed the effect may be great enough to cause oedema and may have the effect of reducing the rate of growth in the child. A peripheral problem of this type also gives rise to autonomic defects involving the control of blood vessels and sweat glands. Skin changes corresponding to this occur. Atrophy of the skin may develop causing it to become dry, scaly, thin and more vulnerable.

Disorders of the spinal cord will interfere with the autonomic control of the blood vessels and may have a general effect on the patient's ability to give correct blood pressure adjustments. The higher the level of cord injury the more severe the effect. This is seen most dramatically in paraplegic and tetraplegic cases.

Hypotonia will also give rise to defects of muscle pump activity although the effect may not at first be noticeable because it is more general and there is no 'normal' for comparison.

RESPIRATORY PROBLEMS

The patient may show paralysis in the respiratory muscles and will then obviously have respiratory difficulties. Those who have paralysis or severe hypotonia in the throat musculature will also have difficulty, since the inspiratory movements tend to suck the walls of the pharynx inward unless muscle tone braces against this effect. Thus the patient may choke for this reason or because the throat muscles are inco-ordinate in swallowing so that inhalation of food occurs.

Respiratory movements may be so impaired as to make speech difficult and coughing impossible. Communication is therefore a problem and lung secretions gather.

The patient showing rigidity may have impaired respiratory function due to the difficulty in obtaining thoracic mobility.

SPEECH DISORDERS

These may be the direct result of respiratory problems, due to paralysis of speech muscles, or due to more complex problems of dyssynergia, spasticity and speech perceptual problems. A patient is said to be *dysphasic* when he has inco-ordination of speech and is unable to arrange his words in correct order. He is said to be *aphasic* when he is unable to express himself in writing, speech or by signs and is unable to comprehend written or spoken language. There are many different forms of aphasia and each one is very distressing to the patient.

DISTURBANCE OF EXERCISE TOLERANCE

This is inevitable. Only the most minor neurological changes would leave this undisturbed. The dysfunction of normal movement necessitates uneconomical substitute movements which undermine exercise tolerance. If this is not apparent because the patient is relatively immobile due to his disorder, his exercise tolerance will be reduced because of lack of exercise. The chairbound patient who is wheeled about by relatives, quickly loses such exercise tolerance as he had because his circulatory and respiratory mechanisms are not put to any stress. Added to this he may be inclined to overeat and will put on unnecessary fat which will further reduce his condition of tolerance.

Any patient whose respiratory capacity is reduced must have diminished exercise tolerance.

Since there are many reasons for this problem they should be noted by the physiotherapist who may be able to minimise them in some cases.

PAIN

This is a factor in neurological cases but is not so prevalent as might at first seem likely. Pain can only be felt if there are pathways to convey the sensation.

Pain is most likely to occur in irritative lesions when the threshold of pain reception is low. Thus pain is a feature of neuritis. Other reasons are those connected with raised intracranial pressure giving rise to headache and throbbing sensations.

Some patients with lesions in the thalamic region show intractable thalamic pain which is difficult to understand until it is appreciated as a centrally placed lesion and is not due to damage in the peripheral area from which the pain is interpreted as coming.

Discomfort and pain from habitual bad posturing also occur and patients who have sudden waves of increase in muscle tone will complain of pain.

Referred pain

This is a term used to denote pain interpreted as arising from an area which is not, in fact, the site of the trouble. For example, pressure on the roots of origin of C5 and 6 can give pain which is referred to their dermatomes, myotomes and sclerotomes. The patient will complain of pain over the deltoid area, lateral aspect of forearm and over the radial side of the hand. He may complain of deep pain over the scapula, lateral aspect of humerus, radius and over the bones of the thumb. The site of this problem is, in this case, in the cervical region but the patient suspects disease or injury where he feels the pain. This type of referred pain is often called root pain.

Referred pain does not always relate to surface structures but may also relate to viscera. For example, in cardiac disease pain may be referred to the left shoulder.

It is well known that pain in the otherwise normal individual will give rise to protective muscle spasm and abnormalities of movement and posture. It must, therefore, be appreciated that pain will do the same to the neurological case provided the nervous pathways are available to react. Thus the abnormality induced by pain will be superimposed upon those already existing.

Causalgia

This is a term used to describe a severe sensation of burning pain which accompanies some peripheral problems. The patient shows hyperaesthesia or increased sensitivity, trophic changes and over-activity of the autonomic supply of the area.

The pain is aggravated by exposure to heat or cold and also by emotional crises. Because of the hyperaesthesia the patient protects the affected area to an extreme degree and does not move it at all. Even cutting the fingernails, if the hand is affected, may prove too painful and gloves, shoes and stockings and other items of clothing may be intolerable.

The skin shows atrophy and scales, and vascular changes occur ranging from vasoconstriction to vasodilation. The skin appearance will relate to the condition of the vessels. If vasoconstriction is present the skin is mottled and cyanotic and usually moist due to activity of the sweat glands. If the vessels are dilated the skin will be pink, warm, dry and later may become very glossy.

Muscle atrophy and joint stiffness are frequent in these cases and osteoporosis may be evident.

The exact cause of this condition is not fully understood. It is known to occur when the peripheral injury is incomplete and may be due to deflection of nerve impulses from efferent nerves to afferents so that more impulses are reaching the posterior nerve roots. This could happen in a nerve crush situation where the traumatised area may form a kind of pseudo-synapse between various nerve fibres. It is generally thought that the autonomic disturbances are secondary to the hyperaesthesia.

LOSS OF CONSCIOUSNESS

We are said to be unconscious when we are unaware of sensations such as seeing, hearing, feeling, tasting, smelling. The reticular arousal system in the mid-brain and subthalamic region awakens the cerebral cortex to the reception of sensations. If this formation is damaged or if the cortex is diffusely damaged we may lose consciousness.

Sudden changes in movement may cause temporary loss of consciousness by causing torsional strain on the mid-brain. Space-occupying lesions like tumours and haemorrhages may press upon the mid-brain either directly or indirectly.

The reticular arousal system is very sensitive to deficiencies of oxygen and also of glucose and these may therefore bring about unconsciousness.

It is most important to realise that there are various levels of unconsciousness and that many patients who are apparently totally unconscious are, to some extent, aware of their external environment. They do not appear to be aware of it because they cannot react, but they may have a level of consciousness which makes them semi-receptive.

Careless management of such a patient could be detrimental to his recovery. He may hear discouraging information about himself or be treated in a way which he may resent. He should always be talked to when he is being handled and in an adult manner so that he may as far as possible understand what is happening around him. The physiotherapist should never talk about the patient in front of him.

EPILEPSY

This is a recurring disturbance of cerebral activity in which there is a sudden flood of discharge of impulses from neurones which have, for some reason, become uninhibited. If the area affected is near the reticular arousal area consciousness may be lost. Exact events depend upon the area affected.

Seizures may be major or minor in nature and may complicate many neurological problems, particularly those related to head injuries and tumours.

LOSS OF NORMAL FUNCTIONAL INDEPENDENCE

This is likely in most neurological problems except the most minor. In slowly progressive disorders loss of function appears late since, subconsciously, the patient substitutes for each disability as it appears. In sudden disorders functional loss is dramatic, since the patient has suffered sudden physiological trauma which requires time for adjustment in addition to the psychological trauma associated with sudden disability.

Many patients show rejection of the area most severely affected or at least disassociation from it and they manage as best they can with what is left. Sometimes this is a necessity but there are occasions when such a drastic adjustment is detrimental to the ultimate result and should therefore be discouraged.

Simple functions may be lost because of lack of balance reaction or postural fixation.

The patient may not be able to move around in bed, transfer himself from bed to chair, dress, wash or feed himself.

If functional independence is permanently lost a great burden is placed upon the relatives and on the community as a whole. The patient may live an excessively confined life and have, therefore, limited horizons. This must be avoided and dealing with this aspect plays a large part in the patient's treatment programme.

Urine retention and incontinence

These distressing problems may complicate some of the more severely affected patients.

Sphincters may remain closed leading to retention of urine,

which eventually leaks out due to overfilling of the bladder. Such a condition often gives the appropriate stimulus for flexion withdrawal and may increase flexor spasticity.

The recumbent position added to urine retention may lead to back pressure into the kidneys with further complications. It is always wise to allow such patients to adopt a vertical position periodically to relieve this effect.

Incontinence of urine may lead to skin breakdown since, inevitably, the skin will become soggy and more vulnerable.

Some patients may develop 'automatic' bladder-emptying mechanisms but others may have to have some permanent help in the management of the problem.

There may also be problems related to defaecation although these can often be managed by careful control of the intake of food and fluids in addition to developing a routine of timing of likely bowel activity.

Chapter 5

The Myotatic Reflex

by G. L. KIDD MSc, PhD

This chapter has a dual objective. It will outline current thinking on the myotatic reflex, the element of postural control and, arguably, of all motor co-ordination. It will offer also to physiotherapists an example of how the other sub-divisions of neurophysiology should be approached in study by illustrating how one should move away from a restrictive basis on neuro-anatomy and toward a more dynamic emphasis on the interaction between systems of neurones, and on the processes of neural adaptation.

THE REFLEX

In context, a reflex is an element of motor organisation which allows a certain kind of stimulus to evoke a specific kind of motor response. A reflex belongs to the 'most automatic' category of movement. It may be compared with a skilled, voluntary movement categorised as 'least automatic'.

Neurological tradition has it that the 'most automatic' movements are allowed by the 'lower level' of motor control, the segmental reflex pathways of the spinal cord. The 'least automatic' movements originate in, or are directed by, the 'highest level' of control in the sensori-motor cortex of the cerebrum. At that level the programmes of movement are expressed and subsequently modified by the cerebellum and by sensory feedback systems. As it will be shown, too strict an adherence to neurological tradition is not always to the best advantage of the physiotherapist.

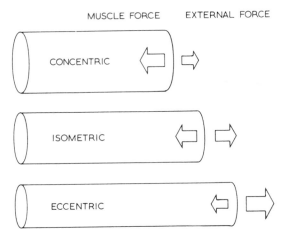

FIG. 5/1 The balance between the external force applied to a muscle and the force developed by a muscle as a consequence determines the mode of muscular action. Where the magnitude of the force is indicated by the size of the arrows, a superior muscle force allows the muscle to shorten on excitation. The muscle action is concentric. Where muscle and external forces balance there is no change in overall muscle length. The muscle action is isometric. Even though a muscle is excited, a superior external force can stretch it. The muscle action is eccentric

THE MYOTATIC REFLEX

To define stretch of a muscle as 'a certain kind of stimulus' is far too academic for the purposes of physiotherapy. What should concern us is not an increase in muscle length, but the superiority of a force being applied to a muscle over the force being generated by that muscle (Fig. 5/1). The superiority of the external force does indeed lead to stretch of the muscle, but an appreciation of the importance of force imbalance leads to an understanding of the pathological changes in the myotatic reflex due, for example, to paresis or spasticity.

THE RESPONSE OF A MUSCLE TO A SUPERIOR EXTERNAL FORCE

The ways in which a muscle will yield to superior and steadily maintained external force deserves thought. Consider the effect of

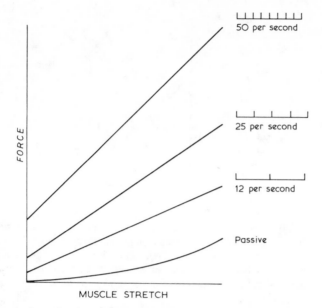

FIG. 5/2 Stretch of a paralysed muscle is opposed by a force generated by the passive elasticity of the muscular tissues. Activity in the muscle fibres generates an active change in muscle elasticity. Electrical stimulation of the nerve to a muscle at 12, 25 and 50 stimuli per second mimics natural muscle activity

applying force to a paralysed muscle (Fig. 5/2). The force is opposed by the passive elasticity of the muscle but, in the example shown, the external force is always superior and the muscle stretches. The passive elastic force in the muscle continues to oppose the external force.

A more realistic condition is seen when the external force is applied to a muscle excited artificially through its nerve by electrical stimuli. In this way natural muscular activity is simulated. Under these conditions, as the frequency of steadily maintained electrical stimulation increases, a given amount of stretch to the muscle is opposed by increasing muscular force. In other words, the elasticity of muscle shows a marked stiffening as the muscle becomes increasingly active (Fig. 5/2).

We have considered so far only the steadily maintained application of external force, the condition found, for example, in antigravity muscles in a static upright posture. But naturally the force

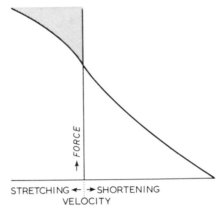

FORCE

STRETCHING ← : → SHORTENING
VELOCITY

FIG. 5/3 The force developed by an active muscle is related to the velocity at which it is able to shorten against an external force (the curve to the right of the vertical force-axis). When a muscle under constant excitation is stretched it shows an increment of active elastic force to oppose the external force (the curve to the left of the vertical force-axis)

is applied to a muscle so that its magnitude changes with time. Examine Figure 5/3. The relationship between the force developed by a muscle and its form of mechanical action under constant, natural excitation are well known. This force-velocity relationship shows that the faster a muscle shortens, the less is the force it develops. Conversely, a muscle develops maximum force (during isometric contraction) when its velocity of shortening is zero.

By extending this familiar graph to include the less familiar negative velocities of shortening (you may prefer to think of a muscle, although active, being lengthened by a superior external force) the muscle generates an increment of force to oppose the external stretching force. The filled region of the curve in Figure 5/3 to the left of the vertical axis shows this.

It can therefore be seen that without involving any of the afferents of the myotatic reflex arc a wide range of elasticity changes can be generated in a muscle to oppose external force. The changes occur as the muscle becomes involved in differing levels of activity. The additional control of active muscle elasticity by the myotatic reflex arc gives great versatility to the postural mechanisms.

THE RECEPTORS AND THE AFFERENT LIMB OF THE REFLEX ARC

Paradoxically, the stretch reflex operates not to allow stretch of a muscle but to prevent it, by absorbing kinetic energy, and by balancing exactly the external force by reflexly modifying the elastic force of active muscle. The receptor in which the reflex originates is the muscle spindle. The term 'spindle' is descriptive and serves little useful purpose. All sensory receptors should be thought of in terms of what they do, and not in terms which only describe their appearance.

Sensory receptors are *transducers*. They will transduce or change the energy form of the stimulus to one able to excite the terminal of the afferent axon.

Usually, the receptor has to *amplify* the stimulus energy to produce sufficient electric current flow for excitation.

In doing so the receptor *measures* the amplitude of the stimulus, and *encodes* the measurement for transmission to the central nervous system.

From elementary neurophysiology it may be recalled that an action potential has an all-or-nothing characteristic. The magnitude of a peripheral action potential is related to the properties of the axon over which it is travelling. A large and a small stimulus, providing they are both above threshold, generate in an axon identically sized action potentials. The magnitude of a stimulus is encoded by the receptor as a pulse interval code, with the times between action potentials carrying all the information and the size of the potential ensuring certain transmission to the central nervous system (Fig. 5/4).

The two forms of receptor ending in the spindle, the primary ending and the secondary ending (previously called annulospiral and flower-spray) are wrapped around and applied to delicate and feeble muscle fibres. This form of muscle fibre is restricted to the structure of the muscle spindle and is referred to as *intrafusal*.

The receptor endings respond to any stimulus which distorts their form. Anything which opens the coils of the primary endings or attempts to shear the secondary endings from their attachment to the intrafusal muscle fibres generates an afferent discharge to the central nervous system.

The intrafusal muscles are under a motor control separate from the control on the main musculature of the body. The intrafusal muscles are unable themselves to generate sufficient force to act

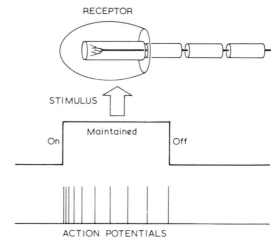

FIG. 5/4 A sensory receptor ending receives a stimulus that is rapidly applied, steadily maintained and then rapidly withdrawn. The receptor generates a train of afferent action potentials with all-or-nothing characteristics. The information on the importance of the stimulus is encoded in the time interval between potentials. The importance of 'stimulus on' is signalled by potentials separated by a short time interval. The physical magnitude of the stimulus is not encoded, only the importance of the stimulus to the system within which the receptor is operating

directly upon joints, and can do so only by influencing the excitability of the spindle receptor endings, by modifying greatly the excitability of the myotatic reflex arc, and by applying a power assistance principle and recruiting the strength of skeletal muscle into a response.

The afferent activity of the myotatic reflex travels over axons in the Group I and Group II conduction velocity range. They are therefore contained in the fastest afferent conduction systems of the body. Activity from both primary and secondary receptor endings participate in the myotatic reflex, with the former being the most important. (Further discussion will be limited to the response of primary endings, and Matthews (1972) should be consulted for additional information.)

THE ANALOGUE SYNAPTIC EFFECT

A most important component of the myotatic reflex arc is mono-synaptic in structure, with the reflex afferents terminating directly on the motor neurone. It contributes strongly to the phasic myotatic reflexes, the jerk reflexes for example, which can be elicited by a tendon tap. A polysynaptic reflex system provides a neuronal circuit which adds support to tonic myotatic reflexes, and the interneurones between muscle spindle afferents and the motor neurones are the point of convergence of supraspinal excitatory and inhibitory effects.

Illustrating the analogue synaptic effect by specific reference to

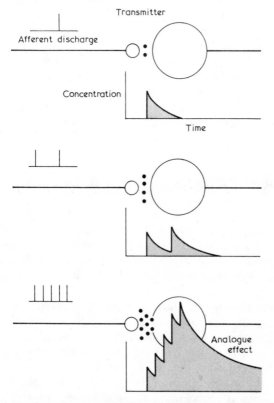

FIG. 5/5 A single action potential invading the synaptic terminals on a motor neurone releases a 'quantum' of transmitter. The concentration of transmitter on the motor neurone membrane rises rapidly and decays slowly with time. A second potential at the synapse produces a higher concentration of transmitter than did the first because of a summation effect. A train of potentials produces on the motor neurone membrane a copy or analogue of the importance of the stimulus which excited the receptor

the monosynaptic myotatic reflex, an action potential of an afferent axon will invade synaptic terminals applied to the basal dendrites and cell bodies of motor neurones. Membrane channels are opened by the action current flow, and calcium ions enter the terminal causing the release of a 'quantal amount' of excitatory neurotransmitter. The molecules of transmitter bind to membrane receptors situated post-synaptically on the motor neurone. Here they cause a localised depolarisation of the motor neurone which lasts until the transmitter is removed.

The time course of action of transmitter is longer than the duration of an action potential, and usually outlasts the time between two action potentials in an afferent train (Fig. 5/5). The 'quantum' of transmitter released by a second action potential can therefore add its effect to the tail of a preceding one.

The discharge of afferent activity during muscle stretch can in this way create, in terms of concentration of excitatory transmitter at membrane receptors on motor neurones, an analogue or copy of the importance of the stretch to postures or movements underway.

MOTOR NEURONES AND THEIR DISTRIBUTION

The motor neurones of the spinal cord occupy, bilaterally, two columns, 40cm in length in the adult and 0.5mm in diameter. These form Lamina or Nucleus IX in the Rexed nomenclature. Each column contains 200 000 motor neurones, with 150 000 innervating skeletal muscles and 50 000 innervating intrafusal muscles.

The motor neurones show a range of diameters. Cell bodies with a range between 100 and 25 micrometres (μm) are classified as alpha-motor neurones. Those with a diameter between 40 and 15μm are gamma-motor neurones. It is possible that the population overlap represents beta-motor neurones (see below).

Within the anterior horn of the spinal cord the motor neurones have a distinct topographical localisation. Motor neurones supplying the muscles of the neck and trunk are located medially, whereas those supplying the muscles of the limbs have a lateral location. The cervical and lumbar enlargements of the spinal cord accommodating respectively the supply to the musculature of the arms and hands, legs and feet. The distal, finely controlled muscles of the hand are controlled by motor neurones situated more dorsally and caudally in the segmental nuclei.

THE HENNEMAN SIZE PRINCIPLE AND THE ORDER OF RECRUITMENT

Studies of the electrical properties of motor neurones have shown that because of the higher input resistance of the dendrites of small motor neurones they tend naturally to be more excitable to spinal and to descending reflex excitation. This gives the smaller gamma-motor neurones a spontaneous, tonic activity of 30 to 50 impulses per second. Larger alpha-motor neurones have levels of spontaneous activity between 0 and 10 impulses per second. On receipt of increasing natural excitation, small motor neurones are recruited first and fire steady trains of action potentials. The largest alpha-motor neurones are the last to be recruited, and when active fire intermittent bursts of high frequency action potentials. A system of specific neuronal address by the corticospinal tract adds a higher direct control to Henneman recruitment. This is a most important aspect of neuronal organisation and reference should be made to the detail of Shepherd (1974) and Phillips and Porter (1977).

THE PATTERN OF MOTOR NEURONE DISCHARGE AND THE CHARACTERISTICS OF THE MOTOR UNIT

A remarkable match exists between the size of the cell body of a motor neurone, its position in the recruitment series, the pattern of action potentials it discharges and the metabolism and the mechanics of the muscle fibres which comprise the motor unit. Small diameter motor neurones which discharge on steady, natural excitation a maintained pattern of low-frequency action potentials innervate muscle fibres with Slow mechanical characteristics and a fatigue resistant Oxidative metabolism. By comparison, larger motor neurones firing irregular bursts of action potentials innervate muscle fibres with a Fast mechanical action energised by a rapidly fatiguing Glycolytic metabolism.

The two forms of motor unit are called respectively SO- or Type I motor units, and FG- or Type II motor units. An intermediate form with FOG characteristics is found in most muscles. In this form a Fast mechanical action has an Oxidative energy supply which almost meets the demands of a dominant Glycolytic metabolism.

The forms of motor unit are not immutable. There is opportunity for change of characteristics, with transition from FG- towards SO- being the most likely to occur. This has been demonstrated in experiment by exchanging surgically the innervation of muscles with differing mechanical and metabolic characteristics. The transition has been shown also to follow the electrical stimulation of FG- with patterns of stimuli which stimulate or copy the discharge of motor neurones innervating SO- muscles. There is no opportunity here for discussing further this important feature of neuromuscular physiology and reference should be made to Vrbova, Gordon and Jones (1978); Pette (1980) and Guba, Marechal and Tokacs (1981).

CENTRIFUGAL SETTING OF SPINDLE RECEPTOR RESPONSE: THE FUSIMOTOR SYSTEM

A functional as opposed to an anatomical classification of the peripheral motor systems serves better in application to physiotherapy. We can usefully re-examine the alpha-, beta- and gamma-classifications introduced above.

The largest alpha-motor neurones innervate skeletal muscle fibres exclusively. The motor units so formed act during fast, phasic movements and during the phasic myotatic reflex. The entire population can be functionally classified as phasic skeletomotor units.

Smaller alpha-motor neurones innervate tonic skeletomotor units, active during the tonic myotatic reflex.

Beta-motor neurones have axons which branch to innervate both SO- skeletal muscle fibres and the intrafusal fibres of muscle spindles. They, too, are also active during the tonic myotatic reflex. They form the skeleto-fusimotor system.

The larger gamma-motor neurones give a motor end-plate innervation to the polar extents of the intrafusal muscle fibres. Unlike the beta-motor neurones, gamma motor neurones do not innervate skeletal muscle fibres in addition to intrafusal fibres.

They and the smallest gamma-motor neurones, which provide a trailing motor terminal at the equator of the intrafusal muscle fibres, form the fusimotor system.

The skeleto-fusimotor and the fusimotor systems have three functions in the setting of reflex excitability and motor control.
1. To regulate the gain of the myotatic reflex (the magnitude of

the force developed reflexly to oppose stretch in relation to the external force used to generate stretching).

2. To modify continuing voluntary movements perturbed unexpectedly by opposing forces.

3. To form an efferent pathway for the extrapyramidal motor system to relay controls for habitual movements which will mix uniquely with novel and external mechanical influences at the level of the muscle spindles in the muscles involved.

It is the first function which concerns us here. (Details of the complex motor and sensory innervation of muscle spindles and their role in reflex control should be sought in Matthews (1972).)

SETTING OF THE MYOTATIC REFLEX GAIN

The skeleto-fusimotor and fusimotor systems modulate the afferent discharge from the primary and secondary endings of the muscle spindles. They act in the manner of the controls on a transistor radio.

Beta- and large gamma-motor neurones are dynamic in control. They act as a dynamic fusimotor system, 'tuning' the spindle receptors by increasing the viscosity and stiffness of the intrafusal muscle fibres around which and upon which the sensory endings are placed. The spindle sensitivity to the rate at which itself, and of course the muscle fascicle in which it is situated, is being lengthened is in this way selected (Fig. 5/6). In the analogy of the radio the spindle receives a different programme.

The small gamma-motor neurones increase the sensitivity of the spindle receptors to a steadily maintained stretch. They increase the position sensitivity of the receptors. In our radio analogy, the 'loudness' of the receptors is turned up. With the radio the sound can reach a larger audience. In the spinal cord a greater recruitment of motor neurones into reflex action occurs. The force then generated by the muscle innervated appropriately opposing and balancing the external stretching force.

THE ROLE OF INHIBITION

In the past too much emphasis perhaps has been placed on the powerful monosynaptic excitatory component of the myotatic reflex. Its priority command of the motor neurone and the speed with which it can operate are undoubtedly important but they

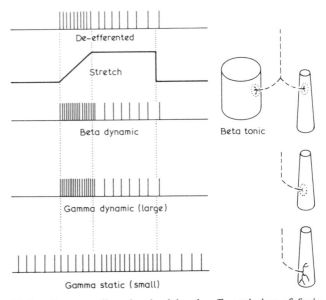

FIG. 5/6 A primary ending deprived by de-efferentiation of fusimotor influence responds to a gradually increasing stretch which is then maintained, by discharging a pattern of afferent action potentials. The higher frequency of discharge seen during stretching than during maintained stretch indicates a dynamic sensitivity. Excitation of intrafusal muscle fibres by beta-or by large gamma-motor neurones increases the dynamic sensitivity of the ending. The skeletomotor component of the beta-motor neurone innervates an SO motor unit. Excitation of the intrafusal muscle fibres by small gamma-motor neurones increase the static excitability of the receptor ending, and at the same time reduces the dynamic sensitivity. The relative positions on the intrafusal muscle fibres of the motor terminals of the three divisions of the fusimotor system are shown to the right

should not detract from the polysynaptic component and certainly not from the interplay of inhibitory events which are so important in postural mechanisms. We do well to recall Sherrington's statement in his first paper describing central inhibition:

Desistence from action may be as truly active
as is the taking of action.

Three inhibitory events co-operate in the myotatic reflex:
1. Recurrent inhibition
2. Autogenous inhibition
3. Pre-synaptic inhibition.

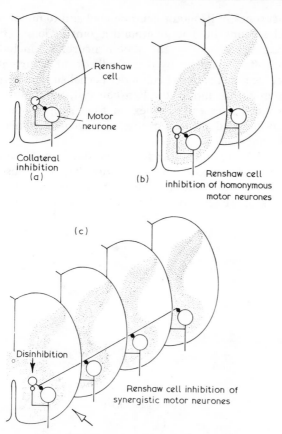

FIG. 5/7 (a) A collateral inhibits its motor neurone through the agency of a Renshaw cell. This is more than a simple negative feedback mechanism. (b) The Renshaw cell applies the recurrent inhibition also to homonymous motor neurones occupying the same pool as the motor neurone of origin of the inhibition. (c) Synergistic motor neurones occupying pools throughout several spinal segments are similarly inhibited. Inhibition of the Renshaw cells of one segment (arrowed), effectively releases from inhibition or disinhibits a set of motor neurones and releases a posture or movement performed in synergy

With recurrent inhibition each action potential discharged by a skeletomotor neurone traverses an axon collateral in addition to conducting over the main axon to the muscle fibres. The collateral excites an interneurone, the Renshaw cell, which applies inhibitory terminals to the motor neurone of origin of the activity, to motor neurones in its motor neurone pool and to motor neurones of muscles acting in synergy around a joint or joints (Fig. 5/7).

Reflexes operating on the motor neurones, including the myotatic reflex, maintain by this 'feedback' or recurrent inhibition a set, or reflex pattern held under partial suppression. A control system able to inhibit the Renshaw cell, the inhibition of an inhibitory cell releases the reflex set from suppression, and the pattern is inserted into a posture or movement. This event is called *disinhibition*.

The tendon organ, another force transducer in the muscle, inhibits the skeletomotor neurones controlling the muscle via a Group Ib afferent axon and inhibitory interneurones. This receptor is far more sensitive to force developed by the muscle than

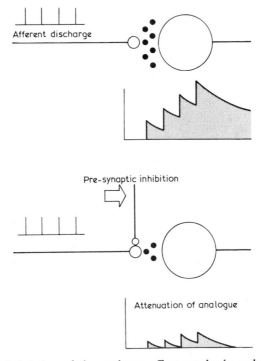

FIG. 5/8 Modulation of the analogue effect can be brought about by pre-synaptic inhibition. An afferent volley invading excitatory synaptic terminals releases transmitter and generates an analogue effect (Fig. 5/5). Activity in a synapse on a synaptic terminal reduces the amount of transmitter released by an identical afferent volley. The pre-synaptic inhibition attenuates the analogue

it is to a stretching force applied externally to the muscle. This gives it a role in reflex co-ordination more subtle than is revealed by 'jack-knife' inhibition.

Tendon organs on the tendon slip, into which the muscle fibres of single motor units insert, respond to the force generated by the action of a single skeletomotor neurone. In, for example, the tonic myotatic reflex the active muscle force generated applies again an inhibition to the motor neurones responsible (see recurrent inhibition, above). Should the muscle fibres of the motor unit fatigue and so generate less force, the tendon organs detect the decrement and part of the inhibition they generate centrally is released. The now less inhibited motor neurones increase their rate of action potential firing and the muscle force is restored.

In the foregoing description of the analogue effect generated at the synapse the 'quantal' nature of transmitter release was discussed. A form of inhibition, or more exactly disexcitation, exists where the amount of transmitter released at a synapse is reduced by the action of neurones which depolarise the synaptic terminal (Fig. 5/8). These synaptic endings on synaptic endings provide pre-synaptic inhibition. This must be compared with the more frequently described post-synaptic inhibition where an inhibitory cell releases an inhibitory transmitter which binds to a membrane receptor on the neurone to be inhibited.

This form of control is the second centrifugal control we have met. The first, the fusimotor system, modulates the excitability of the receptor endings of the muscle spindle. The pre-synaptic control determines what proportion of the afferent discharge so modulated is to be involved in synaptic activity in the motor neurone pools.

Some indication of the importance of this control is shown in Figure 5/9 which describes the effectiveness of the peripheral and central structures which influence synaptic transmission from the receptor endings involved in the myotatic reflex.

SUMMARY AND A SYNTHESIS

The myotatic reflex has been defined and discussed in a way which extends it from the simplistic, monosynaptic 'knee jerk' type of stretch reflex to a harmony of reflexes operating within a myotatic synergy. All the neurophysiological consequences of stretching a muscle act in a complementary and integrated fashion.

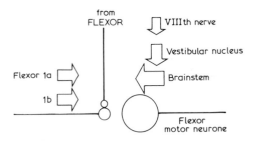

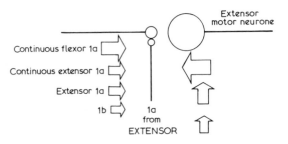

FIG. 5/9 Monosynaptic terminals on both extensor and flexor motor neurones are powerfully influenced by pre-synaptic inhibition. The magnitude of the effect is indicated by the size of the arrows. Central structures providing pre-synaptic inhibition are shown on the right; peripheral structures on the left. The symbols of central structures influencing extensor motor neurones relate to those influencing flexors

A polysynaptic supraspinal effect, mediated notably by the vestibulospinal system, adds an excitatory drive able to generate tonic, postural contractions to those which are limited and phasic.

The action potential pattern discharged by motor neurones, by its action on the structural adaptability, or *plasticity*, of muscle fibres of the motor unit, ensures an appropriate match of metabolism and mechanics to the motor demands made upon the muscle.

In discussing the richness of inhibitory interplay in the motor neurone pools of the reflex arcs, a population of neurones, the Renshaw cells, emerged linking spinal and supraspinal systems. Bonding homonymous and synergistic motor neurones into a remarkably integrated and versatile system for postural control. A stable posture can melt to allow a flowing volitional motor act, only to set again momentarily as a calculated modification of an ongoing movement is put into effect. But the symphony of tone and movement can become discordant, the co-ordination disappear.

DISTURBANCE OF THE MYOTATIC REFLEX

In the light of contemporary human neurophysiology we can see further than the classical explanations of disturbances in reflex muscle tone. It is no longer sufficient to talk only of imbalance in Sherrington's descending excitatory and inhibitory systems. These, in the normal nervous system, summate in the spinal interneurones to give an edge of excitation, and provide facilitation of reflexes of a higher order than spinal.

Facilitation, as its name plainly states, does not initiate any motor act, but it does 'make easier' the operation and integration of the spinal segmental, intersegmental and supraspinal repertoire of reflex actions. We cannot dismiss such an imbalance altogether. The release of the vestibulospinal excitation on the polysynaptic myotatic arcs by lesion or insult in inhibitory tracts and nuclei does contribute greatly to the disruption of reflex muscle tone.

We need to look closely too at some older views on the part played by the fusimotor system in the generation of such tonic imbalances as are found in the spasticities.

As techniques of human microneuronography (where recordings are made of the discharge of single afferent and efferent axons in conscious human subjects and patients) heightened fusimotor activity plays little part, except possibly during the early stages of the developing hyper-reflexia, in the hypertonus of spasticity.

Further techniques in human neurophysiology enable measurement of reflex interplay at the spinal level. (These techniques and the application of the information coming from them to diagnosis and therapy are most important. Teachers in particular should read Desmedt (1983).) Hoffmann reflex testing (a form of monosynaptic reflex excitability determination) and a comparative analysis of the tonic vibratory reflex (where the receptor endings of the muscle spindle are excited when vibration, and not stretch, is applied to the tendon of the muscle) allow measurements of the relative contributions of Renshaw cell and presynaptic inhibition. They show both to be involved in the generation of spasticities, and that the latter should be given a much more prominent place in the philosophy underlying diagnosis and development of new techniques in physiotherapy than it has at present.

Powerful increases in the effectiveness of pre-synaptic inhibition have been described during the a-reflexic 'shock' which follows spinal transection. In spasticities profound decreases in spinal pre-synaptic inhibition are believed to contribute to the hyper-reflexia. The muscle spindles may not be driven by heightened fusimotor activity, but an inordinate proportion of their discharge enters into the myotatic reflex pathways.

Spinal reflex circuits deprived of a balanced supraspinal facilitatory influence attempt to redress the abnormal synaptic influence on the motor neurone by an act of collateral sprouting. Collaterals from the axon terminal of a descending, with a contribution from peripheral afferent pathways from the muscle spindle, place new excitatory synaptic endings upon the motor neurone. The gradual failure of the spinal inhibitory mechanisms over a number of years is believed to underly the development of a spastic state. The plastic rearrangement of spinal reflex connections due to collateral sprouting is comparably slow. If, as seems likely, the synaptic endings formed by the collateral sprouts lack pre-synaptic inhibitory terminals, the hyper-reflexia of spasticity has an explanation.

CONCLUSION

There is as yet no complete analysis available of the neural circuitry and action of the myotatic reflex. In this chapter no attempt has been made to introduce controversy, or to explore the extent of 'long-loop' myotatic reflexes involving brainstem nuclei and cerebral cortex. It has barely touched upon the neuronal and muscular plastic adaptation that is so important in the maturation of normal motor activity, in the development of symptoms of motor pathology, in the response of a patient to physiotherapy, and in the consequent acquisition of improved motor skills (Bach-y-Rita, 1980). In neurological diagnosis and treatment, physiotherapy has a new philosophy to adopt and new techniques to employ. To do so it must look energetically to the future, and not with fondness on the past.

REFERENCES

The following books refer to the suggested in-depth reading mentioned in the text.

Bach-y-Rita, P. (1980). *Recovery of Function: Theoretical Considerations for Brain Injury Rehabilitation*. Hans Huber, Bern.

Desmedt, J. E. (1983). *Motor Control Mechanisms in Health and Disease*. Raven Press, New York.

Guba, F., Maréchal, G. and Tokács, O. (1981). *Mechanisms of Muscle Adaptation to Functional Requirements*. Pergamon Press, Oxford.

Matthews, P. B. C. (1972). *Mammalian Muscle Receptors and their Central Connections*. Edward Arnold, London.

Pette, D. (1980). *Plasticity of Muscle*. de Gruyter, Berlin.

Phillips, C. G. and Porter, R. (1977). *Corticospinal Neurones*. Academic Press, London.

Shepherd, G. M. (1974). *Synaptic Organisation of the Brain*. Oxford University Press, Oxford.

Vrbová, G., Gordon, T. and Jones, R. (1978). *Nerve-Muscle Interaction*. Chapman and Hall, London.

Chapter 6

Principles of Assessment

by H. W. ATKINSON MCSP, HT, DipTP

Assessment is a key factor in the subsequent planning of short- and long-term objectives in the therapeutic programme of any patient referred to the physiotherapist. This does not conflict with any diagnostic examination conducted by the medical practitioner and its purpose is to enable the therapist to appreciate the nature and extent of the patient's difficulties in adapting to the day-to-day environment. It indicates the steps to be taken either to help the patient to return as quickly as possible to his previous level of functional ability or assist him to make the best of the current situation and adapt his quality of function to an existing state.

In assessing the patient it is important for the physiotherapist to appreciate her own personal limitations, as well as those of her profession, so that she recognises the need to request the assistance of more experienced colleagues or members of other disciplines who may have specialist knowledge which is beyond the scope of physiotherapy. In this way, a clearer picture of the total problem will be obtained and the patient will benefit from an interdisciplinary approach.

Most patients with a neurological disorder have complex problems and it is not always possible to make a full assessment in any one session. Additionally, a characteristic of some conditions is that of variation from day to day, and misjudgement of the extent of the difficulties could occur if the assessment is completed on a 'good' day or a 'bad' day. Most workers find that new facts are learned about the patient all the time and that approaches have to be adjusted frequently.

It is usual to have an initial period of assessment to clarify the most important features of the case and then to undertake intermediary assessments at intervals appropriate to the difficulties seen in the individual patient. A final assessment should always be made, and its findings recorded, prior to the discharge of the patient. Such records should be stored for retrieval in the event of the patient returning at a later date for further assistance.

Emphasis in this chapter will be placed on the assessments most suitably made by the therapist and will indicate areas of overlap and where the input of the specialised knowledge of another discipline would be helpful. Some or all of the points included should be considered, depending on the nature and extent of the problem.

THE MEDICAL AND SOCIAL HISTORY OF THE PATIENT

Prior to assessing the patient the physiotherapist should have studied the medical history to extract any relevant details found during the medical examination which will already have taken place. It is important to be aware of any tests the patient has experienced, and the results of such tests, which may have led to confirmation of the diagnosis. The therapist should be able to learn from the notes the impression gained by the medical practitioner and also any social details which are available. The social history is very relevant to the therapist's programme of management and gives some indication of how much family support can be expected in the event of the need for relatives to assist in the therapeutic programme at home. Additionally, such factors as recent bereavements or other personal tragedies should be noted as they may affect the patient's current emotional and behavioural state and may also have an influence on the physical condition and projected improvement of the patient. In studying the patient's notes only relevant material should be extracted and recorded but care must be taken to see that potential hazards are not overlooked. For example, a history of coronary disease, diabetes, focal fits, must be noted so that the management of the patient within the physiotherapy department takes due consideration of any problems which could arise because of these features.

A GENERAL IMPRESSION

To obtain a general impression of the patient's physical and mental condition it is best to create as informal a situation as possible. If the therapist is community based this is perhaps easier than when the patient is a hospital outpatient. A social type of visit and introduction can be made during which the physiotherapist can note the general condition and attitude of the patient and his relatives, friends or nurses (depending on the environment). It should be noted whether the patient is ambulant, chairbound or confined to bed and whether he requires assistance in any of these. His general appearance should be observed for build, postural attitudes, muscle atrophy, skin colouration, signs of obvious ill-health or malnutrition. The overall condition of skin, nails and hair can tell a great deal about the physical condition of the patient and should not be overlooked. The possibility of pressure sores should be noted for future attention during the more formal inspection of the patient.

The physiotherapist should try to gain a general impression of the mental state of the patient, his attitude to his disability and the attitude of those who are fulfilling a supportive function. The relationship and social interaction between the patient and those taking care of him can be an important part in the motivation of the patient and if it is seen to be constructive and helpful may be used to advantage by the therapist.

DISCUSSION

Discussion can occur separately or in conjunction with other sections of the assessment. It must include the problem as seen by the patient, how it interferes with his daily life and family responsibilities. The patient's viewpoint is likely to be very different from that of the medical practitioner and the physiotherapist and must never be ignored. If the patient indicates a particular difficulty which is worrying him, it is important to pay particular attention to this and, where possible, take steps to alleviate the problem when fulfilling the immediate short-term objectives. In this way the patient's anxieties will be reduced, the therapy will be seen to be of some value, thus ensuring future co-operation.

The discussion should bring to light the patient's hopes and fears for himself and his family as well as his grasp of the real situation. Many patients take months, or even years, to come to terms with severe physical handicap and the physiotherapist must not automatically expect him to fully appreciate the nature of his problem or have realistic long-term expectations. During the discussion the therapist should find out relevant details of the patient's occupation; in doing so she must be aware that a return to employment may not be possible and should be careful to avoid holding out any false hopes to a patient. Notice should be taken of any pain or discomfort manifested by the patient and he should be asked whether he has any pain, how he would describe it and where it is felt. The patient must be given time to tell his problems in his own way and the therapist must avoid asking questions in such a way that they suggest an expected answer.

While the discussion is occurring the physiotherapist can note other important factors. Problems of speech or hearing can be detected, the ability to interpret speech and reply quickly can be noted, respiratory control, salivation, deglutition and facial expression difficulties can be observed. The physiotherapist can note whether the patient is able to make automatic postural adjustments while conversing, whether he uses gestures to supplement speech; and other features which will become obvious to the therapist as experience is gained in interviewing patients. The viewpoint of relatives, nurses and helpers can be helpful in completing the picture but, unless the patient is incapable of answering for himself because he is too young, unconscious or otherwise severely handicapped, they should be discouraged from acting as spokesman on the patient's behalf.

However, the point of view of relatives and other helpers is invaluable. The patient's interpretation of his ability to cope may be unrealistic and the relative will be able to clarify any points of detail. Additionally, the patient's attitude of co-operation and participation may be totally different in the home to that demonstrated in the physiotherapy department and this information is of great importance to all concerned. Another way in which relatives can help is by giving the therapist an insight into the patient's character, interests and capabilities prior to hospitalisation. For example, if an intelligent, mentally alert and active elderly person sustains a cerebrovascular accident his previous capabilities will not be at all obvious to the physiotherapist who may see only a pathetic and confused patient of doubtful intellect, who can only communicate by waving his unaffected arm in an agitated manner and who drools all the time. Some insight into the patient's interests and capabilities can only be of benefit to all concerned, since topics of his interest can be discussed in the patient's presence and his desperate efforts to communicate and overcome his state of confusion are more likely to be successful.

ASSESSMENT OF THE 'SENSORY' MECHANISMS

Sensory activity and interpretation is vital to normal functional activity. Knowledge of the environment, a good body image and the relationship of the body to other structures in the environment are essential factors in the production of efficiently coordinated movements. It is, therefore, important for the physiotherapist to take the sensory modalities into consideration when making an assessment of the patient.

Assessment of hearing

This is not really the province of the physiotherapist but it is important for her to know whether the patient can hear ordinary speech or whether this is difficult. She also needs to know whether he can hear himself moving against the bedclothes or chair or his feet on the floor, since the ability to do so makes a difference to his ability to move in a co-ordinate manner and with assurance.

If any serious defect is detected, or the physiotherapist feels that there is a difficulty which may affect the patient's ability to fully comprehend and interpret sound, it may be necessary to request that the patient is seen by an audiologist.

Assessment of eyes and vision

Although this is the province of the highly qualified specialist, it is helpful for the physiotherapist to know whether the field of vision is limited or full, whether the pupils are able to react to light and whether there are inco-ordinate movements of the eyes such as nystagmus.

It is also important to know whether the patient has normal vision or requires the help of glasses to enable him to see near or distant objects. If the eyes are to be used to help in the production of movement it is important to know how much they can be expected to help. The medical notes may give most of the information that is required and should be studied carefully.

Visual fields can be roughly tested by holding two different coloured pencils some distance apart and asking the patient how many he can see. If he only claims to see one then the one he can see can be identified by colour (provided he is not blind to colour). This gives some indication of the visual field. The pencils can be moved about to find the extent of defect of field and the search can be narrowed down to the field of one eye by masking the other.

There is also the possibility of double vision and this can be assessed by holding up one object and asking how many the patient can see. If the patient has difficulty of convergence of the eyes he is likely to show double vision which can be distressing and make him insecure. Covering one eye will prevent double vision from being too troublesome and can be used to help patients who have no hope of correcting the problem in any other way.

The help of the ophthalmologist or the orthoptist may be necessary to complete this part of the assessment.

Skin sensation

It should be noted whether the patient can distinguish between different types of sensation such as blunt and sharp, hard and soft, hot and cold.

It is possible to map out areas of defect on line diagrams of either the whole patient or the part requiring attention.

Two-point discrimination can be assessed for some patients but it must be remembered that this is variable in accordance with the area being examined. In the normal person two-point discrimination is better on the palmar aspect of the hand than it is on the dorsum. Thus one must expect discrepancies even in the normal individual. By two-point discrimination is meant the ability to distinguish two distinct areas being stimulated at any one time and noting how close the stimuli can be to each other before they are interpreted as one.

Vibration

This can be applied by a vibrator or by a tuning fork and is detected as a sensation by receptors in skin and bone. Because vibration has been found to have an important influence on muscle activity this is an interesting test to try. After the vibration stimulus has been given muscles working over the vibrated area may be seen to contract although they have not been stretched or stimulated in any other way. It is thought that the vibration is transmitted to the muscle spindles via the bone and gives a rapidly repetitive mild stretch stimulus. This may, incidentally, be one reason for the need for compression force of weight-bearing (giving a vibration) if one wishes to encourage co-contraction of muscles over a joint.

Joint position

This should be checked carefully and it may be done in various ways:

1. The patient may have the movements of a joint named for him – e.g. 'this is called bending the elbow and this is stretching'. Then the joint may be put through a passive range of movement while the eyes are closed and the patient asked to state whether bending or stretching is occurring. When moving the joint passively the physiotherapist must not indicate change of direction by moving her hands as the patient could otherwise detect discrepancies in direction because of this and give a false impression of his ability.

2. If the patient is sufficiently co-ordinate he could be asked to keep his eyes closed and to move a free limb into the same relative position as a limb being moved by the physiotherapist.

3. His limbs and trunk could be positioned by the physiotherapist and the patient could be asked to draw a pin man diagram of his position or to put a 'bendy toy' into a similar position. A 'bendy toy' is a toy doll made of sorbo rubber round a malleable wire frame which can be bent to any shape. These last methods do more than test joint sensation – they test body-image interpretation and are suitable for only certain disabilities.

Body image

Body image is built up by reception of visual impressions, skin sensation, joint position, pressure distributed through and received by skin, joints and muscles, information received via the semicircular canals, impressions of muscle tension and muscle length and contact of one part of the body with another to establish relationships. Thus, some of the assessments already made will assist the therapist to assess the patient's body image. Other methods include the naming of different parts of the body, aligning them differently and asking the patient to realign them; distributing the patient's body-weight differently and asking him to redistribute it; putting a 'bendy toy' into a position similar to that of the patient and asking him if this is similar to his position and then changing the 'bendy toy' to another posture and asking for a comparison is yet another approach.

Perceptual problems

Clinical psychologists and occupational therapists have a great deal to offer on this aspect of patient assessment. The ability to orientate the body in relationship to the space it occupies is an important factor in body image and movement and the patient needs to be able to interpret the different heights, depths and widths of structures. For example, patients with spatial perceptual difficulties may well roll off the bed on to the floor because they are unappreciative of the height relationship of the bed to the floor. Patients with this sort of problem are not always understood by the physiotherapist, and are dubbed clumsy, careless and unintelligent by relatives and friends. Some patients may have difficulty in distinguishing between themselves and the furniture they are using, and many elderly patients, even without other obvious neurological symptoms, may try to climb out of a chair over its arms instead of via the normal route.

Perceptual problems lead to difficulty with all functional activities and are very noticeable when the complex activities of dressing and undressing are required. The patient may not be able to find his way into his shirt, trousers or pullover and may spend a long time trying to discover the hole through which his head should pass, or even distinguishing between the holes and the material of the pullover. Physiotherapists must appreciate when these problems exist and be prepared to request the help of other disciplines when assessing the extent of the problem. The perceptual problems indicated in this paragraph are gross and easily recognised but many patients demonstrate very mild forms of difficulty which need careful and precise assessment if the patient is to achieve the most relevant help from the appropriate discipline. Simple sensory re-education is not enough in these circumstances and a concerted effort is needed by all the relevant team members if the patient is to progress.

Stereognosis

This is the ability to recognise objects by feel and manipulation. It requires the ability to feel with the hands and to assess size and shape by the position of the joints. It also involves the ability to move the hands over and around the object.

It can be checked by putting objects into a patient's hand or hands while he is blindfolded and asking him to state what they are. Everyday articles should be chosen such as money, buttons, pens, etc.

Another method would be to put a number of simple articles into an opaque bag and ask the patient to bring out only the pen or coin or button.

Closely allied to stereognosis is the ability to recognise texture of material and weight of identical-looking objects. Thus the patient may be asked to identify different materials such as wool, silk, paper, wood. The patient may do so by moving his hands over the material or having the material placed into or moved over his hands or other part of the body. Identical looking objects but with different weights may be arranged in order of heaviness. This requires touch, pressure and joint sensation as well as some interpretation of the muscle activity needed to support the weight.

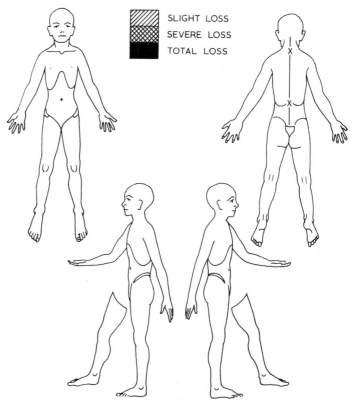

SLIGHT LOSS
SEVERE LOSS
TOTAL LOSS

FIG. 6/1 Chart for recording afferent information

Areas of lost sensation should be recorded and also any areas of paraesthesia should be noted. Numbness and tingling give false sensation and dull sensory perception and so need to be taken notice of as they are indicative of disturbance occurring in sensory pathways (Fig. 6/1).

JOINT MOBILITY AND SOFT TISSUE LENGTH

The available range of movement in the joints should be noted. In some cases the range should be accurately measured but in most cases of neurological disorder this is not really necessary.

Passive and active range should be assessed since many patients cannot move the joints because of muscle weakness, hypotonia or hypertonia. When assessing the passive movements available the physiotherapist should remember to check the biological length of two joint muscles as well as individual joint ranges.

If the patient is known to be spastic it should be remembered that certain positions of the head and neck could make movement of joints less available. For instance, supine lying could make hip and knee flexion very difficult for either the patient or the operator.

The physiotherapist should try to ascertain the reason for limitation of movement, note any fixed deformity and also any habitual posturing.

VARIATIONS IN MUSCLE ACTIVITY

Here the physiotherapist is looking for flaccidity, hypotonicity, hypertonicity and the fluctuations associated with athetosis and ballismus.

Some information will already have been gained if the other assessments mentioned above have been carried out. However, discrepancies in muscle activity can also be assessed in the following ways:

Passive movements

Relaxed passive movements may give the following information:
1. That the muscles are flail and are allowing movement to occur with no opposition and may even be allowing an excessive range of movement to occur. If many muscles are involved the

limb may feel heavy as there is no support from normal muscle activity.

2. That the muscles are showing excessive opposition to stretch. If they are showing spasticity they may show the clasp-knife phenomenon and will certainly oppose movements away from the spastic patterns. If they are showing rigidity all movements will feel stiff and the cog-wheel phenomenon may be detected.

Passive movements should be performed both slowly and quickly to detect any difference in the response of muscles to slow and quick stretch.

If the muscles are found to be flail they may be hypotonic or atonic. However, quick passive movements to joints controlled by the hypotonic muscles may initiate a sluggish stretch response which is not available in atonic muscle.

Palpation

Handling of muscles in varying states of tone can give helpful information. The *atonic* muscle usually feels non-resilient, soft and atrophied. The term flaccid means 'relaxed, flabby and without tone' (*Stedman's Medical Dictionary*, 24th edition). However, as it is inclined to be used carelessly by medical practitioners, nurses and therapists, students are advised to avoid the use of this term and substitute the more precise terms where they are appropriate. The *hypotonic* muscle feels soft but not really non-resilient. It does not usually show much atrophy. The *spastic* muscle feels tight and hard particularly if it is put slightly on the stretch. Its tendon may be felt to stand out from underlying structures. Muscles showing rigidity feel solid and the limbs are rather leaden to move about.

Reflex testing

This is a common method of assessing muscle tone and the condition of the various neurological pathways.

Superficial reflexes may be tested by scratching the skin over an area and watching for muscle contraction. If the skin of the abdomen is stroked the abdominal muscles contract. If no response occurs there is either an interruption of the lower reflex pathway or a state of central shock in which the motoneurone pools are not receptive to stimuli. The response may be exaggerated if flexor spasticity is present, sluggish if there is hypotonia, and difficult to see if there is rigidity because the muscles will not be adequately relaxed to start with.

Scratching the sole of the foot has a similar effect. There is a withdrawal from the stimulus involving dorsiflexion of the foot. In the normal situation the great toe of the mature individual will plantar flex while the rest of the foot dorsiflexes. However, if hypertonicity of a spastic nature is present there will be dorsiflexion of the whole foot accompanied by flexion of knee and hip. This is often called a Babinski sign. In hypotonicity the response will be sluggish and in the case of flaccid dorsiflexors there will be no response of these muscles but there may be flexion of knee and hip if these muscles are working and the limb is free to move. Again, as for the abdominal reflexes, if there is a state of spinal shock the reflex will be absent.

Tendon reflexes may be tested by tapping the tendon of a muscle. This does not stretch the tendon but, by putting a momentary kink into its shape and by vibrating it, the muscle fibres attached to the tendon are suddenly stretched. The normal response to this is for the muscle fibres to contract together giving a jerk of tone in the muscle. Reference is, therefore, made to the knee, ankle and elbow jerks. In these cases the patellar tendon, tendo calcaneus and triceps tendon are struck once with a tendon mer and the appropriate response is awaited. The lower limb, foot and forearm must be free to move if the full effect is to be observed. This method can be applied to any muscle tendon but these are the ones most commonly tested.

If there is no response there may be interruption of the motor pathway between the spinal cord and the muscle indicating a flaccid paralysis of the muscle. It is possible also that sensory interruption has occurred which may or may not mean flaccid paralysis depending upon whether the motor pathway is also involved.

No response will occur if there is a state of spinal shock which may occur temporarily in injuries to the brain or spinal cord.

If the response is exaggerated it means that an excessive contraction of muscle occurs, then some hypertonicity of a spastic nature should be suspected.

A pendular or oscillating response indicates hypotonicity and lack of postural fixation to steady the limb after the initial jerk. The limb swings back and forth several times before settling down.

If hypertonicity of a spastic nature is suspected the physio-therapist should look for dominant reflex patterning and could well make use of her knowledge of the tonic postural reflexes to assess the severity of the condition. By placing the patient in the various postures which will most readily elicit a static reflex response, she can assess the dominance of the reflexes by the spastic patterning which occurs or by the increase in tone she feels in the muscles. For example, if the patient is placed in supine lying and the tonic labyrinthine reflex is therefore allowed free rein, the patient showing spasticity will show an increase in extensor tone and flexion will be difficult. If the head is then flexed forwards there may be more extensor tone in the lower limbs but an increase in flexor tone in the upper limbs indicating a symmetrical tonic neck reflex patterning.

Head turning may give extension of the limbs on the side to which the face is turned and flexion of the others indicating the influence of the asymmetrical tonic neck reflex. It should be noted that full patterning into spastic patterns may not necessarily occur. There may be a simple, slight increase in tone into the patterns, or movement out of the patterning may just be made slightly more difficult in the milder cases. Figure 6/5 indicates the patterns created by these reflexes.

Fluctuations of tone as seen in the athetoid, chorea and ballismus case can usually be readily seen as involuntary movements.

ASSESSING FUNCTION

The ability to function normally depends upon the patient's ability to respond to the demands of the environment and to his own needs quickly, efficiently and effectively. To do this he must be able to receive and process sensory information (as has already been indicated earlier in this chapter) and to be able to react to this information by producing well co-ordinated bodily movements. The ability to achieve this state depends upon the availability of a mature and healthy nervous system and healthy muscles working over mobile joints in a pain-free manner. Damage to the sensori-motor activities of the nervous system, or in the muscles or joints, will inevitably lead to impairment of function by either the production of abnormal and, possibly, uneconomical movements or, total loss of functional ability. Thus assessment of function must include not only *whether* the patient can achieve a function, but *how* he does so. The quality of the functional activity as well as the fulfilment of the function is important.

Assessing quality of function

Several factors need to be taken into account if quality of function is to be assessed adequately. These are:
(a) the versatility of movement permutations available
(b) the ability to balance
(c) the ability to co-ordinate
(d) the muscle power available
(e) speech, feeding and swallowing
(f) respiratory control.

Movement permutations

By this is meant the ability to mix the flexion and extension components suitably in order to achieve a balance of activity which leads to functional use. It will be remembered that the spastic pattern of extension in the lower limb is most commonly extension, adduction and medial rotation of the hip, extension of the knee and plantar flexion of the foot (Brunnstrom, 1970). The reversal of this is flexion, abduction and lateral rotation of the hip, flexion of the knee and dorsiflexion of the foot. Mature movements involve a mixture of these two synergies so that the hip does not have to adduct every time it extends but can abduct if this is more appropriate. The observant therapist needs only to think of a few basic activities to appreciate that they require a mixture of flexion and extension in any one limb. The swing phase of walking requires dorsiflexion of the foot in combination with knee extension and a strong hand grip requires flexion of the fingers with extension of the wrist.

A quick method of assessing the patient's ability to produce suitable permutations of movements is to progress them through a few functions which relate to fundamental starting positions, all of which require good movement permutation. Consider the lying position:
(a) Can he lie on his back with his legs abducted a little and alternately medially and laterally rotate them?
(b) Can he roll from supine to prone, leading with different parts of his body, e.g. head and neck, arms, lower limbs, and does his body *spiral* as he rolls?

(c) Can he take up crook lying with his knees and feet a little bit apart and not touching each other?

(d) Can he 'bridge' from crook lying? (Fig. 6/2.)

(e) Can he raise his arms and point to the ceiling, protracting his shoulder girdle as he does so and also extending his fingers?

It must be remembered that disturbance in movement permutation need not necessarily be the result of a neurological problem but may be orthopaedic, traumatic or painful in origin.

Assessing balance

Good balance requires a well-integrated nervous system with adequate afferent information, mobile joints and sound muscles. Faults in any of these factors will influence the patient's ability to balance.

The ability to balance needs to be assessed in various postures and during movements from one posture to another. The earliest balance activity involves balancing the head over the upper trunk in prone lying and supported sitting, whereas a very advanced balance activity could be walking, carrying a tray full of glasses while avoiding and talking to people who are passing by! Obviously circus artistes perform many more advanced balance activities but few of us aspire to their heights.

Thus it would take a complete volume to assess every posture and movement for balance. However, having selected a position for assessment suitable for the patient the following procedure may be adopted:

(a) How much help does he need to maintain the position?

(b) Test his conscious balance responses by applying pressure and telling him to 'hold' or saying 'don't let me move you'. Give pressure in various directions and note his stability.

(c) Try the same approach with his eyes closed. If he has been relying on eyesight he will be less stable or may fall when his eyes are closed.

(d) Let him have his eyes open and test his automatic reactions to balance disturbance. Ask him to let you move him and tilt him backward, forward, sideways and rotate him – all gently – so as to disturb the position of his centre of gravity. Notice whether he moves his head, trunk, upper limbs or lower limbs or all of them to maintain his equilibrium. Try disturbing his balance this way by moving him at the shoulders, or using his arms as handles or by using his legs. The reaction you will

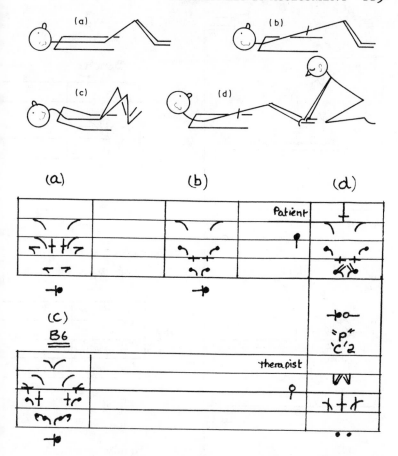

FIG. 6/2 The 'quality' of the activity of crook lying-pelvic lifting (bridging). (a) Starting position; (b) A good pelvic lift – well co-ordinated with mature muscle synergy; (c) A 'grotesque' attempt to achieve a pelvic lift using the symmetrical tonic reflex effect of cervical extension to assist. The pattern of flexion and abduction of the lower limbs with feet drawn up under the knees is typical of this sort of attempt; (d) Another attempt to achieve a pelvic lift, using the same reflex, but the effect of cervical flexion being enlisted to assist the patient to press the feet towards the helper who is blocking them so that the extensor effort causes the pelvis to lift.

((c) and (d) are examples of two poorly synergised efforts and therefore demonstrate a poor quality of pelvic lifting. There are many variations to these abnormal efforts and therapists must be able to observe and analyse them correctly if they are working for quality of movement)

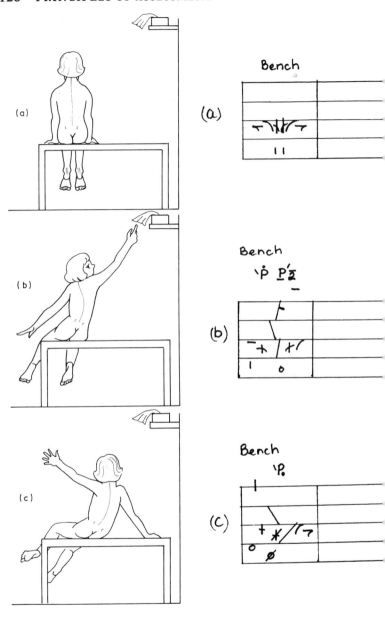

FIG. 6/3 An important series of balance reactions to lateral displacement of the trunk

get will depend upon what is available to the patient and what part of him you have left free to react.

(e) Try the same reactions with his eyes closed. Be careful to prevent injury should his ability be poor in this situation. Record the reactions you obtain and relate them to those which should be obtainable. For example you do not expect stepping or hopping reactions if you have tested the patient in sitting.

(f) Now test his reactions when carrying out a movement of some part of the body. For example in sitting, movements of the arms require balance adjustment. Try this with the eyes open and then closed.

(g) Objective activity test. This requires the use of the position for a function such as dressing or any simple activity which takes the patient's mind off balancing and puts it on to the fulfilment of purposeful activity (Fig. 6/3).

The various reactions obtained will depend upon the condition being examined. If there are many flaccid muscles exaggerated reactions will be seen in the normal parts of the body as compensation. If there is hypotonicity balance will be precarious, reactions slow to occur but exaggerated when they do occur and of rather a primitive nature (putting hand down on to a support and using a wide base) (Figs. 6/4 and 6/5).

If there is spasticity, disturbance in balance will give exaggerated reactions to any normal part and spastic patterning of the rest of the body.

If there is rigidity, balance reactions will probably be almost entirely absent except for forward stepping and protective extension. The reactions will occur very slowly.

It must be remembered that balance reactions may be altered by joint stiffness and account must be taken of this in any patients who are likely to have limitation of movement.

Assessing co-ordination and precision

Well co-ordinated purposeful movement requires (1) a variety of movement permutations, (2) good balance reactions, and (3) the ability to stabilise one part of the body while moving another part so that movement occurs smoothly. In assessing (1) and (2) a large part of (3) has already been examined. However, smoothness of movement needs to be checked, the ability to move the trunk on the limbs and the limbs on the trunk needs checking, and the ability to stop and start movement is very important.

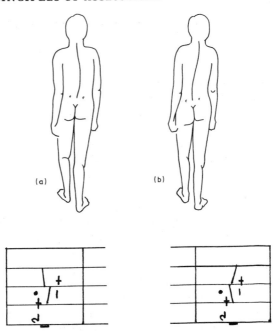

FIG. 6/4 Lateral displacement of trunk during weight-bearing on the right lower limb. (a) Shows the balance reaction of lateral tilt of the pelvis to the right giving a gentle 'C' curve of the trunk to distribute weight; (b) Shows the balance reaction of lateral tilt of the pelvis to the left (i.e. drop on unsupported side) with increased compensatory curve in the upper torso to ensure that weight falls over the right lower limb. An 'S' curve is the result. (a) and (b) are both within normal limits and occur to a varying degree during the normal gait pattern and from individual to individual.

This ability to transfer weight laterally is vital to gait to enable correct weight transmission and to release the non-weight-bearing limb for forward swing when the centre of gravity is displaced forward

This can be done by examining the patient's ability to move from prone lying to supine and from supine to prone in a slow smooth manner stopping and starting on the way. If suitable, he may be required to take up side sitting from prone lying and then proceed to all-fours, kneeling, half kneeling and standing with stops and starts throughout. While doing this, precision and smoothness are being checked and any tremor, overshooting or lack of precision is noted. These are gross co-ordinate activities

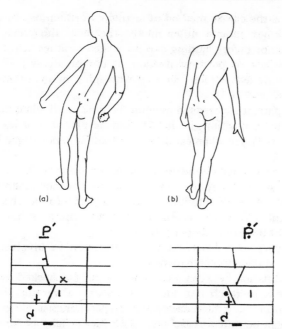

FIG. 6/5 Two examples of abnormal weight transmission over the right lower limb. These postures are gross accentuations of those illustrated in Figure 6/4 and are commonly seen in the physiotherapy department when, for either orthopaedic or neurological reasons, the control of the posture of the pelvis over the lower limb is defective. The balance reactions of the upper torso and upper limbs are extreme and mechanically and physiologically inefficient. Both of these postures can be seen as manifestations of the Trendelenburg sign and are the two most common ways in which patients distribute their weight over one limb in this circumstance

and provided the patient is capable of coping with the various positions and movements they make a good starting point.

It should be remembered that slow movements are very often more difficult for the inco-ordinate patient and so both fast and slow movements should be assessed.

More detailed checks can be made regarding the abilities of the patient by placing him in a very stable position and asking for free movements of the limbs of a precise nature. The *finger to nose test* is the classic method of testing co-ordination. In this the inco-ordinate patient either misses the nose altogether or has much tremor before landing and he strikes it rather heavily. This indicates lack of postural fixation of the proximal joints. The patient with sensory loss shows a worsening of symptoms if the eyes are closed.

If the patient succeeds in moving the limbs well when the trunk is in a stable position, it should then be placed in a less stable position so that mechanical proximal fixation is no longer helping the patient.

The movements should be checked for smoothness, ability to stop and start, ability to occur as a whole and not be broken up into joint by joint activities. Later they should be checked as purposeful actions in which the patient's mind is not on the movement but upon the purpose of moving.

Obviously such functions as walking must be involved if the patient is sufficiently able to do so.

Co-ordination between hand and eye can be checked by asking the patient to reach out and take objects of various sizes and shapes and to give them back to the physiotherapist. Objects such as balls can be rolled to the patient for him to take as they arrive, later they can be thrown to him and smaller balls can be used. Shapes and sizes and co-ordination can be tested by asking the patient to put objects of certain shapes through appropriate slots. This requires extremely good hand co-ordination, co-ordination between hand and eye and also sensory perception.

The effect of hypertonicity on functional activities

Hypertonicity (spasticity and rigidity) will have a profound effect on movement permutations, balance, co-ordination and precision and may be clearly seen in any general functional test. Attempts are being made to measure and quantify hypertonicity and particularly the spastic variety. However, success in this field is hampered by the fact that spasticity is a very variable phenomenon and will be affected by any or all of the following factors:

(a) *External stimuli*: Noise, discomfort and activity around the patient will increase muscle tone.

(b) *Condition of bladder and digestive organs*: Discomfort and distension will incline towards increased flexor tone.

(c) *Environmental temperature*: Chilling increases tone.

(d) *State of general health*: If the patient feels generally unwell and restless the tone may be increased.

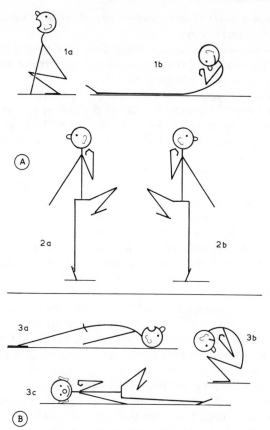

FIG. 6/6 Diagrams to represent the patterns of bias placed on muscle tone by the primitive tonic reflexes. Students should note that the effect may not be strong enough to actually produce these postures but increased tone *towards* these postures may be detected.

A. The effect of the tonic neck reflexes. These relate to neck postures and may be activated by stimulation of cervical joint and muscle receptors: 1(a) and (b) = symmetrical tonic neck reflex effect; 2(a) and (b) = asymmetrical tonic neck reflex effect

B. The effect of the tonic labyrinthine reflexes. These relate to the stimulation of the receptors in the inner ear by the force of gravity: 3(a) and (b) = the effect of 'supine' and 'prone' postures of the head; 3(c) = the effect of a 'lateral' posture of the head.

Students must realise that patients may often show combinations of these effects and the resultant tone detected may also be influenced by other factors as indicated in the text

(e) *Emotional states of fear, anxiety, apprehension*: These give rise to an increase in tone.

(f) *The position of the cervical spine*: Primitive tonic reflexes can be stimulated and bring about specific patterns of increase in tone in the spastic patient (Fig. 6/6A).

(g) *Position of the patient in relationship to gravity*: The relationship of the labyrinth of the ear to the pull of gravity and the pattern of pressure on the body exerted by body-weight can strongly influence the pattern of hypertonicity present in the spastic patient (Fig. 6/6B).

(h) *The degree of effort (physical or mental) required from the patient*: The physiological irradiation of this effort through the central nervous system will act as a trigger to the already over-excitable or under-inhibited stretch reflex circuits.

(i) *Handling ability of the assessor*: Clumsy, careless handling may produce many of the problems listed above and may also elicit pain. Pain will give rise to an increase in flexor tone. Thus, exact measurement will always be inaccurate except at the precise moment of measurement.

Bearing these points in mind, it is possible to classify hypertonicity in relationship to functional 'bands' so long as it is appreciated that within any one time-span, in the case of spasticity, the patient's condition may move out of one band into another.

If this approach is used, the therapist must realise that the assessment relates to the degree to which the hypertonicity is interfering with the ability of the affected parts to participate in functional activities. Thus, the pattern and quality of movement used to accomplish the function is important. The bands suggested for this purpose are detailed on page 143.

ASSESSING VOLUNTARY MUSCLE ACTION

Physiotherapists have always been concerned with assessing voluntary action of muscle and the terms power, force, strength and torque have been used to describe what is being measured. There is much confusion over the definition and use of these terms and sooner or later physiologists, biomechanical engineers, physiotherapists and medical practitioners will have to adopt a common language so that the present loose application of debatable terminology does not interfere with interdisciplinary communication (Laird and Rozier, 1979). The classic method of assessing muscle action is to relate the ability of the muscle to move the appropriate part of the body against the force of gravity. The Medical Research Council assessment gradings from 0–5 are assigned for recording purposes as follows:

0 = No contraction felt or seen.

1 = Flicker of activity either felt or seen.

2 = Production of the movement with the effect of gravity eliminated.

3 = Production of the movement against the force of gravity.

4 = Production of the movement against the force of gravity and some additional force.

5 = Normal muscle activity.

It is usual to start assessing for grade 3 and be prepared to move up or down the scale. Obviously the specific action of the muscle to be tested must be known since positioning the patient must be related to the effect of gravity on the movement to be produced.

It is important to note that a muscle can only give its best performance if its synergists are also participating. For example, deltoid is an abductor of the arm and requires a stable shoulder girdle if it is to be successful in this action. It particularly requires the activity of serratus anterior and trapezius as fixators of the scapula to prevent the inferior angle of the scapula from swinging medially as the arm tries to move sideways. Unless these muscles work with deltoid it is unlikely to succeed in producing abduction.

If the physiotherapist is testing a weak deltoid it is important that she checks the abilities of the synergists and fixators to see that the weak muscle gets adequate chance to show its abilities.

If the scapula is not fixed by the patient's own muscles then steps must be taken to fix it manually or mechanically before assessing the power of deltoid. This is true of all muscles – deltoid has only been taken as one example.

There is usually not much difficulty in coming to conclusions about grades 2, 3 and 4 in this method of assessment. Grade 1 can be difficult and so can grade 5. Before deciding that no flicker is available and therefore scoring '0' it is wise to try maximum facilitation and see if some activity can be encouraged. In that case grade 1 can be awarded provided it is made clear that it was only achieved with maximum facilitation. Grade '0' should never be awarded until maximum facilitation has been tried and failed.

For grade 5 the muscle must be compared to the normal side if there is one. It must be remembered that different activities use different levers and that movements against gravity can be done as weight-bearing and non-weight-bearing activities. Thus, for instance, the hip abductors cannot be graded as 5 unless they can function correctly to prevent a dropping of the pelvis towards the non-weight-bearing side (Trendelenburg's sign) while receiving weight in walking, running and jumping (if these last two are applicable to the age of the patient being examined).

These readings can be charted.

It is obvious that this approach to assessment of voluntary muscle activity is fraught with human error and many attempts to quantify more accurately have been made, using such pieces of equipment as grip dynamometers for finger and hand activity, spring balances, dead weights and pulley and weight circuits for bigger muscle groups, and electronic gauges for static muscle action. None of these methods has proved to be overwhelmingly successful and the original standard method still holds good for practical purposes.

However, biofeedback equipment, using surface electrodes, can be invaluable in detecting early activity in superficial muscles and will confirm the presence of a muscle flicker as well as more obvious activity. Accurate placement of the electrodes is essential as artefacts do occasionally mask the true picture.

Myometers of various kinds are now available in some physiotherapy departments and in physiological research laboratories. These range from small, simple to operate, electronic devices which can be easily stored and transported to the patient, to the more complex, multirecording devices which are best kept in one area and the patient transported to the apparatus. Such devices will, if used correctly, accurately assess static muscle action, and some will measure dynamic activity.

A high degree of accuracy in measurement is not always essential and a proper perspective on the value of numerical recording methods for voluntary muscle action and indeed, any other section of patient assessment must always be taken.

The methods of assessing voluntary muscle action indicated above offer a very 'orthopaedic' approach and are not always so applicable to the neurological problem. They are most relevant to the lower motor neurone situation where there is disturbance in the final common pathway for control of muscle. When the problem is more central, the difficulty of channelling voluntary impulses to the appropriate lower motor neurones can become so complex that the value of the test is minimal, gravity being, in some respects, the least of the patient's problems.

OTHER IMPORTANT ASPECTS OF ASSESSMENT

Everyday variations in environment are important. Collaboration with the occupational therapist is essential and both disciplines can help each other in this area. In many cases a home visit may be required and, in some instances, a visit to places of employment may be needed.

Home visits

Home visits are sometimes necessary in order to enable the management team to assist the patient to cope with their physical disability, or to assess the suitability of discharge when recovery has not returned the patient to normal. The most satisfactory teamwork for home visiting is carried out by the social worker, occupational therapist and physiotherapist, each of whom will be assessing the situation from their own viewpoint and with different objectives in mind. Many areas cannot afford the luxury of a visit by all three disciplines and sometimes one person alone may have to suffice. In this event the most pertinent objectives must be clearly defined so that a member of the most relevant discipline carries out the visit. However, as that one person may have to consider the three aspects it is important that the selected visitor has sufficient experience to see the problems relating to other disciplines and to be aware of her own limitations of judgement in these areas, so that she does not experience undue difficulty in reporting back and seeking appropriate advice.

It could be loosely stated that if all three disciplines visit one patient the physiotherapist should be looking to see how the patient's physical abilities could be improved to adapt him to his home. This is not always easy to assess unless the patient is actually seen in his own home as sometimes the design of the home and the layout of furniture and equipment are such that very specific joint range and muscle power requirements are needed and certain patterns of movement may be essential for the safe conduct of some activities.

The occupational therapist would probably be looking to see how the home and equipment could be adapted to suit the patient's needs, while the social worker should be looking to the social problems and support services which may be required to enable the patient to retain independence.

All workers should bear in mind that further physical treatment (at home or hospital), housing and equipment adaptations and support services are costly and, while their chief responsibility is to the well-being of their patient, indiscriminate expenditure of a wasteful nature is ultimately detrimental to the health service as a whole and may have an adverse effect on the well-being of other patients.

THE CRITERIA TO BE OBSERVED WHEN UNDERTAKING A HOME VISIT

The purpose of a home visit is to assess the patient's ability to function independently within the home and its environment, and should take into consideration (a) activities essential to basic daily living; and (b) leisure activities and social pursuits.

If functional impairment is evident: To assess the nature and extent of the problem and consider whether further therapy (such as joint mobilisation, muscle strengthening or movement co-ordination techniques) could enable the patient to ultimately overcome his handicap without the addition of aids and appliances and without permanent structural alterations being required.

In the event of a more severe degree of handicap: To assess the need for aids, appliances and even structural alterations to the home. It is important that patients and relatives are not confused and agitated by excessive gadgetry and home alterations while ensuring that basic needs are catered for adequately.

POINTS TO CONSIDER WHEN MAKING HOME VISITS

Three main questions should be in the mind of the visitor:
1. If the patient's condition is such that he cannot fit into the existing home environment at the time of the visit, is there any possibility that further specific remedial therapy will enable him to do so eventually?
2. If the ultimate result is still likely to be unsatisfactory, is it possible to adapt the home to meet the patient's needs?
3. If the patient and the home cannot be fully adapted to ensure functional independence, would certain supportive services bridge the gap and enable the patient to live at home and are there services available?

The answers to these three points will assist in the formation of the long- and short-term objectives underlying the management of the case.

The visit should include:

(1) An appraisal of the degree of limitation of function of the patient in the home.

Certain activities may have to be actually carried out by the patient if the visitors are to be satisfied that the manœuvres used are safe and effective. Discussions should also be held with the patient and, if appropriate, relatives and friends sharing the accommodation so that specific difficulties are clearly defined. The tactful guidance of the visitors is required to remind patients of difficulties they may (in the excitement of the moment) either have forgotten or about which they may feel some embarrassment in discussing. During this discussion the visitors should also be assessing the equanimity between patient and relatives and whether appropriate co-operation is likely to be obtainable.

(2) A tour of the house and, if available, the garden.

This is best done with the patient showing the visitors around as far as possible, because some of the difficulties will be immediately obvious to the visitors and other relatively minor points which could easily be remedied may be noticed.

When touring the house the following points should be among those noted:

(a) Access to the house.

(b) Width of doorways.

(c) Width of corridors.

(d) Type and condition of flooring.

(e) Position of lights, switches and power points.

(f) Type of staircase including its position in the house, number of steps per flight, angular, spiral or straight: width of stairway, position and height of handrails, depth and height of step and approximate size of landing area above and below.

(g) Position of bathroom in the house in relationship to kitchen, living room and bedroom. The size of the bathroom and the arrangement of its equipment should be noted particularly if the patient is wheelchair bound. Manoeuvrability of the wheelchair in the bathroom should be assessed on the spot and appropriate transfers should be seen. Appropriate measurements of heights, widths, and so on, of bathroom equipment should be taken and recorded. The patient should be asked to explain or demonstrate any particular difficulties experienced when using the bathroom facilities. The need for temporary or permanent aids should be discussed.

(h) The bedroom and bedroom fitments should be noted including the position of the bed, its stability, access to it and type of bed used. Appropriate measurements should be taken and note should be made of the accessibility of a light switch to the occupant of the bed. Again, the patient should be consulted about difficulties such as getting into and out of bed, and also in getting from bedroom to bathroom. If need be, a demonstration should be requested so that the therapists can see how each discipline could adapt the treatment programme of the patient to make life easier. The need for a temporary or permanent aid of some kind should be discussed.

(i) Access to the living room and ability to cope with furniture and equipment here is important, including the use of the television, radio and stereo equipment, if any is present.

(j) The kitchen should also be visited and examined in detail for safety, arrangement of equipment, appropriate size, and so on. Measurements should be taken if any alterations are likely to be needed. Accessibility of kitchen equipment to the wheelchair patient is particularly important and if the patient offers to make the visitor a cup of tea this should be accepted so that some of the difficulties can be observed as a first hand experience. Discussion must take place to enable the patient to voice his own difficulties and the need for aids and adaptations should be discussed.

(k) Accessibility of the garden and garden facilities. If the patient is interested in gardening, details of problems must be discussed. Absorbing hobbies are very important and any measure which can be taken to continue this warrant consideration.

(l) Laundry facilities should be discussed and, if need be, demonstrated.

(m) Accessibility of shops, delivery facilities and ordering methods should be considered, particularly if the patient lives alone. It may be advisable for one of the visitors to go to the local shops to assess the difficulties.

(n) Library facilities are important. The local shops may include a small library but, if not, a travelling library may exist which could call. The provision of large print books and tape cassettes for the visually-handicapped patient warrant investigation.

(o) The proximity and quality of the neighbours should be considered when visiting a person who lives alone. Co-operative and kindly neighbours can alleviate the difficulties of a disabled person enormously.

RECORDING OF MEASUREMENTS

All measurements taken should be clearly recorded and diagrams to illustrate areas measured should be used if these clarify the points to be made.

A small plan of each floor of the residence can be helpful as can a plan of specific room layouts. The pattern of furniture arrangements in bedroom, bathroom and kitchen can often dictate the pattern of functional movement required from the patient. If the visit by the physiotherapist is to enable her to plan a future exercise programme so as to help the patient to function in the existing environment then the specific pattern of functional movement required must be known. Equally, if the occupational therapist is to plan her management effectively, and perhaps supply aids and equipment to assist in the production of effective movement patterns, she must know exactly the demands made upon the patient.

In a situation of this kind it is *essential* that the two therapists work in close consultation with each other. Disharmony between disciplines can only lead to disaster for the patient. There is no place for interdisciplinary rivalry when a patient's well-being is at stake.

Following these investigations it should be possible to conclude:

1. How the patient's physical condition and mental attitude can be improved to overcome the problems.
2. How much in the way of temporary or permanent 'small aid' assistance is needed.
3. Whether any minor or major structural alterations are required as permanent measures.
4. The need for supportive services such as home help, laundry care, district nurse attendance, meals-on-wheels.
5. Whether it should be recommended that the patient is offered alternative housing or, in the case of private ownership, advised to move to a more suitable residence.
6. Whether it should be recommended that the patient requires residential care.

THE REPORT

When a joint interdisciplinary visit has been made, it is customary for a joint agreed report to be written which includes recommendations. The report should be signed by all the disciplines concerned.

If one member alone has carried out the visit a report should be made and signed by that person. However, any recommendations which could involve the other disciplines should only be made after consultation with the appropriate members of that discipline.

The report should include:

1. A verbal report on the difficulties seen and brought to light by the visit. This must be clear, concise and written under appropriate headings.
2. The diagrams, house plans and measurements taken at the time of the visit.
3. The long- and short-term objectives as seen by the visitors.
4. The appropriate recommendations which should be clearly listed.

ASSESSMENT OF SPEECH, TONGUE MOVEMENTS AND SWALLOWING

This is largely the province of the speech therapist but the physiotherapist may need to check some points for herself. The early interrogation will have given some indication of the patient's problems and speech patterns will have been noted.

The physiotherapist also needs to know whether the patient understands the spoken word even if he cannot reply. This can be assessed by asking the patient to make a signal if he understands what is being said. The signal requested must be one of which the patient is capable. It must be appreciated that many patients know what they want to say but can only say one phrase or word which may come out every time they try to speak. Thus they may say 'no' if this is their only word when they mean 'yes' or 'it doesn't hurt' or 'hello'! If this is the case, yes/no signals need to be devised and questions worded so that yes or no is the only answer required.

Tongue movements are essential for speech, mastication and deglutition. The physiotherapist can assess the availability of tongue movements by using any of these functions but if they are absent she may need to use a spatula or ice cube to encourage tongue movements while urging the patient to co-operate. It must be remembered that the tongue musculature is attached to the hyoid bone and if the synergists which control the position of the hyoid bone are not working control of tongue movements will be difficult. The infra- and suprahyoid muscles are important and may be paralysed. Equally, a patient with poor head control may well have infra- and suprahyoid synergy difficulties.

The ability to swallow involves complicated synergy of tongue, infra- and suprahyoid muscles and pharyngeal activity coupled with the maintenance of the closed mandible and closed lips. The muscles need power and co-ordination to be able to achieve the function.

Swallowing is most easily carried out in an upright position and is much more difficult if the patient is either recumbent or if the neck is extended.

It is important to remember that repetitive swallowing is self-limiting so the patient should not be asked to repeat the activity very often in quick succession.

RESPIRATORY FUNCTION

This may seem remote from neurology but it must be remembered that respiratory capacity depends not only upon lung field and thoracic mobility but also upon the muscle power and co-ordination of the respiratory muscles which include those of expiration as well as inspiration. Measurements of vital capacity using a spirometer can be recorded by means of a graph and give some idea of the power of the muscles and mobility of the thorax. Consecutive measurements at intervals give an idea of progress or rate of deterioration. A measurement of forced expiratory volume is one method of assessing the power of the expiratory muscles. This group includes the abdominal muscles.

Thus, a functional assessment by a physiotherapist must include specific tests, as appropriate to the patient, bearing all the areas indicated in mind. Such functions as the ability to move about in bed, transfer from bed to chair, chair to toilet seat and bath, dressing, walking, climbing stairs and manage in the home environment, cope with rough surfaces, cross roads, get on buses and even drive a car, can be assessed. Centres do exist where potential drivers can be advised, assessed and try their skill. Banstead Place in Surrey offers this facility and is prepared to accept patients referred for assessment from anywhere in the United Kingdom. In some cases it may be necessary to conduct not only a home visit to the patient but also a visit to his place of employment.

ELECTRICAL TESTS

Strength duration curves

These are done as part of the assessment of a patient suffering from a peripheral nerve lesion. Representative muscles of the affected group are stimulated by stimuli of different durations ranging from 300ms pulses down to 0.01ms. As is mentioned in Chapter 7, page 181, denervated muscle is only capable of responding to the longer duration stimuli because the shorter stimuli are too fast for muscle tissue unless very high intensities are used. The shorter stimuli are usually only transmitted via a nerve supply and thus only the innervated muscle can respond to such stimuli.

The term strength duration relates to the duration of the stimulus and the strength of the stimulus applied. More intensity is required for the shorter duration stimuli to produce a contraction even when there is a nerve supply. Thus a characteristic curve can be graphed relating stimulus duration and intensity applied to the contraction obtained (Fig. 6/7).

It is usual to attempt to obtain a minimal perceptible contraction using a long duration stimulus and then progressively shorten the stimulus duration. If the contraction disappears, the intensity is increased until a contraction of the same degree is obtained, a reading is then taken and recorded. This goes on until the shortest stimulus is reached. However, if the muscle is denervated the long duration stimuli only will be successful and no amount of increase in intensity for the shorter stimuli will produce a contraction. Thus the graph will not be complete for the denervated muscle.

A muscle containing some innervated and some denervated fibres will show a special type of curve with a 'kink' in it. It is a mixture of the short graph for the denervated fibres and the long graph for the innervated group (Fig. 6/7c).

Accurate strength duration curves are only obtainable after 21 days following injury. This is because denervation takes this time to be completed.

Rheobase is a term used to describe the lowest intensity which can produce a muscle contraction when a long duration stimulus is applied.

Chronaxie is a term used to denote the duration of stimulus which requires an intensity equal to twice the rheobase level, before a contraction is obtained.

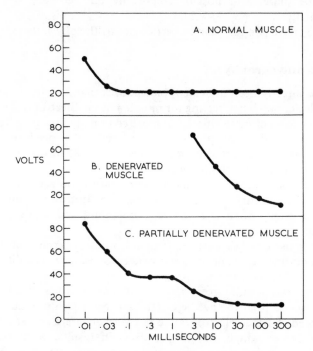

FIG. 6/7 Strength duration curves

As a muscle becomes innervated the chronaxie should gradually be a shorter duration of stimulus and move to the left of the graph.

Nerve conductivity

This is sometimes done to assess whether a nerve which has suffered compression is degenerating or not. The nerve is stimulated directly by a short duration stimulus along its course. When it is stimulated it conveys impulses to the muscles it supplies (provided it has fibres to carry them) and the muscles contract. If this is carried out at intervals from the time of injury the nerve will at first be hypersensitive and require a very low intensity. Later it may require more and, if it is degenerating, it will not conduct after about the 14th day. If, however, it does continue to conduct after 21 days the nerve has not degenerated and the injury is only a neurapraxia. In this case voluntary movement may be difficult or absent temporarily but recovery is likely eventually.

The above two tests can be carried out by the physiotherapist.

Electromyography

As has already been indicated, biofeedback may be used to assess muscle activity when testing for muscle power. Electromyography is also a form of biofeedback but more commonly uses penetrating electrodes and so constitutes a minor surgical procedure. It is most usually conducted by a physician and will record and amplify electrical activities in muscle.

A muscle is electrically silent when there is no activity in the fibres. This occurs when it is fully relaxed. It creates sound and gives a graph when it is active. The sound and graph give a distinctive pattern.

If a muscle is fasciculating (which it does in certain muscular disorders and at certain stages of denervation), there is a different sound and visual pattern.

Such tests require great accuracy if they are to be valid since it is essential that the needle electrode is exactly in the muscle to be tested. Surface electrodes are not very accurate and there are many factors which can give artefacts in results. A shortwave machine working in the vicinity, for example, can cause interference if it is of unsuitable wavelength.

RECORDING THE RESULTS OF THE ASSESSMENT

It is important that the physiotherapist records the findings as clearly as possible so that the initial assessment can be compared with those occurring later and progression or regression noted. The final assessment is very important for future reference, should the patient re-attend for further help at a later date.

There is no standard method or recording the results of the assessment although many workers are using the method described as Problem Oriented Medical Recording (POMR) or their own interpretation of this method. Workers using this method pay particular attention to formulating treatment objectives in relationship to the patient's view of his problems. Whatever system is used for recording findings there are various methods of storing the information and these may include:

(a) *Written records:* These should be in a logical sequence, concise and emphasise only the important points. Excessively lengthy notes will discourage the reader and unless the handwriting is very clear will be difficult to interpret.

(b) *The presentation of charts:* These may be used to record some aspects of assessment such as mapping out areas of sensory impairment, quality and quantity of functional independence, muscle power, strength duration curves from electrical tests, etc. Some examples of charts are indicated at the end of this chapter.

(c) *Notation:* Movement notation may be used to analyse posture and movement very effectively and the recording method gives three-dimensional information in terms of space, and a fourth dimension in terms of time. The quality and rhythm of the movement can also be recorded very accurately and easily interpreted by anyone skilled in the method of notation used. Notation is a written language of movement in the same way as written music is a language. Benesh Movement Notation particularly lends itself to the clinical situation and uses a five-line stave, representing body areas, to plot the information. Some examples have been included in the illustrations for this in the next chapter and, additionally, Figure 6/8 illustrates the use of notation to describe two different gait patterns which may be seen. Students should note the length of the verbal description required to equal the information given by the notation in these examples. The particular values of notation are: the effect it has on developing the analytical and observational skills of the notator; the easy storage of the information; and the need for minimal equipment (manuscript paper and pencil).

(d) *Video-recording:* This is a rather more sophisticated and expensive way of recording movement and storing the information. It does, however, have its uses in that it can be played back to the patient for information and for therapeutic purposes and can be presented to the medical team during clinical discussion sessions. In itself it does not encourage the development of analytical skills or observational activity in the therapist or medical practitioner, requires specialist equipment for both filming and 'playback', is expensive and takes up a considerable amount of storage space.

(e) *Electrogoniometers, polarised light goniometers and isokinetic dynamometer:* These are all instruments to which the patient can be either attached or exposed and which can be linked to

FIG. 6/8 Benesh Movement Notation.

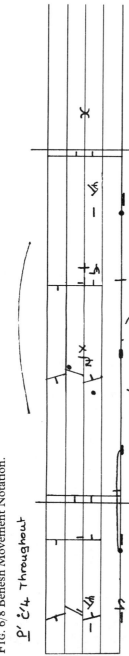

A. A gait pattern used by a young hemiplegic patient walking without any aid

The starting position indicates that the patient is bearing weight on the left foot which is plantigrade and the right foot is in front and touching the floor on the ball of the foot, which is plantar flexed and turned laterally. Both knees are straight. The pelvis is tilted to the left and rotated to the right, the upper torso is tilted to the right. The head is tilted to the left and rotated to the left. These last postures are compensatory for the pelvic posture and are 'righting' postures. The right scapula is protracted and depressed, the hand touching the front of the body and the wrist is flexed, forearm pronated and hand clenched. Left arm hangs at side. As weight is taken on to the right foot it flattens on to the floor and left heel is raised, the spine straightens but the rotational components and scapula protraction remain. The left foot steps forward normally but as the right foot follows it slides on the floor with knee straight circumducting as it proceeds, the pelvis tilts and the spine resumes its righting patterns but the right scapula retracts and elevates, and the elbow flexes behind the body, forearm supinates with hand and wrist still flexed while the left hand swings behind body. When the right foot gets in front of the body, it is in plantar flexion and the spine straightens as the pelvis resumes a normal posture; the scapula protracts and depresses, elbow remains flexed by side of body and the forearm adopts a neutral posture. Finally, weight is transferred on to the right foot which is still turned laterally, the right hand lowers and is pressed against the front of the body, pronated, fingers and wrist flexed. The left hand hangs by the side and the left foot is ready to take the next step. The cycle begins again

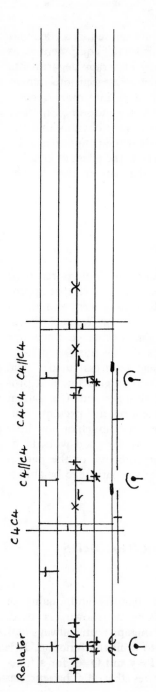

Rollator

C4C4   C4||C4   C4C4   C4||C4

B. This is the gait of a spastic diplegic patient, using a Rollator

The starting posture indicates that the patient is standing on the balls of the feet in plantar flexion, the feet are slightly apart and the lower limbs are medially rotated, the knees are slightly flexed and close together, the pelvis is tilted forward and the neck is also flexed. The elbows are flexed anterior to the body and the hands are supported by the Rollator in front of the body. Before beginning to 'walk', the patient lifts the head and extends the neck. The gait is one of rotating the pelvis to the right as the left foot slides forward on the floor, the head compensates by rotating to the left. The left knee crosses the midline after sliding against the right knee to get in front of it. The Rollator swings to the left as the step occurs and the left elbow becomes posterior to the body and the left hand is in the coronal plane. The right arm moves forward with the Rollator. The next step is the reverse of the above, and then the cycle begins again. The Rollator takes a weaving course

computers so that the findings can be analysed, recorded and printed out for future reference. This sort of equipment is, at present, not generally available in physiotherapy departments but is to be found in units undertaking research into human movement and may well eventually move into more general clinical use. It is expensive, requires space and some expertise and has the disadvantage of making it very obvious that the patient is being assessed – particularly if the patient has to be attached to the equipment – and this has the effect of creating an unnatural movement pattern in the patient until he becomes accustomed to it.

CONCLUSION OF ASSESSMENT

When the assessment has been made and the findings recorded the patient's profile should be looked at carefully so that appropriate treatment aims and objectives, both long-term and short-term, can be formulated. In all cases, the short-term aims will change as time progresses and as each aim is achieved a new one will be required. The long-term aims and objectives need to be reviewed periodically as the patient may progress further than originally expected. It is better to set one's sights low and progress, than to aim too high only to be disappointed. If a patient is heavily handicapped, it is wise to have a relative present at his final assessment so that the relative knows how much or how little help the patient needs at home. It is easy for good work to be undermined by relatives who are overprotective to the patient but, at the same time, it is important for the patient to be able to obtain the help he does need.

CHARTS, GRAPHS AND OTHER RECORDS

Charting functional independence

The same chart can be used to plot quantity and quality of independent function provided the key, as shown, is used. Thus, when observing the function the therapist must always look also at the quality of movement used to fulfil the function. It is quite possible for a patient to receive $I = 5$ and $Q = 2$ for a function. Such a recording simply indicates that the patient has

	Independence (I)		*Quality* (Q)
0	Not possible and cannot be achieved by one helper	0	Not possible and cannot be placed passively
1	Can be achieved by one helper	1	Can be passively placed
2	Can participate a little with one helper	2	Grossly abnormal
3	Needs some help	3	Abnormal
4	Needs 'stand by' for safety	4	Some abnormality observed
5	Independent and safe	5	Normal

achieved the function independently but has demonstrated grossly abnormal movement patterns.

The chart can also be used to indicate the nature of the abnormality in the comment column.

Hypertonicity bands

These can be used to classify both spasticity and rigidity and relate to the degree to which the hypertonicity interferes with the quality and quantity of functional independence. When using this method it must be appreciated that because of the many factors influencing the spastic type of hypertonicity, it is likely that within any one period of time the patient's condition may move out of one band and into another. Suggested 'bands' are:

A. *Minimal hypertonicity:* This level of hypertonicity has to be 'looked for' and is often missed by people who have not made a careful study of human movement. The patient is totally independent, the hypertonicity does not appear to interfere with functional activity. Stress situations and fast changes in equilibrium requirements may demonstrate a minimal excess of tone. Tendon reflexes may be slightly exaggerated and this is particularly noticeable if the patient is placed in reflexogenic postures. The patient may be considered to be 'clumsy' by his colleagues.

B. *Mild hypertonicity:* This is more noticeable in gross functional activities and reflexogenic postures. The patient is independent for most activities but fine skills are disturbed and tendon reflexes exaggerated. Finger movements are clumsy and lack precision. Balance reactions of the trunk are poor and the limbs disinclined to become involved. If the hypertonicity is spastic in nature the knees weight-bear in hyperextension.

C. *Moderate hypertonicity:* Depending on the extensiveness of distribution the patient may require 'stand by' help for some activities and be unable to accomplish fine skills without considerable help. Function of the affected area is noticeably impaired and the patient adopts a specific posture consistently. In the case of the spastic variety, the patient is able to use the affected limb(s) to act as props in transfer situations.

D. *Severe hypertonicity:* This patient is very dependent upon assistance from relatives and helpers unless the distribution of increased tone is very localised. The hypertonicity prevents participation in functional activities but does permit the affected parts to be positioned in wheelchairs or similar support. The patient can only assist with transfers to a small extent and the affected parts are really 'passengers'. The patient can, however, be manoeuvred for essential nursing procedures. This type of patient is in danger of developing pressure sores if the hypertonicity is widely distributed.

E. *Very severe hypertonicity:* This also prevents participation in gross functional activities of the areas involved. If generalised, it may prevent head control and therefore seriously disturb feeding, communication and socialisation. The affected parts strongly resist positioning of the patient in suitable patterns in a wheelchair, bed or any other type of support. Nursing procedures are very difficult and may require two or three people to cope adequately. The patient is likely to have pressure sores, develop severe, fixed deformities of joint position and if the head and neck are involved he is in danger of choking and suffocating. The spastic variety of hypertonicity may give rise to dislocations or subluxations due to extreme force of uneven muscle pull.

It must be clearly understood that these bands relate to the degree to which the hypertonicity interferes with the quality of function and the pattern of the activity must be carefully observed. It is possible to function independently or almost independently with quite severe hypertonicity if it is sufficiently localised. Therefore, the therapist must take note of the degree to which the affected part participates economically to the function in order to 'band' the result.

The bands described above are not a standardised, fully researched approach to the subject. They are the criteria used by the author to classify degrees of hypertonicity. Their use has been indicated on the following chart.

Sample functional chart (bed assessment only illustrated)

FUNCTION	I	Q	COMMENTS
Bed assessment			Hypertonicity, spastic both lower limbs – $C \leftrightarrow D$ Upper limb, head and neck and upper torso function good
Move up	5	3	
Move down	3	3	
Move to left	3	3	
Move to right	3	3	
Bridge	O	I	
Turn in body width to left	3	3	
Turn in body width to right	3	3	
Sit up to left	4	3	
Sit up to right	4	3	
(and so on)			

Sample chart for charting voluntary muscle action using Medical Research Council grading

Muscle group	Grade	Comments
Hip abductors	3	
Hip flexors	5	
Hip extensors	5	
Hip medial rotators	3	
Hip lateral rotators	5	
(and so on)		

The above example refers to *joint movement* rather than specific muscles. The alternative might be:

Muscle	Grade	Comments
Gluteus medius and minimus	3	
Psoas major, iliacus	5	
Gluteus maximus	5	
Biceps femoris	5	
Semimembranosus and tendinosus	5	
(*and so on*)		

REFERENCES

Brunnstrom, M. (1970). *Movement Therapy in Hemiplegia: A Neurophysical Approach*. Harper and Row, New York.

Laird, C. E. and Rozier, C. K. (1979). Towards understanding the terminology of exercise mechanics. *American Journal of Physical Therapy*, **59**, 3.

McGuiness-Scott, J. Benesh movement notation series. *Physiotherapy*, 1981 and 1982.

BIBLIOGRAPHY

Coates, H. and King, A. (1982). *The Patient Assessment: A Handbook for Therapists*. Churchill Livingstone, Edinburgh.

Gowitzke, B. and Milner, M. (1980). *Understanding the Scientific Bases of Human Movement*. Williams and Wilkins, Baltimore.

McGuiness-Scott, J. (1984). *Movement Study and Benesh Movement Notation*. Oxford University Press, Oxford.

Chapter 7

Principles of Treatment

by H. W. ATKINSON MCSP, HT, DipTP

Many factors influence the management of patients suffering from neurological disorders. There are many views on appropriate action and treatment, some of which are complementary while others may conflict to some extent.

The greatest conflict occurs when the need for urgent independent function is taken as top priority when perhaps a little delay in independence could lead to more adequate adjustment of the patient. There are arguments for both sides. It must be remembered that, while early functional independence may de-congest hospital wards and outpatient departments, this approach inevitably encourages the development of undesirable abnormalities of movement. These are substitutes for those normal activites which have now been temporarily or may be permanently made unavailable.

If a patient's potential is really quite good, given adequate time to redevelop along more normal lines, it may be quite seriously detrimental to him to allow substitute abnormalities to become a habit. Compromise is not always the answer since the result is often that of 'falling between two stools'.

Thus, the teamwork between consultants, nurses and therapists in addition to other workers is vital. There is nothing more detrimental to the patient than conflicting views between the team members dealing with his own particular case.

DISTURBANCE OF AFFERENT INFORMATION

This can complicate the progress of the patient considerably and must always be taken into consideration.

Loss of afferent information

This may be local and specific if the problem is a peripheral one or it may be diffuse if the problem is more centrally placed. In either case there is much in common from the physiotherapist's point of view.

INJURY TO THE AFFECTED AREA

This is an important aspect in the management of such cases since cutaneous loss, in particular, is likely to make the patient vulnerable to cuts, burns from fire and steam, frictional abrasions from contact with harsh surfaces and pressure sores from prolonged contact with a supporting surface.

All patients with this problem should be made aware of this danger and it is the job of all concerned with the patient to ensure that he fully appreciates the dangers.

Obviously avoidance of injuries is to be encouraged and the patient should be told to use substitute measures to enable him to detect hazards. His hands are particularly vulnerable if they are involved since it is hard to avoid injury when the hands are so often used as tools. He must always use his eyes to detect hazards and beware of likely problems ahead of their occurrence so that complications do not arise.

Frictional abrasions and pressure sores can be avoided by adequate padding of areas likely to be subjected to friction and by care over the tying of such things as shoelaces if there is sensory disturbance in the skin of the lower leg and foot. The application of sheepskin cushions and mattresses for the more heavily disabled is valuable so that the patient is 'cushioned on air' trapped in the wool. Ripple beds and frequent turning are necessary for the severely handicapped patient.

To some extent the patient should be responsible for his own safety. He must be warned to inspect his skin for signs of injury and to take steps to relieve pressure whenever possible. For instance the patient who is confined to a wheelchair should endeavour to lift himself up in the chair by using his arms to relieve the weight and pressure on the buttocks frequently. He will most particularly need to be reminded to do this if he has lost sensation in the buttock region since he will not then receive the uncomfortable stimuli which would normally encourage him to change position.

LOSS OF BODY IMAGE AND REJECTION OF THE AFFECTED AREA

This can be quite a difficult problem and to achieve any measure of success it is important to remember that we develop a knowledge of body image by being able to move, touch and feel objects in close proximity to us and by being able to touch different parts of ourselves. It will be remembered that, as far as the hands are concerned, contact with the face, nose, mouth and hair is important. Thus we may be able to prevent loss of body image and rejection of parts of the body by using passive movements which are directed in simulating some of the more natural activities, e.g. taking the hands to the face and running the fingers through the hair, allowing the affected area to come into contact with more normal parts of the body and vice versa.

The patient may be positioned so that he can see the affected part and have his attention drawn to it frequently.

In some problems this aim of treatment is more important than in others. Permanent rejection is unlikely to occur in the localised peripheral problem but it is very common in the more centrally placed lesions.

If rejection and loss of body image have already occurred by the time the patient is receiving physiotherapy then the task is much more difficult to deal with. Sometimes exaggerated application of stimuli helps and heavy compression force repeated with the affected limb in a weight-bearing position may help. Constant handling of the area and helping the patient to simulate normal activities with the affected limb may be of value. Much patience and tolerance is needed in these cases.

If the patient is accepting an abnormal position as being normal, this must be pointed out to him and explained in such a way that he understands. Recent activities with video equipment seem to indicate that this can be very helpful for some patients who can see their own difficulties more clearly when they view a video film of themselves in action. However, care must be taken before exposing a patient to his own image in this way as some may find the experience unduly disturbing. Provided the patient is suitable, the re-educational effect of this method is likely to be greater than that achieved by the use of mirrors as the patient is not looking at a mirror image of himself and need not be carrying out the activity while he is watching it. Thus, all his attention can be put into studying his movements and comparing them with those he sees in other people. It is, of course, possible to correct the patient while he is being filmed and he can see himself in the monitor at the same time. If this method is used, it must be remembered that patients are more accustomed to seeing mirror images of themselves than video images and it takes them a little while to adjust to the new concept.

Mirrors are, of course, cheaper and more commonly used but the mirror image can be confusing and is not suitable for all patients. Those with visual perception problems or with severe disorientation may not find them helpful and the elderly and confused patient may be totally disturbed and not relate the mirror image to himself at all. Thus, both video filming and the use of mirrors must be considered very carefully before the patient is subjected to them and if they are not fulfilling their purpose, should be discarded. If, however, they are found to be helpful and the patient has appreciated his problems he should then be encouraged to work towards correction.

In cases of defects of sensory perception of this kind and in cases where loss of ability to move inevitably encourages the immediate adoption of abnormality, the patient must be treated as early as possible to avoid bad habits taking hold. For example, a patient who has had a cerebrovascular accident of such severity that he awakes as a hemiplegic, starts to develop abnormalities *as from that moment*. He substitutes and quickly accepts disability on that side of the body which for a time is virtually useless to him. Very soon it seems 'normal' to carry that half of the body as a passenger and to depend solely upon the non-affected side. This will be perpetuated unless some measures to prevent this occurrence are taken very quickly.

DISORIENTATION DUE TO FAULTY INFORMATION

This can occur if afferent information is not completely cut off so that faulty impressions are being received. For instance, some patients may have diminished touch and pressure sensation. If this occurs in the soles of the feet it gives rise to a 'cottonwool' sensation when the foot contacts a hard surface and very little sensation at all if a soft surface is contacted. This can make life very difficult for the patient. He may develop the type of gait which involves lifting the knee high and forcing the foot down hard on to the floor in order to obtain an exaggerated effect. This method of walking also makes a noise which tells the patient when he has landed. He may also have to look where he is walking all the time.

In this type of problem, substitution would have to be encouraged particularly if the disorder is permanent. Such a patient may have to be advised against wearing cushioned soles and heels since he cannot hear these land on the floor. He may have to wear studded shoes which make more noise than normal when he walks. He would have to be encouraged to use his eyes as substitute sensory organs.

As far as possible his high-stepping, exaggerated weight-bearing should be avoided since this could cause joint injury.

There are special methods of helping the movement problems of such cases. These will be considered under the heading relevant to movement abnormality.

Vertigo is another problem associated with faulty afferent information. As was stated in the previous chapter the patient may feel giddy and nauseated due to disorientation of the position of the head in space. The fault lies usually in the vestibular pathways or in the vestibular organs themselves. Any movement of the head or even of the eyes may make the patient feel symptoms. Impressions from the eyes and vestibular apparatus are so closely associated with each other that disturbance in one can give problems to the other.

The patient may have to be trained to rely upon the information he is receiving from his joints and skin and from his eyes since these are more reliable than the vestibular impressions. This takes time and while help from certain drugs is available to the patient, helping to reduce the feeling of nausea, he will still need help in movement activities.

Such patients frequently show a very fixed posture of the head and shoulder girdle because movement of the head is known to trigger off the symptoms.

The more unfortunate patient may well have vertigo in addition to faulty position sense. This makes life very difficult since substitute information is less available. Many patients with multiple sclerosis show these mixed problems and they may also have defective vision to complicate their problem even further.

The method of approach to the movement problem associated with vertigo will be considered under the appropriate heading (p. 188).

SENSORY RE-EDUCATION

Many patients with sensory difficulties respond to sensory re-education methods which may include the factors indicated under the section on loss of body image but may also include other methods of stimulation such as contrast baths, whirlpool baths, exposure of the part to soft and hard surfaces and different textures of materials – rough hessian, satin, cotton, wool, fur and towelling – and asking the patient to note the difference and possibly attempt to identify the materials without the use of their eyes. The provision of identical looking objects but with differing weights can be very useful and are very cheap and easy to provide. It is easy to fill small plastic bottles or medicine containers with different substances to make them heavy or light and ask the patient to try to arrange them in order of weight.

Shape and size can sometimes be difficult and patients can be encouraged to handle objects of identical shape but a different size such as a large beach ball and a small tennis ball and compare the two. A hoop or a quoit can be used to provide apertures through which the balls can pass and the patient may be given the opportunity to select the appropriate ball for the aperture. This may later be transferred to the selection of head and arm apertures in the clothing of the patient.

These suggestions can be endless and relate to different types of problem. Occupational therapists have many ways of handling the patient with perceptual difficulties and the physiotherapist should be prepared to consult with the occupational therapist whenever possible so that the two disciplines complement and supplement each others efforts for any one patient. It is very easy to undermine the activities of a member of a related discipline who is also treating the patient. This must be avoided at all costs and frequent consultations should occur between all disciplines concerned. No one is entirely self-sufficient as far as patient treatment and management is concerned; there is no room for interdisciplinary rivalry and knowing when to ask for help and advice is a key factor in successful teamwork.

DISORDERS OF MOVEMENT

The average person has very little appreciation of the complexity of performing an apparently simple function. All the necessary reactions are built in so smoothly that the timing and synchronisation of muscle and joint activity escapes notice. Throughout activity movement occurs against a background of malleable postural tone adjusted to maintain the equilibrium of the individual in all eventualities. In this way movement flows in a smooth, coordinate and purposeful manner.

Even less appreciated is the importance of afferent information.

If there is no appreciation of the position in space the necessary steps to alter it cannot be taken. Moreover, if inadequate information is forthcoming during the performance of the movement it can be nothing but crude and wide of the mark since no corrective measures can be taken.

For normal function to occur the nervous system must be in sound order from the receiving, correlative and transmission aspects. There must be adequate mobility available in the joints of both the trunk and the limbs and the muscles must be healthy and able to respond to the activities of the nervous system. It is only under these circumstances that appropriate muscle synergy will be forthcoming giving the common movement patterns associated with normality.

The more common movement patterns incorporate a balanced mixture of the movements seen in the more primitive mass flexion and mass extension patterns. Primitive mass flexion and extension patterns may be seen in the young child but even these are more refined than those seen in the patient whose central nervous system is grossly disordered.

The tiny child does have some control over his reflex mechanisms which gives him the ability to modify these effects to some extent. Although the normal child does show a poor vocabulary of movement when compared with the normal adult, he does have the basic foundations upon which to build the permutations of movement with which we are familiar in the mature individual. Skilled activity is dependent upon mature movement permutations and therefore mature muscle synergy.

Since all human beings are built along essentially the same lines and all require to be able to achieve similar basic functions, certain movement permutations are common to all. During the development of these permutations the child repeats a movement until it can be achieved with ease, thus illustrating the phenomenon of physiological facilitation. Repetitive use of a neuromuscular pathway lowers the threshold of synapses involved and makes it easier for the pathway to be brought into use. Thus the pathway is said to be facilitated.

Since movement involves excitation of some muscle groups and inhibition of others, it is important to remember that we are facilitating both excitation and inhibition when we facilitate a neuromuscular pathway so that a movement occurs. The word 'facilitation' means 'to make easy' and it is in this context that the word will be used throughout this chapter.

The physiotherapist who undertakes the problem of movement

re-education in a disabled person is accepting an enormous responsibility. Not only must she be able to detect and assess the degree of, and type of, abnormality presented, but she must have the necessary knowledge and skill to guide the patient towards normality while recognising the limitations set by the nature of the disorder.

FACILITATING MOVEMENT AND ENCOURAGING FUNCTION

Many ways of doing this have been developed over the last 30 to 40 years and, initially, eminent workers developed their own approach in an isolated way and were not always sufficiently in communication with each other to permit free exchange of ideas. Thus, different schools of thought have developed, each with its own individuality but there are several common, and now acknowledged, themes which run through all of them. The various approaches can perhaps be compared to the activities of an orchestra in which the different sections develop their own theme and together produce the whole effect. Some parts of the symphony are restful while others are stimulating depending on the way in which the sections develop their theme. The clever conductor works his orchestra according to the effect he wishes to have and according to the work they are playing. A clever physiotherapist selects the methods of facilitation she uses according to the effect they will have and the patient to which they are applied. Thus, the more knowledge she has of the methods available, the more variation she has to hand to achieve her aims. There is not really a standardised 'right way' to treat a patient. The 'right way' for any patient is the method which, in his individual case, achieves realistic objectives.

All facilitation methods are directed at improving the quality of movement and the quantity of function but, before embarking on an exacting programme of facilitation techniques, it is wise to ensure that all members concerned in the management of the patient agree with, and understand, the short- and long-term objectives of the therapy. Unless this is clear from the start a great deal of confusion can ensue and the patient can suffer from conflicting advice, comments and general management.

The long-term aim may be to achieve functional independence with maximal economy of effort and minimal joint and muscular strain. This may necessitate a short-term policy of general improvement of quality of movement within the capacity of the specific nervous system. Thus, a delay of achieving total independence in the interests of better quality of function may be necessary. This approach is seen to be eminently suitable when handling patients with many years of useful life before them and in the treatment of young children during their developmental years. Additionally, patients who have a large area of undamaged nervous system still available to adapt to the changes of activity required and who, themselves, are able to exert the necessary self-discipline and patience will be suitable candidates for this approach. The plasticity of the nervous system is such that younger people have the greatest chance of organising or reorganising their nervous system to function appropriately even when it has been quite severely damaged, whereas the older nervous system may have lost some plasticity and be less adaptable in the event of injury or disease. However, it is unwise to automatically assume that the elderly nervous system will not adapt at all. Many workers report evidence to the contrary although most people agree that the elderly have greater difficulty than the young. This approach is generally considered to be 'expensive' in therapists' time because unskilled therapy is unsuitable and so the patient requires the help of a therapist, skilled in facilitation techniques, for a comparatively long time.

At the opposite end of the scale is the approach sometimes adopted to restore functional independence as quickly as possible, regardless of the quality of movement used and irrespective of the basic biomechanical principles involved in economy of joint and muscle activity. It is true that outstanding levels of functional independence can be achieved in the presence of gross abnormality. The essentials for this are motivation on the part of the patient, necessity as far as the patient and relatives are concerned and the ability to put in hard physical and mental effort to overcome the difficulties as they present themselves. This approach does empty the hospital beds because the patient is quickly made 'ambulant' or adapted to a wheelchair existence. In terms of immediate economy and, in some cases, of self-respect, this may be desirable. This is particularly so in the very elderly, senile person where independence can all too easily be totally lost forever and may also be the only approach to take if the damage to the nervous system is extensive and absolute as in some spinal injury cases. This approach only requires skilful physiotherapy for a limited period of time, since most of the practice sessions can be conducted by less skilful staff under the supervision and guidance of a skilled therapist. Later, relatives and friends, or the patient working alone, can achieve the desired results. It is important for therapists to realise when the work they are doing is relatively unskilled and could be equally well carried out by an unqualified person. Reluctance to shed the first-hand relationship to the patient must be avoided when this stage is reached, so that the time-consuming activities can be taken over by the less skilled leaving the therapist more available for duties appropriate to her specialist skills. The therapist who feels 'threatened' by an intelligent but unqualified helper needs to look inwardly. She may find that she is not availing herself of the specialist skills of her qualification.

In applying these two extremes of approach to the real situation, most therapists adopt a compromise attitude in relationship to the availability of 'back-up' support, the specific needs of the individual patient and the demands of the patient care system operating at the time. Whatever approach is made, facilitation techniques are available and are selected and adapted to fulfil the agreed objectives of the team.

The assumption in this chapter is that an appropriate level of functional independence is the long-term aim and that this will be achieved by fulfilling an initial short-term aim of improving the quality of function.

To carry out effective facilitation techniques it is essential to have a basic appreciation of:

1. The patterns of motor activity which are recognised as 'normal'.
2. The importance of the pattern of 'sensory' input to the programming of motor output.
3. The value of accurate 'feedback' information.
4. The relevance of the stretch reflex mechanism and factors influencing its activity.
5. The normal developmental milestones.
6. The phases of learning related to the acquisition of motor skills.

The selection and implementation of appropriate facilitation techniques for a specific patient requires an appreciation of the nature and disturbance to the nervous system and:

1. The way in which this disturbance has caused deviation from the 'normal' patterns of activity.
2. Whether and how it has altered the pattern and perception of afferent information and, therefore, altered the programming of motor output.

3. Whether accurate feedback is available to the patient.
4. What factors, if any, are having an adverse effect on the stretch reflex mechanism.
5. Whether certain developmental milestones have been 'lost' or 'missed out' and need reinstatement or initial instatement before real progress can occur.
6. How the phases of motor learning can best be applied to the acquisition of skill in the individual concerned.

Two more questions must be considered:

1. How does the rest of the team view the problem – including the patient? Will they feel able to support the therapist's approach and reinforce its effect by co-operating in full?
2. What are the patient's expectations and will he/she be able to sustain the co-operation needed to fulfil the short-term goals as they present themselves?

Thus, the assessment of the whole patient and his environment is essential to ensure maximum possible success.

Methods of facilitation

Students would be well advised to study the works of Signe Brunnstrom, Dr and Mrs K. Bobath, Margaret Rood, Dr Kabat, Margaret Knott and Dorothy Voss, Temple Fay, Doman and Peto, Cotton and Kinsman and a suitable bibliography is listed at the end of this chapter.

THE SELECTION OF PATTERNS OF MOTOR ACTIVITY

All facilitation methods involve the use of motor patterns of activity because functional movements occur in pattern and are seen as a balanced mixture of the flexion/extension synergies of activity. Sound patterns of movement give a cosmetically 'good' and co-ordinated appearance, fulfil the functional needs of the individual efficiently and minimise the biomechanical stress involved. They are thus economical, efficient and look safe and co-ordinate. Students should study carefully the patterns of movement described by Signe Brunnstrom as comprising the total flexor and extensor limb synergies of mass movement. All functional movements involve balanced mixtures of these synergies and never involve the total flexor or total extensor group alone (Figs. 7/1 and 7/2).

Patterns described by Dr and Mrs K. Bobath tend to relate to

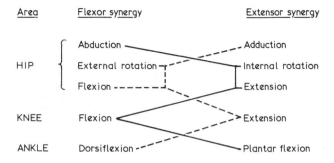

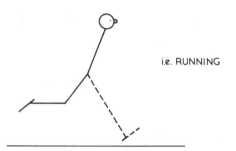

FIG. 7/1 Balanced mixtures of the basic limb synergies – running

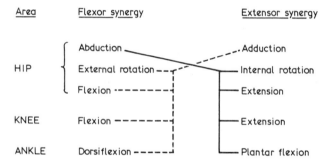

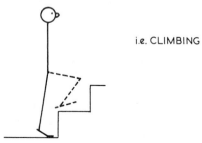

FIG. 7/2 Balanced mixtures of the basic limb synergies – climbing stairs

the developmental milestones of movement and are very fundamental to the basic functions of locomotion. The proximal components of these patterns relate closely to those described by
Knott and Voss but offer more variation distally.

Although Margaret Rood does not define the movement patterns so explicitly as other workers she encourages components of
activity which can be related to the other systems.

Any student who wishes to successfully facilitate movement
must become an astute observer of detail in motor patterns of
activity. Pay attention, therefore, not only to the gross and obvious movements but, more particularly, to the subtle alterations
of body-weight distribution during the fundamental locomotor
activities. If the patterns of response to altered weight distribution
are ill-controlled, skilled movements are unlikely to be successful.

THE PATTERN OF SENSORY INPUT

This has a profound effect on motor output in that the orientation
of the individual in space depends upon the information received
from the bone, muscle and joint receptors, skin, eyes and ears.
The pattern of vision, sound, equilibrium, acceleration, pressure,
stretch, traction or compression has the effect of programming
the postural mechanisms of the body in such a way that a pattern
of muscle tone specific to the input is achieved.

Physiotherapists need to become conversant with the effect of
various types of stimulus so that they can effectively encourage
or discourage certain types of response. For example, pressure on
the ball of the foot is likely to cause the 'push-off' effect of plantar
flexion of the foot because this is part of the positive supporting
reflex mechanism, whereas pressure under the heel may well
stimulate dorsiflexion of the foot as an equilibrium reaction.

Traction to a limb will most likely encourage flexion, whereas
compression may more readily elicit extension. Studies made by
Margaret Rood indicate that profound attention to detail of afferent stimulation may well be the key to many movement problems.

All methods of facilitation agree that the posturing of the head
and neck are of great importance because of the receptors in
cervical joints and inner ear. These have an important bearing on
posture and tone and the activity of these structures and their
associated reflexes may have to be suppressed or encouraged
according to the needs of the patient. Whatever the problem, it
is generally agreed that control of head and neck posture is vital
to successful facilitation of movement for the following reasons:
(a) Certain positions of the head and neck trigger off undesirable

reflex activities which give rise to total flexor or extensor synergies and therefore lead to danger of deformities, pressure sores and general 'stiffness' of the patient. Thus, the overall mobility of the patient is reduced if head control is lost and the patient is 'at risk' from infection, dislocations, subluxations, and such like.

(b) Functional feeding reactions require control of head position and independent activity of tongue, cheeks and lower jaw. Head control is essential for effective swallowing and reduces the incidence of choking, gagging and vomiting.

(c) The cough reflex is more effective if head posture can be controlled. Thus, food inhalation is less likely.

(d) Eye focus is more possible and spatial orientation is thus facilitated.

(e) Without head control, speech cannot be co-ordinated and other facial methods of communication are difficult.

(f) A patient who can see a little, spatially orientate himself and communicate is more likely to remain mentally alert.

(g) All the above factors contribute to social acceptability of the handicapped person.

ACCURATE FEEDBACK

When carrying out basic or complex skills, it is essential to know whether success is the likely outcome. Adjustments cannot be made to the motor output if there is no monitoring of the skill while it is being performed. Patients with normal sensory input are in a position to judge the likely result of their efforts to some extent. This is true unless they have become adapted to an abnormal pattern of movement and are attempting to move away from it towards the more normal. In this event they will not be able to judge clearly as the normal movement will actually feel abnormal.

Such patients, and those with sensory disturbance may need the help of the therapist to obtain accurate feedback. It is essential, therefore, that the therapist only praises the outcome of an activity when it is satisfactory and not just because the patient has 'tried hard'. If the patient has 'tried hard', and the movement is poor, praise will lead to a repetition of the same 'poor' movement and the therapist will be guilty of facilitating poor movement. Biofeedback equipment may also be useful in helping the patient to monitor their activities. It will not, however, totally substitute for a good physiotherapist.

THE STRETCH REFLEX MECHANISM

This is well known to all therapists and its activities are vital to the production of appropriate background of postural tone and the production of fine skilled movement. Factors creating abnormalities in the stretch reflex mechanism have a devastating effect on the production of normal movement patterns. Most facilitation procedures are directed at the stretch reflex mechanisms with a view to controlling them more effectively by having an inhibitory or excitatory effect according to the needs of the patient. In many cases it is necessary to inhibit in some areas and activate in others so that the correct balance of inhibition/excitation is achieved.

Postures of rest and patterns of activity are directed to programme the correct balance of activity in the stretch reflexes and are assisted by the application of manual and verbal skills. These skills and techniques are listed at the end of this subsection.

THE NORMAL MOTOR DEVELOPMENTAL MILESTONES

A knowledge of these is valuable when attempting to develop the fundamental equilibrium and motor skills in a patient and, in particular, when treating children.

When treating adults it is sometimes apparent that the nervous system has regressed to a more primitive level and some milestones have become temporarily 'lost' or forgotten. In this case a knowledge of human movement development can often help the therapist to assist in the reinstatement of a particular skill. Additionally, the ways in which children learn and repeat activities throw guidelines to the therapist who may wish to emulate some of these methods when treating her patients.

THE PHASES OF LEARNING RELATED TO MOTOR SKILLS

Under normal circumstances the patterns of movement developed by the individual occur naturally by trial and error learning during the early years of life as the central nervous system matures. As each pattern demonstrates a functional outcome to the child, so it is repeated again and again until it is automatically produced when circumstances are appropriate. The pattern is by this time stored in the central nervous system for future reference. The system of learning has been very gentle and the cerebral cortex may have played very little part in the process. This form of learning movement patterns and storing them is often called subcortical learning.

In this way basic patterns of equilibrium, locomotion and

fundamental function are learned and, provided the pathways used are undisturbed and the bones, muscles and joints remain in good order, these patterns remain with us forever.

The more advanced skills, however, have to be learnt at a higher level and involve, at first, maximum use of the cerebral cortex in order to achieve, even marginal, success. During the learning process many extraneous activities may occur which are quite unnecessary to the skill and may even be detrimental to its ultimate success. These 'associated activities' have to be curtailed and inhibited by the individual until either they no longer occur or no longer interfere with the successful outcome of the skill.

Time and repetition are needed in quantity before such skills become part of the 'make up' of the individual. The patterns of activity are ultimately stored and available when required and, when this occurs, the skill 'looks easy' to the observer and the person carrying out the skill has the ability to vary the skill in order to produce an effect – something which is not available during the basic learning phase. By the time the skill has reached this 'automatic' level the patient has passed through the cognitive phase and the fixation phase described so clearly in Turnbull (1982) and Dunkin (1981). In facilitation of movement these factors are of importance because in some cases the loss of basic locomotor patterns may not be profound. In this instance, a programme of activity which 'revives' and 'revises' these patterns, with as little involvement of the cerebral cortex as possible, may well reinstate the lost patterns with little effort on the part of the patient, leaving time and energy available to concentrate on the more difficult tasks.

In other situations it may be necessary to skilfully 'programme' the patient with sensory input so that the most likely output is a good functional movement pattern using minimal cortical involvement to finally achieve the desired effect. This sort of approach is particularly valuable to the patient showing hypertonicity of a spastic type.

In yet other circumstances it may be necessary to bring the whole activity up to a cortical level and make total demands on the patient's volitional concentration and effort in a repetitive manner, patterns of activity only becoming more automatic in the long term.

The various approaches to neuromuscular facilitation make it possible to encourage motor learning in a variety of ways from the 'least cortical' methods to the 'most cortical' methods and it is up to the therapist to select the approach she uses according to the needs of the patient at any one time.

Some manual and verbal skills used in facilitation techniques

The skills indicated below are used to varying degrees by all workers involved in facilitation techniques. The reasons why they should have this effect are not always known and there is room for a great deal of research in this area. However, whether the reasons are understood or not therapists have found the skills listed below to be of value:

Selection of 'resting' postures: To minimise the effect of unwanted tonic reflex activity.

Application of cold: Prolonged immersion of the muscles – or packing in towels soaked in ice cold water – to have the effect of reducing muscle spindle activity. The application of brief cold stimuli to appropriate dermatomes – to have a stimulating effect on corresponding myotomes.

Relaxed passive movements: Using slow stretch and rotational components of mature movement patterns – to reduce activity of muscle spindles.

The use of reflex inhibiting patterns of movement: Assisted active and free active. These are given to encourage appropriate sensory input from mechanoreceptors and muscle spindles which will help to 'programme' the central nervous system to more appropriate motor output.

Specific relaxation techniques: To produce inhibition of muscles or muscle groups by influencing the bias placed on muscle spindles through the Golgi tendon organs, for example, hold, relax techniques.

Initiation of movement: Using reversals of patterns to encourage inhibition of the antagonistic patterns as movement is commenced in one direction. On completion of this movement the previous antagonists are stimulated to become agonists by the phenomenon known as successive induction.

Brushing over relevant dermatomes: To activate corresponding myotomes.

Touch over relevant dermatomes applied as stroking, clapping and pressure on the skin: To activate corresponding myotomes.

Compression through joints, preferably via weight-bearing surfaces of the skin: To have the effect of encouraging extension and/or co-contraction.

Traction through joints: To have the effect of stimulating a flexion' response.

Stretch to muscle: Short sharp stretch stimulates primary receptors in the stretched muscle. Slow steady stretch may well have an inhibitory effect by minimising the activity of primary receptors and by stimulating a Golgi tendon response. The pattern of stretch is important because:

(a) A slow stretch of postural extensor muscles will stimulate the secondary receptors in the muscle spindles. In these muscles the afferent fibres of the secondary receptors are thought to have an inhibitory effect on the muscle stretched and an excitatory effect on its antagonist. This effect, added to the effect of gentle excitation of the primary endings may then result in co-contraction of muscles as needed in 'stance' situations.

(b) Stretch of trunk muscles and, in particular, rotational and side flexion stretch encourage righting and equilibrium reactions which may help to inhibit tonic postural mechanisms. This effect may also be seen in the limbs if stretch incorporates rotations.

(c) The brief stretch stimulus applied within a spastic ('reflex') pattern will stimulate the reverse 'reflex' pattern. Thus, stretching the lower limb towards flexion, abduction and lateral rotation will stimulate an extension, adduction and medial rotation response.

If, however, the stretch stimulus is applied towards a mature pattern the response is likely to be towards the mature reversal of the pattern. Thus, a stretch of the lower limb towards flexion, adduction and lateral rotation will stimulate an extension, abduction and medial rotation response.

(d) Stretch may be applied directly by the therapist or by the effect of gravity as in 'tapping' techniques.

Specific vestibular stimulation: Rocking, inverting and rotating the patient may have the effect of reducing hypertonicity and, in some cases, of stimulating more normal postural activity. These effects can be achieved by the use of a hammock, rocking chair, rotating the chair or supporting the patient over a large therapeutic ball which can be moved in various directions. Some workers have also reported useful results following the use of a trampoline.

Commands and timing of commands for volitional effort: A movement may be made strongly 'volitional' by the type of command given and the emphasis placed upon it. In certain cases, when maximum effort is required, strong use of the voice and brief instructional commands are essential. In other situations a more gentle and less emphatic approach is more suitable.

Pressure over the muscle belly: To have the effect of activating muscle spindles - possibly by distorting the shape of the muscle fibres and creating a 'stretch' situation.

Vibration applied to the muscle: This may have an excitatory effect on muscle spindles (vibration applied to bone via weight-bearing areas seems to induce co-contraction possibly because the bony vibration is transmitted to muscle on all its aspects). The frequency and nature of vibration appears to decide whether excitation or inhibition is the outcome.

Use of irradiation of nervous impulses: Strong volitional effort in a mature movement pattern has the effect of creating central excitation and causes many motor neurone pools to 'fire off' - particularly those conditioned by the starting position to have a low threshold. Thus, associated movement is likely to be seen in other limbs which can be valuable. This effect is used when it is desired to initiate activity in lower motor neurones which have a high threshold. The weak muscle is not worked specifically, initially. Instead a stronger area of the body is exercised so that the effect of irradiation will activate the motor neurone pool of the weakened muscle. When activity is initiated this way the weakened muscle is then directly exercised in an appropriate movement pattern. This technique is not so successful in central nervous system disorders because the associated reactions produced in this instance tend to occur in spastic patterning. This is probably because the tonic reflex mechanisms frequently lower the threshold of these motor neurone pools to such a level that they are too easily activated and dominate the patient's responses.

Limb shaking: Traction and shaking the limb from the distal end appears to have an inhibitory effect. The reason for this is not clear.

All methods of facilitation use these skills in various ways according to the patient's needs.

The methods of facilitation described by Knott and Voss and designated 'Proprioceptive Neuromuscular Facilitation Techniques' have been given specific names and are conducted in exact patterns of movement which have to be carefully learned and practised by the therapist before skill in their application can be developed. The names given to techniques described by this method are:

Reversals of antagonists – isotonic and isometric
Rhythmical stabilisation
Timing for emphasis
Repeated contractions
Hold relax
Slow reversal hold relax
Contract, relax
Rhythmic initiation.

These techniques often involve resistance and strong volitional effort and are most suitable for the treatment of lower motor neurone problems and ataxic patients, but can be adapted to give great benefit to other groups if used by a skilled worker.

The methods used by Rood, Bobath and Brunnstrom involve the use of most of the techniques described in this section with different emphasis placed on the value of each technique. Rood places emphasis on brushing, icing and the stimulation of joint receptors and secondary endings in muscle spindles (see Chapter 8), while Dr and Mrs Bobath emphasise reflex inhibiting patterns of activity, the development of righting and equilibrium reactions and the use of key points of control. They also particularly emphasise the need to appreciate the dangers of strong volitional effort in some patients which can lead to pattern abnormalities and the development of undesirable associated reactions detrimental to progress. Brunnstrom uses the primitive reflexes more positively at first and changes her tactics as the patient progresses. She also uses more conscious volition than Bobath and Rood.

Temple Fay and Doman place emphasis on the use of more

primitive patterning initially and encourage reptilian and amphibian patterns of movement before working towards the more sophisticated patterns of the mature human being. They also emphasise, more positively, the need for constant repetition and the importance of stimulating the patient intellectually as well as physically. The methods advocated for the brain-damaged child involve teamwork by relatives and friends who 'pattern' the child for many hours each day, the therapist acting primarily as an innovator and consultant. Even less therapist-centred and more patient-based are the methods advocated by Peto (and described clearly by Cotton and Kinsman (1983)) entitled 'Conductive Education' in which the therapist 'conducts' a group of patients encouraging them to both verbalise their activities and produce the movements as they do so, starting with relatively simple movements and progressing to more complex and very functional activities. The interested student should keep a flexible and open approach to all these methods as each has something valuable to offer. Many workers use an eclectic approach and, of course, add ideas of their own. (The methods used by Levitt, Carr and Shepherd, and Sullivan, Markos and Minor, are examples of their type of development on facilitation techniques.)

The physiotherapist who is interested in neurological problems should try to be familiar with all these approaches, study and keep up to date with advanced neurophysiology and develop her own variations on facilitation methods.

Bearing these points in mind the following pages indicate how some of the more common neurological problems may be approached.

THE PROBLEM OF HYPOTONIA AND ATONIA DUE TO PERIPHERAL NERVE PATHOLOGY

This may be seen when there is disorder in the peripheral system. On referring back to Chapter 4 it will be noted that such a state of affairs is usually the result of damage to the motoneurone pools of the anterior horns or to fibres passing peripherally from these motoneurones towards the muscles they supply. If all the motoneurones supplying any one muscle or group of muscles are completely destroyed then the muscles concerned will be completely paralysed, become flaccid and show atrophy in which muscle bulk is markedly reduced offering no protection to underlying structures.

If the damage is complete and irreversible, no amount of physiotherapy will restore muscle action. However, if only part of the motoneurone pool is affected, leaving intact those cells which have a higher threshold of stimulation, certain physiological factors may be applied to increase the excitatory effect on the motoneurone pools. In this way the remaining cells and their fibres may be made to convey impulses to the muscle, by the process known as *recruitment*. Similarly, if the cells or fibres of the motoneurone pools have suffered temporary damage they may eventually regain their ability to conduct impulses to the muscles. This may, at first, be difficult because they may have a raised threshold of activity.

These recovered neurones may also be encouraged to become active more readily by the physiotherapist exploiting her knowledge of physiology so that the use of these pathways is facilitated.

In this instance the physiotherapist has to make use of all the methods she can devise to have an excitatory effect upon the offending motoneurone pool or pools so that each effect can be added together or summated to reach the threshold of excitation.

Methods of excitation which are suitable

THE USE OF NORMAL MOVEMENT PATTERNS

This involves the use of muscles which commonly work with the muscle which is flail. This is of value because the neuromuscular pathways commonly used are facilitated during the developmental process by repetition. Volitional impulses are conveyed to the motoneurone pools of the whole pattern. Neurones influencing one motoneurone pool in the pattern are thought to branch and also influence the other associated motoneurone pools. By this spreading of effect the motoneurone pool of the weakened muscle will receive maximum volitional stimulation.

USING THE EFFECT OF STRETCH STIMULATION

The stretch stimulus applied to the muscles involved in the whole pattern will, by branching of the afferent nerves, stimulate the motoneurone pools of each other as well as those of their own muscle. The excitatory state of the motoneurone pools including that of the weaker member of the team will be increased for a brief period of time. If to this effect, is added volitional effort (by summation) the excitatory influence may be enough to cause the lower motoneurones to conduct impulses to the muscles showing weakness.

RESISTANCE

This is, in effect, a kind of continuous stretch applied to a working muscle and thus is a facilitatory method. The degree of resistance applied should be as great as the muscle can overcome and *no greater*. In some instances suitable resistance may be appreciably high whereas in other circumstances it may be as little as frictional opposition offered by the joint being moved. The term maximal resistance is often used and this must always be related to the available power in the muscle under treatment.

THE USE OF TRACTION FORCE

Traction is applicable if the movement pattern to be produced is that of flexion. It simulates the natural influences upon such movements which are basically a withdrawal from the pull of gravity. This effect summated to stretch, resistance and volition will further alter the excitatory influence upon the motoneurone pools.

THE USE OF APPROXIMATION (compression through the joints)

This is a postural stimulus associated with extension and is thus suitable in any situation in which a weight-bearing stimulus could be applied. The extension patterns are most suitably facilitated by the application of approximation. This stimulus, like traction, could be applied to summate with resistance, stretch and volition.

THE USE OF TOUCH

This should be applied over the working muscles and/or to the surface against which the movement is to occur. This supplies skin stimulation which acts as a guidance to the movement and facilitates activity in the motoneurone pools.

THE USE OF VISUAL AND AUDITORY STIMULATION

A well-voiced command facilitates volitional effort. The patient's eyesight is of particular value if sensory information is otherwise a problem.

The timing of the use of stretch, traction or compression and the use of auditory stimulation is of vital importance. These should all be applied together, simultaneously, if they are to offer maximum facilitation to the patient's volitional effort. Use is made of both spatial and temporal summation. Misuse of the timing of the application of various stimuli can lead to a reduction in effect.

THE USE OF COLD

Short duration applications of cold in the form of crushed ice over suitable dermatomes can be used to cause excitatory influences to occur at the appropriate motoneurone pools. A time lag is usually necessary between the application of the stimulus and expecting a result so, consequently, this is a stimulus which can be applied prior to the other methods and it will then be able to add its effect by summation with the other stimuli.

THE USE OF BRUSHING

This can be applied to encourage excitation if it is carried out briskly over the appropriate dermatome. Usually there is a delay in response of up to 20 minutes, so this can be applied prior to the other stimuli.

THE USE OF RIGHTING AND EQUILIBRIUM REACTIONS

These can be applied if the patient is placed in such a position that balance is rather difficult. The postural and equilibrium mechanisms will influence the motoneurone pools of the muscles concerned in implementing the reaction and if these include the weakened group of muscles the influence applied may well have the necessary excitatory effect.

To use these reactions effectively the physiotherapist must have a knowledge of the most common reactions and which patterns of muscle activity they are likely to stimulate. It is possible to add to this effect by applying approximation through the appropriate limb or limbs and trunk and by commanding the patient to 'hold' while counter pressure is applied in different directions.

THE USE OF OTHER PARTS OF THE BODY AS A PRELIMINARY PROCEDURE

When other parts of the body are used, strongly associated reactions can be seen in those parts not being directly stimulated. This may occur because the nervous pathways controlling the movement influence the motoneurone pools of counterbalancing muscles or other associated groups. This is another form of spreading. Thus, if the affected muscle is in the right leg, it would be quite feasible to work the left leg or either of the upper limbs or even the head and neck or trunk first in order to have an irradiation effect upon the motoneurone pools of the affected limb.

THE USE OF REVERSAL PATTERNS

Sherrington found that the flexor withdrawal reflex was stronger if the extensor thrust reflex preceded it. The phenomenon became known as that of 'successive induction'. This phenomenon also seems to relate to volitional movement. If a movement is preceded by the exact opposite one the final pattern is produced more strongly. Thus it is physiologically sound to precede a flexion pattern by an extensor one in order to obtain a stronger flexion pattern. This method would be reversed if it was desired to use this phenomenon to facilitate extension.

Emphasising the weaker team members

When using the above methods to facilitate activity in the weaker members of a muscle team it may be found that the weaker member does show activity. This should then be exploited. One method of doing this is to maintain activity in the muscles concerned in the rest of the pattern by making them hold the pattern strongly. The weaker member of the pattern should then be stimulated, by stretch and command, to participate concentrically, repeatedly through a suitable range. In other words, the total pattern is held in a suitable range and movement is only allowed to pivot about the joints controlled by the weaker member of the team. This approach is often called 'timing for emphasis'.

Let us take an example: the weakened muscle group is that supplied by the musculocutaneous nerve of the upper limb. Thus biceps brachii, brachialis and coracobrachialis muscles are involved. The most appropriate movement pattern for involving these muscles is called the flexion, adduction and lateral rotation pattern of the upper limb which would be combined with elbow flexion. In this pattern the wrist and finger flexors would be used and flexion would be accompanied by radial deviation. The forearm would supinate, the elbow flex and the shoulder flex, adduct and laterally rotate so that the hand would be carried towards the face and may progress obliquely across. The scapula would protract and laterally rotate carrying the upper limb into elevation across the front of the face.

Let us suppose that the efforts of biceps and brachialis as elbow flexors are to be emphasised. The patient is commanded into the pattern with the physiotherapist using the appropriate grasps, traction and stretch stimuli. The biceps and brachialis may be participating weakly and may need help to produce the elbow flexion. At the point in range where they offer the most activity the patient would be commanded to hold the pattern and pressure would be applied to make the shoulder, wrist and finger muscles hold a strong static contraction while stretch stimuli and command to bend the elbow would be repeated again and again to get maximum effort out of biceps and brachialis as elbow flexors. As appropriate, the range of the holding of the pattern may be changed until the two muscles are participating well throughout.

It may, of course, take many treatment sessions to achieve full-range participation.

Such an approach may be applied to any muscle group involved in any pattern and may even be used to facilitate a weak pattern of one limb as a whole by making the other limb, limbs or trunk hold appropriate patterns while the weaker limb is encouraged to move through some range. This method of approach is exploiting the spreading effect of branching neurones which influence their own specific motoneurone pools and those of associated groups. Thus, volition directed to the weaker groups may be more effective since the excitatory threshold of these motoneurones has been, to some extent, prepared and lowered.

The above methods form an ideal way of (a) initiating activity in the weakened groups of muscles and (b) of building on the activity obtained. This second point is very important.

When trying to initiate activity the physiotherapist must be prepared to go to a great deal of trouble to obtain the maximum facilitation and may have to try several methods before a result is achieved.

When activity is seen to occur the physiotherapist must exploit it to the full and try not to lose any ground she has gained. Thus repetition is vital. The more often the volitional impulses are able to cross the synapses and be transmitted the more readily can they effect a crossing. Thus, once activity is seen it must be repeated again and again until it becomes relatively easy to produce. Progress is then made by reducing facilitation and expecting an equally good action to be produced.

Once the weakened member has been made active, encouragement should be given to getting it involved in as many functions as are appropriate so that it is no longer allowed to become a passenger but has to participate.

These methods are particularly appropriate in the lower motoneurone problem because they make use of strong volitional effort in addition to other stimuli. Since there is nothing wrong with the 'computer' system but only with the external connections strong volition is unlikely to lead to undesirable associated movements. In fact, as has been said before, the associated movements may be highly desirable in this case and can be exploited to good effect.

When the weakened muscles are participating well in pattern with minimal facilitation, muscle strengthening techniques of a standard variety may be used quite effectively. Progressive gravity-free to weight-resistance exercises may be given either in patterns or in a more isolated manner to build up muscle power and endurance. Deep pool therapy may be of particular value. Movement patterns may be produced quite effectively in deep water and the efforts of the patient may be directed to moving the limbs about the stationary body or the body about the limbs.

Pool therapy is of particular value if the patient has large muscle groups involved, when the limbs and trunk may be particularly heavy and unwieldy in a dry land environment. If, however, the muscle weakness is associated with severe reduction in afferent information, as may be the case in polyneuritis, then deep pool therapy may not be so appropriate. Many patients of this type find the weightlessness and lack of sensory information which is associated with immersion in a deep pool, very frightening. They already have sensory loss and do not know their position in space when gravity is being fully effective. If they are then put into a pool where the effect of gravity is minimised then disorientation may be intensified to an alarming level. Each patient must be considered as an individual and assessed and treated to his best advantage.

In this section emphasis has been placed upon the exploitation of physiological factors while using movement patterns. The patterns which are most effective are those described by Dr Kabat, Margaret Knott and Dorothy Voss. They are of a diagonal nature and include rotational components which are of great importance (see Bibliography pages 217–19).

The patterns used are described through full range and are most commonly used through full range during certain aspects of treatment. This gives maximum facilitation. Functional daily activities which include these movement patterns through a lesser range are also encouraged in the patient's treatment programme. Eventually, it is hoped that the patient will gain maximum participation of the affected muscles without having to have maximum facilitation on their motoneurone pools.

It is important to note that the use of movement patterns themselves only offers some help to the affected motoneurone pools.

Much more is to be gained by exerting the additional physiological influences which can summate with the patient's volitional efforts to produce the movement pattern. In other words the patterns are there to be used, they are not sufficient in themselves.

The techniques described can be applied to straight movements, and even to individual muscle action if the physiotherapist so desires but they are not as effective used in this way because the patient is really using a pattern of muscle synergy which is new and alien to him, and pathways which have therefore not been physiologically facilitated during their early developmental processes.

Following this account it may be helpful to consider one lower motoneurone problem in a little more detail. Let us consider that the patient has had an axillary nerve lesion and that the deltoid muscle is at present not participating at all in any movements although the nerve injury has not been severe enough to disrupt completely the continuity of the nerve fibres. The problem is one of neurapraxia and the nerve fibres are showing a very high threshold of activity.

To deal with this satisfactorily the physiotherapist must have a knowledge of the functional significance of the muscle and how it participates in many simple daily living activities.

Deltoid must be recognised as having the following functions:

1. It is an abductor muscle of the upper limb.
2. Its anterior fibres flex and medially rotate the humerus.
3. Its posterior fibres extend and laterally rotate the humerus.
4. It commonly works with trapezius and serratus anterior to elevate the upper limb.
5. It becomes involved in any functional activities in which the arm is taken away from the side of the body.
6. It counters traction force applied by gravity to the upper limb by supporting the humerus up into the glenoid cavity. It is helped in this function by biceps brachii, triceps (long head), coracobrachialis and the smaller rotator cuff muscles in addition to the clavicular portion of pectoralis major.
7. It helps to stabilise the shoulder in weight-bearing activities and is particularly active if weight is being taken on one arm in the prone kneeling position when it acts as a supporter of the shoulder girdle in the same way as the hip abductors support the pelvic girdle when the opposite limb is taken off the ground. It may be seen working strongly in side sitting

particularly if the body is being pushed away from the supporting arm. It moves the arm away from the body or the body away from the arm if the hand is fixed.

8. It becomes involved in balance reactions when the body is pushed sideways. One upper limb may move outwards to be placed upon a support at the side of the individual while the other may lift sideways in an effort to readjust the overall position of the centre of gravity. In both instances deltoid is involved.

9. It becomes involved in stabilisation of the non-weight-bearing arm when hand skills are being carried out. It may be felt and seen to be functioning in many fine skills of the hand as a stabiliser and/or adjuster of the glenohumeral positioning.

10. It is involved in turning over movements, when moving up and down the bed and from side to side, walking with free swinging arms, carrying the shopping, doing the hair and putting on the hat.

In fact there are so many functions which involve this muscle that a book could be filled with an account of them.

The physiotherapist must have a knowledge of these functions and also a knowledge of the most appropriate movement patterns which may help to facilitate early activity. Probably the most appropriate patterns are the flexion, abduction and lateral rotation pattern and also the extension, abduction and medial rotation pattern.

Method of approach

1. Make the patient aware of the reason for his movement difficulties. This can be done by comparing the activities of the affected limb with those of the normal side.

   The patient may also be shown, by using mirrors, the lack of muscle bulk of deltoid and the trick movements which he is inclined to produce due to lack of participation of the muscle.

2. Make the patient as aware of the muscle as possible. This may be done by using simple methods such as handling the muscle and moving it over the underlying bone using a mixture of kneading and picking up massage manipulations while talking to the patient about the muscle. This, incidentally, distorts the muscle fibres and may be a start to offering sensory input which may help to bring about excitation of the motoneurone

pools. Light clapping over the muscle may also help in awareness and will stimulate the sensory area in the immediate vicinity which may be of value. It is also possible to apply electrical stimulation which will have a similar effect. This will be considered in a later section of this chapter (p. 182).

3. Start trying to initiate activity. This may be done in many ways and the physiotherapist should try many before giving up. Some suggestions are as follows:

(a) Use the normal limb and have the patient in a lying position. Give strongly resisted flexion, adduction, lateral rotation, reversing with extension, abduction and medial rotation patterns. While doing this watch for associated activity in the affected limb. It is likely to produce a reciprocal extension abduction pattern of the affected limb reversing with flexion adduction. There will not be much movement but a pattern of tone may be noticeable. If this appears to bring about extension abduction and medial rotation of the affected limb then give repeated contractions into the pattern on the normal limb which is getting the desired associated action. This may build up the associated activity. Then, without wasting any time, give flexion, adduction and lateral rotation as a resisted movement to the affected limb and follow this immediately with a reversal into extension, abduction and medial rotation. If a result is obtained give repeated contractions into this pattern.

(b) Another possibility would be as follows: Have the patient in high sitting leaning on to the hand of the affected side or in side sitting with the supporting hand being on the affected side. Stroke over the dermatome of C5 and 6 on the affected side with a piece of ice and then work the normal limb strongly by giving resisted flexion and abduction with repeated contractions into the pattern. The cold will take about 30 seconds to be of value so work the normal limb for about 30 seconds and watch the abnormal deltoid all the time. Action of its motoneurone pools is being facilitated because of the effect of the cold, the irradiation effect of voluntary action and the effect of the compression force which stimulates a stabilising action (Fig. 7/3).

If the muscle responds then make the patient hold the normal limb against opposition in flexion and abduction and apply compression force through the shoulder on the affected side. Sway the patient in many directions and ask him to 'hold' his position. This may further activate the muscle.

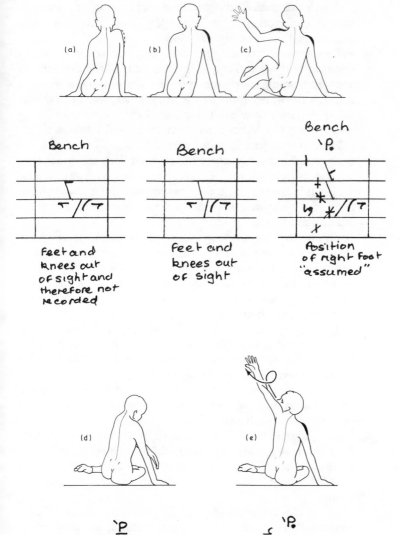

FIG. 7/3 Re-education of the deltoid muscle

There are many other methods which may be used to initiate contraction in this muscle. These approaches are only offered to give a general concept.

4. Follow the contraction which has been initiated into a functional activity. For example in approach (b) the deltoid was used as a stabiliser of the shoulder while weight was put through the upper limb. If the muscle has become active in this way it may be worth using lateral displacement of body-weight to get a balance reaction and stabilisation activity.

Have the patient in high or side sitting. Gently pull the body-weight laterally using the affected limb and place it in a supporting position. Repeat this sideways sway several times and allow the limb to receive a little compression force from the body-weight each time the limb is in a weight-bearing position.

Gradually take the help of the physiotherapist away and displace the body laterally without helping the arm, watching for deltoid activity. As the body sways laterally gravity will help the arm to move sideways but deltoid is needed to prevent over-shooting when the weight of the body arrives on to the upper limb.

The patient can then be encouraged to push himself back to neutral using the arm as a thrusting tool. If he uses too much trunk substitution resistance can be applied to the trunk to make help from the arm a necessity.

At this stage it may not be possible to get full participation of deltoid in these activities, but it should be encouraged to participate as much and as often as possible.

5. Later progress could involve a short period of maximum facilitation as a 'warm-up' method followed by some further functional activities to encourage easy natural usage. This could then be followed by more specific strengthening techniques.

From the moment the patient starts treatment simple functional habits should be corrected and, as appropriate, functional use should be encouraged. For example, the patient with severe weakness in the deltoid muscle may also have had a painful shoulder injury. He will almost certainly have adopted the bad habit of holding his upper arm strongly adducted into his side even if, additionally, it has been supported by a sling. If he has tried to use his hand, he will have steadied his upper arm by, even more firmly, adducting his arm against his body. This habit is very undesirable since it will not only lead to a stiff shoulder joint but will also actively *inhibit* the deltoid muscle and so undermine any progress the therapist may hope to achieve. Thus the habit of 'clamping' the arm to the side must be stopped forthwith and, instead, relaxation, either into the sling or just into a normal postural pattern, should be insisted upon and, indeed, should take priority over every other treatment measure. Unless this re-education of body image and postural pattern occurs quickly the use of any recovery may be seriously delayed.

Similar problems occur when any other muscle group becomes severely weakened and the physiotherapist must become familiar with the most likely pattern abnormalities which are inclined to be associated with weakness of any of the major muscle groups. A sound knowledge of functional anatomy is essential and the therapist must expect to go on developing this knowledge for the whole of her working life.

In the case of the weakened deltoid, early functional activities can be encouraged as soon as a flicker of contraction is available and the patient has learnt to relax the adductors. Relaxed arm swinging, when walking, is one of the earliest early activities and this should become established as a habit as soon as possible. Simple stabilisation of the shoulder *without adduction* during the performance of hand skills should be encouraged next. An example of a suitable situation for the involvement of the muscle in such activity occurs when the subject leans forward to tie up a shoelace while the foot is on the floor or supported on a stool in front of him. In this example the effect of the force of gravity is minimal and deltoid needs only to contract very gently to carry out its stabilisation function successfully.

Balance activities involving the upper limbs may later be added and active participation in rolling activities and weight-bearing on elbows and hands can be expected as the muscle becomes more active. The therapist must make a real effort to help the patient involve the muscle in suitable ways. The patient cannot be expected to do this automatically. He will have had to substitute for deltoid deficiency for so long that he will not necessarily realise that he is continuing to do so and neither will he know when, or how, to involve the muscle without a great deal of help. In the author's view this part of the re-education programme is more important than any of the progressive strengthening exercises recommended, since regular involvement in every-day activities will automatically improve the overall performance of the muscle group as a whole. Strengthening exercises, alone, do not guarantee involvement of the muscle in daily activities.

Specific strengthening could include repeated contractions with emphasis on deltoid in appropriate patterns through different ranges. It could include the use of pulleys and weights as resistances to the pattern of movement and progressive resistance could be applied.

Strengthening could also involve pool therapy in which the limb is abducted, flexed and extended, using the influence of buoyancy as a support or resistance. On the other hand the limb could be held stable by the physiotherapist and the patient asked to move the body-weight away from the limb, the body being supported all the time by the water.

Suspension therapy can be used as a substitute for water and can be made very progressive by some enthusiasts.

6. As the muscle gains enough power to lift against gravity it should require less initial 'warm-up' facilitation and should also be expected to participate in anti-gravity functions. Such things as prone kneeling, changing to side sitting on alternate sides use deltoid in fairly easy weight-bearing activities. Crawling forwards is more difficult because the weight-bearing arm has to support the shoulder girdle of both sides and the non-weight-bearing arm has to lift forward against gravity.

Balance reactions may be given in which the deltoid is expected to help in lifting the affected limb sideways and forward in an effort to adjust the overall position of the centre of gravity. Overhead arm and hand activities should be encouraged and light shopping may be carried by the affected limb.

Strengthening techniques should be carried out against the force of gravity and resisted movement patterns may have to be done in the sitting position or some other suitable position so as to involve gravity also. Progressive resistance exercises should include anti-gravity activity.

7. Eventually the patient should not require any preliminary facilitation methods and should be encouraged to participate in sporting and daily activities which will involve the affected limb totally.

The patient may do some activities as a member of a

group in the gymnasium, and have some individual attention but, most important of all, he should be advised on suitable home activities. Eventually he has to manage his own limb entirely. Home activities are always available and should be exploited.

The above outline is not intended to be specific. It is used to give a concept and there are many variations to any one theme. The physiotherapist is not a technician. She must have a concept of aim, try to fulfil it and be observant of results so that she can adjust her method. No patient is exactly the same as any other and no patient can, therefore, be treated in exactly the same way as anyone else with the same problem.

Maximum sensory input in these cases will give maximum motor output. This fact must be exploited in the early stages of treatment and modified as the patient progresses.

Electrotherapy in the lower motoneurone problem

If a peripheral nerve has been injured in such a way that the pathways will be disrupted for a prolonged period of time prior to being able to conduct again, it may be advisable to make the muscle contract artificially. This is in order to maintain its mobility against underlying structures and to minimise the rate of atrophy and loss of bulk by promoting the circulation through the muscle itself. In this way the muscle is maintained in a sound condition until such time as the nerve fibres are able to be functional again.

In order to influence as many muscle fibres as possible it is usual to place an electrode at each end of the muscle belly. Modified direct current is used and trapezoidal pulses of long duration (30–300ms) are given. These pulses are used because they are less likely to stimulate muscles which have a nerve supply, since they rise and fall slowly and the nerves going to the normal muscles will accommodate to them. Muscle does not have such good powers of accommodation and since the electrodes are placed over the muscle which has, at present, no nerve supply this is the muscle most likely to respond. Shorter duration pulses are not suitable as muscle tissue is unable to respond and only those muscles which could receive the stimulus via their nerve supply would be able to contract.

Apart from keeping the muscle in good condition electrical stimulation may also help to keep the patient aware of the muscle and its actions.

It is also possible to use electrotherapy as a re-educative measure. When the nerve has been repaired but voluntary effort is still having difficulty in producing a contraction, it may prove helpful to use the faradic type of stimulus to help in the initiation of activity. In this situation a train of short duration pulses are delivered to the muscle via its nerve supply. The electrodes are therefore placed one over the motor point of the muscle and the other over the nerve trunk or nerve roots. Voluntary effort on the part of the patient is requested at the same time as electrical stimulation is given and the patient is asked to maintain the contraction when the electrical stimulation is reduced or ceases. This is a method of re-education and it can be helpful in certain circumstances.

Biofeedback

Biofeedback equipment has now been developed which uses the basic principles of electromyography and can involve the use of surface electrodes applied to the patient by the therapist. This has the value of feeding back, to both the therapist and the patient, information regarding the successful contraction of muscle during a movement activity. The apparatus is neat and compact and can be strapped to the completely mobile patient without any difficulty. The electrodes are placed over the relevant muscle and the electrical discharges issued by the contracting muscle are picked up and converted into audible signals. In this way the therapist and patient are informed that the muscle is active and success or otherwise can be monitored. The threshold of muscle activity required before a signal is heard can be varied by programming the apparatus to be more or less sensitive to the electrical changes within the muscle. In this way even the patient with extreme muscle weakness can be informed if his effort has been successful. As the muscle participation improves, the equipment can be made less sensitive so that more activity is required to raise a signal. This equipment is not yet available in all hospital departments but, used skilfully, could be of great value to both therapist and patient.

Disorders of movement caused by changes in the central nervous system

THE PROBLEMS OF HYPOTONIA AND ATAXIA OF CENTRAL ORIGIN

Hypotonia and ataxia are so closely allied that they may be considered together. The bias on the stretch receptors is low and there is deficiency of activity of the excitatory extrapyramidal system. This is therefore a central and not a peripheral problem. There is lack of synergy and postural co-contraction of muscles round joints so that precision of movement and stability of posture is lost. Equilibrium and righting reactions are slow in being produced and inclined to over-react when they do occur. Movements are inclined to be slow to start and to be jerky and ill co-ordinated.

The physiotherapist has to attempt to redevelop the patient's movements along more normal lines and to keep him aware of normal movement patterns and normal posture and balance.

It is most advisable to make use of knowledge of developmental sequence in these cases and to encourage the development of postural stability and co-ordinated movements along these lines. The patient should progress from a position in which the centre of gravity is low and the base wide to the use of positions where less stability is offered.

It is very easy to use basic functional positions and movements following the developmental sequence since this inevitably complies with the low centre of gravity and wide base principles of progression.

If approximation is applied in the direction of weight-bearing, the stimulus already being applied by gravity will be reinforced. This tends to encourage extrapyramidal activity and gives rise to co-contraction of the muscles supporting the joints over which the weight is being placed.

The stimulus of gentle swaying may be applied at the same time to encourage activity in the appropriate patterns. This helps to elicit postural and righting reactions. The patient may be asked to participate volitionally by adding instructions which would be combined with manual pressure in all directions. The instructions would be to 'hold' or 'don't let me move you' as rhythmical stabilisations are carried out. These will further encourage co-contraction and combine automatic reactions with volitional effort.

Let us take as an example a patient whose condition is so difficult that he is unable to balance the head in a stable posture over the shoulder girdle because of hypotonia. To start with he would be most suitably positioned into prone lying with the elbows and forearms supported over a small bolster of pillows so that he is in a supported, elbow support prone lying position. If this position is too uncomfortable for the patient because of age or joint stiffness then a supported elbow support sitting could be used as a substitute (Fig. 7/4). In this position all that has to be supported by the patient is the head. The physiotherapist can then help the patient to raise the head and, still assisting, can apply gentle approximation through the head and cervical spine while encouraging the patient to hold the position. She can take her support away and re-apply it in a rhythmical manner to allow gravity to have a frequent momentary influence upon the supporting muscles giving them a repeated small stretch. In this way a co-contraction can be built up encouraging the patient to be responsible for his own head position.

It should be remembered that while applying sound mechanical principles here, sound neurodevelopmental physiology is also

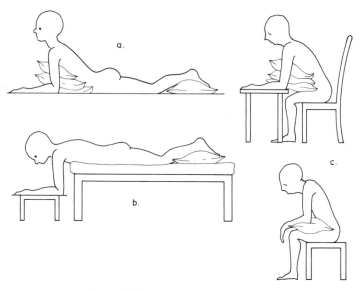

FIG. 7/4 Elbow and forearm supports

being applied since control of the head position first shows itself as head lifting from prone lying.

Progress can be made by encouraging the patient to lift the head actively either by using resisted and commanded movement patterns of extension with rotation reversing with flexion with rotation or by making the patient follow moving objects with the eyes in appropriate directions. Holds should be given in various positions so that the patient learns to maintain suitable co-contraction wherever the head happens to be.

As improvement is noticed the patient can be encouraged to be responsible for the stability of the upper trunk and shoulders. The pillow support is taken away so that the patient is in an unsupported elbow support prone lying. The physiotherapist may need to apply quite vigorous and repeated compressions through the shoulder and elbow at first to gain some activity and then may stimulate the action by swaying the patient's weight from side to side and forwards and backwards to encourage excitation of the co-contracting muscles. It may help to use rhythmic stabilisations again here by pressing on the shoulders and commanding 'hold' and 'don't let me move you'.

When balance on the elbows is fairly secure the patient may be encouraged to rise from complete prone lying into elbow support prone lying and return down again. This requires a remarkable amount of postural and balance control and can be quite difficult for the patient.

The patient can then be encouraged to bear weight on one elbow while using the other limb or pushing on the other hand so that the trunk is rotated towards a more supine position.

Balance activities in this situation can be exploited. The patient periodically is lifted off the almost free hand and pushed down on to it again and made to hold with rhythmic stabilisation. In this way the upper trunk rotation components are now being involved and becoming more able to stabilise.

When the patient has reached this stage it is time to start encouraging head control with emphasis on the flexor muscle groups. The patient may be in a supported sitting position with the head in such a situation that gravity would gently pull it backwards into extension. It can then be worked upon as before encouraging a 'hold' and co-contraction round the neck and shoulder girdle region.

Trunk stability is most important in these cases and the rolling activities from side lying are particularly valuable. Spiral trunk rotation should be encouraged and resisted movements of rolling leading with the head and upper trunk and also leading with the legs and lower trunk should be encouraged, provided the patient does not show signs of going into abnormal patterns. Static holds and rhythmic stabilisations can also be of value to give trunk stability.

The natural progression from here is to make the patient stable in side sitting or in an arm forward support sitting prior to expecting him to be able to take up the position for himself.

The continuing progress would take the patient through prone kneeling, kneeling, half kneeling and standing. In such case the patient should be encouraged to learn to balance in the position before moving into it unaided and before using the position for functional activities.

Patients can be prepared for kneeling by being placed in prone lying with the knees flexed. Co-contraction round the flexed knees can be encouraged by giving compression sharply repeated through the heels and lateral aspects of the foot. In some cases voluntary rhythmical stabilisations may also be used. Half kneeling positions can also be adopted in side lying to accustom the patient to the limb position before being put into a difficult balance situation.

While the above progress is being made it should be remembered that we must also be able to carry out skills with free hands and even free feet and so far the limbs have been used primarily as weight-bearing structures. Thus the patient needs help to move the limbs on the trunk as opposed to moving the trunk over the limbs.

There are many ways of helping the hypotonic patient with this problem. The above approach will help to some extent since it gives the appropriate postural background.

Resisted limb patterns performed against moderate resistance at first quickly and then progressing to slower movements are of value. The emphasis should be placed on smoothness and precision of patterning. Reversals without rest are valuable and starting and stopping with holds in mid-pattern are also useful. At first the trunk should be in a position of supported stability but later progress can be made by making the patient support her own trunk.

The range of the reversals may be gradually reduced and the activity changed to static reversals and eventually to rhythmical stabilisations in different ranges.

It is also possible to train proximal stability for distal movements by using 'timing for emphasis' techniques. The patient is made to 'hold' the proximal part of the patterns while moving the distal parts. Resistance in these cases should be light as it is being used primarily as guidance. Gradually the guidance should be removed and the patient left free to move by himself.

It may be of value to use Frenkel's precision exercises in these cases and, in fact, the principles of these can be added to the above account. Movements in pattern may be done to counting in a rhythmical manner and even mat activities such as moving from side sitting to prone kneeling can be done to counting, using markers on the floor as guides.

When the ataxic symptoms are related to sensory loss as well as to hypotonia, the above suggestions are still applicable but more care must be taken to help the patient with afferent stimuli.

Frenkel's approach may be emphasised more, still using patterns. Mirrors may be a necessity and the patient must be allowed to use the eyes and ears as substitutes for other afferent information. Hard surfaces help this patient more than softly cushioned ones and often the stimuli applied have to be exaggerated to have their effect. Movements carried out to counting or other rhythmical sounds are likely to be more successful than silent performances. All patients showing ataxia have to use cortical control for many of their problems and this can hamper their activities, since movement has to become a conscious activity instead of an automatic one. However, with continuous repetition automaticity can be achieved and automatic balance reactions should be encouraged to occur in a controlled manner.

As the patient gains postural stability he should react in a more controlled manner to gentle, unexpected disturbance of balance. Attempts should be made in all positions to get gentle reactions to body sway, controlled stepping reactions and the use of the hands as a support in standing and sitting only as a last resort. So long as the hands do not have to be used for balance they are free for skills.

It is most important to note that many patients showing hypotonicity may also have an underlying tendency to adopt reflex patterns of movement, mass flexion or mass extension. It is therefore most important to keep a wary eye on the use of volition to see that its excessive use is not encouraging the use of undesirable patterns. If it does, then emphasis on volition should be reduced and more automatic methods adopted to gain the same result.

These patients should not be encouraged to use their upper limbs in 'pulling' functions since this may encourage them to use the arms in a mass flexor manner to pull themselves into standing.

They will never gain balance in this way and for this reason such activities should be discouraged. Thus, such a patient, if confined to bed, should not be supplied with a monkey bar to help him to move around in bed. It will encourage reflex patterning which is undesirable.

Functional activities

As with the lower motoneurone problem, functions within the capabilities of the patient should be encouraged. Suitable functions should be found relevant to the patient's ability. If good movement re-education is to occur, it is most important that excessive demands are not made upon the patient since abnormalities will inevitably appear which might otherwise be avoidable.

Walking will possibly be a goal and this should be encouraged *after* the patient has the ability to balance in standing. At first some support by the hands may be necessary using walking aids of some kind and only when the patient is secure should he be encouraged to walk without using the upper limbs as balance mechanisms.

It must be borne in mind that perfect functioning is unlikely in these cases and the physiotherapist must be aware of the likely limitations. Occupational therapists and physiotherapists can often work well together with these cases provided each respects the other person's aim for the patient. The goal must be discussed and re-set as progress is observed.

The patient's hopes must not be raised excessively and every step forward must be noted by both the therapist and the patient. Every member of the team should be prepared to meet each problem as it arises and no one should expect too much.

There are other problems with these patients but they will be considered under the appropriate headings since they are common to most neurological patients.

Vertigo

Patients with this particular sensory problem have to learn to rely upon joint and skin sensations and those sensations from sight rather than those from the vestibular apparatus. As has been mentioned earlier the giddy sensation and sickness are also accompanied by an active inhibition of movement since movement of the head gives rise to increase of the dizziness and nausea. The head and shoulders show rather a fixed posture and the patient is afraid of movement.

Such is the link between eyes and vestibular apparatus that eye movements may even trigger off the symptoms. Thus the patient need not be moving at all but could be watching a moving object and would have symptoms similar to those which would occur if he had been moving.

Re-education of this patient involves giving him confidence in moving and helping him to take notice only of the reliable sensory or afferent information.

He should be treated at first in a fully supported semi-recumbent position so that head movements are unlikely to occur. Relaxation of the head, neck and shoulders should be encouraged and the patient asked to use his eyes only at first. His attention should be drawn to the sensation of complete support that his position offers so that he is aware of the unlikelihood of moving at that moment. He should look at a stationary object which is a comfortable distance away from him and be asked to focus upon it. When he has it in full focus the object should move slowly while he follows it with his eyes. If he feels dizzy then he should close his eyes and feel the stationary condition of his body. At first the object should only move as far as his eyes can travel but as he progresses head movements may also be involved and, later still, head movements with closed eyes should be encouraged in order to help him to rely only on joint and position sense.

As he progresses the patient may adopt less stable starting positions and exercise the eyes, head and trunk progressively until he can move fairly freely without suffering from excessive symptoms. Gradually he should progress to using hand/eye activities without losing his balance. Such activities as throwing and catching a ball in all directions are suitable. Standing and walking are advanced and the patient must be made accustomed to having objects moving in relationship to him. It is particularly important that stairs are included in his treatment programme, since the sides of a staircase can appear to be moving in the corner of the eye and can give vertigo symptoms in even quite normal people.

As the patient progresses he should be involved in group activities so that people and things are moving about him at the same time as he is moving himself. This does to some extent prepare him for coping with crossing roads and traffic. His treatment is not complete without postural correction and mobility exercises of head, neck and shoulder girdle and at some stage he must be taken in among traffic on foot and given the confidence to cross the road.

THE PROBLEM OF HYPERTONICITY

Spasticity

As described in Chapter 4 the patient will demonstrate at least partial release of certain reflex mechanisms from cortical control and hence difficulty in producing movement patterns other than those produced by the released reflexes. The stretch reflex mechanisms will be extra sensitive particularly in patterns dominated by the released reflexes.

The normal malleable postural background will not be present having given way to stereotyped patterns of a reflex nature. The patient will show poor vocabulary of movement patterns and of quality of control.

There is frequently a lack of synergy, evidence of instability of joint control coupled with lack of righting and equilibrium reactions.

The patient develops a pattern of spasticity related to the dominating reflexes. The reflexes most likely to exert their influence include the tonic labyrinthine, the symmetrical tonic neck reflex and the asymmetrical tonic neck reflex.

These reflex pathways are present in all of us and by the process of maturation of the nervous system their effect becomes integrated into the general control of all our movements. It is only when they are released from integration that they cause disturbance of movement pattern.

A study of these reflexes will show that the position of the head and neck is very important and that if care is taken to control their position and to encourage the patient to control it, excessive domination by the static postural reflexes can, to some extent, be avoided. Careful positioning of the patient can make management easier for the physiotherapist and the nurse and, at the same time, make movement more possible for the patient.

A study of the more dynamic righting reactions is also of extreme value. These reactions enable the individual to obtain the upright position and the spiral movements of the head and neck, trunk and limbs are related to them. It is thought that they may have an inhibitory effect upon the static postural mechanisms. The reduction in spasticity which is seen to accompany trunk and limb rotation may occur for this reason although there is, as yet, no proof that this is so. However, rotation of the trunk and limbs, when trying to reduce spasticity, is a very valuable asset and emphasises the importance of treating the whole patient instead of dealing only with the offending part.

When treating a patient who shows spasticity it is necessary to carry out three important aims:

1. Inhibit excessive tone as far as possible.
2. Give the patient a sensation of normal position and normal movement.
3. Facilitate normal movement patterns.

INHIBITION OF EXCESSIVE TONE

Earlier in this chapter it was pointed out that inhibition could be facilitated as well as excitation. In cases of spasticity it is important to facilitate the patient's ability to inhibit the undesirable activity of the released reflex mechanisms. As has already been mentioned the position adopted by the patient is important since the head and neck position can elicit strong postural reflex mechanisms. Avoiding these head and neck positions can facilitate the inhibition of the more likely reflexes and if the positions have to be adopted, then help in preventing the rest of the body from going into the reflex pattern thus elicited may be required by the patient. The patient cannot, of course, spend the rest of his life avoiding the positions which encourage dominance by reflex activity but, at first, this may be necessary until the patient has developed some control in the suppression of the effect of the reflex activities. As he develops this control then he can be gradually introduced to the use of positions which make suppression of reflex activity more difficult.

As an early introduction to treatment the side lying position, well supported by pillows, is very convenient since it avoids stimulation of the tonic labyrinthine reflex and also, as the head and trunk are in alignment, the stimulation of the asymmetrical tonic neck reflexes. It makes a good resting position for the patient with spasticity and also is convenient for the application of rhythmical trunk rotations of both a passive and assisted active form. These do help to encourage a reduction in tone.

The scapula is also readily available to be involved in the movements. The upper and lower limb of the uppermost side are also easily accessible for any passive, assisted active or automatic movements which may seem suitable.

Side lying is not always desirable because of respiratory problems in the older patient or because of the need to obtain a greater range of movement. Other attitudes are often very satisfactory such as crook lying or even with the knees as high on the chest as possible. These last two are helpful if there is flexor spasticity. As the trunk is rotated the legs are allowed to lower towards the extended, abducted and laterally rotated position. For older patients trunk rotation may have to be encouraged in sitting.

Limb rotations are also very effective in helping to give a more normal control of muscle tone to the patient.

These facts are of help not only to the physiotherapist but also to the nurse who may be concerned in moving the patient in bed or attempting to position the patient so as to avoid the development of deformities.

The important factors in attempting to gain control over muscle tone are:

1. Patterns of movement and posture associated with the released reflex mechanisms must be avoided and discouraged by positioning, guidance and using the inhibitory methods mentioned in this chapter.
2. Conditions which will facilitate control of tone should be given using the stimuli which will encourage normal patterns.

As an example of the above two points let us consider pressure applied to the undersurface of the foot. If it is applied to the ball of the foot it may well stimulate an extensor reflex in which a pathological pattern of extension, adduction and medial rotation of the hip is produced together with plantar flexion of the foot. This would be undesirable in a case of spasticity. If pressure is applied under the heel of the foot then a more useful contraction of muscle is likely to occur giving a suitable supporting pattern. The physiotherapist must become familiar with the stereotyped reflex patterning so that she can avoid permitting them to occur.

It is most important that the physiotherapist becomes familiar with the patterning of normal movements and postures so that she can help her patient to move using them in preference to spastic patterns. Help is needed to facilitate the movements by correcting weight distribution, head and shoulder positioning and encouraging suitable rotational balance activities. The patient may be moulded passively by the therapist into patterns of balance in order to experience or re-experience them (Fig. 7/5). As they are repeatedly moulded they will become accustomed to the movement sensation and may start to help. Provided no undesirable associated activity is produced, the patient should then be encouraged to 'take over' the reaction themselves as their body-weight is transferred.

The lateral weight transference reaction in the illustration is an

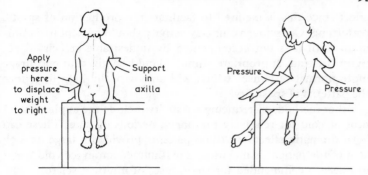

FIG. 7/5 'Moulding' the patient into appropriate trunk reactions as the body-weight is displaced to the right

important preparatory reaction for correct weight transference in standing and walking (see Figs. 6/4 and 6/5, pp. 122, 123). For example, when walking, the right leg cannot be moved forwards unless the left leg is receiving weight correctly and the body is balanced over it. Trunk rotations normally accompany the mature walking patterns as reciprocal balance mechanisms and should be encouraged. Standing from sitting cannot occur unless the head and shoulders are brought well forward so that weight is distributed to the feet. As the patient rises she may extend her neck and trunk too soon and throw her weight back so that she is not successful in reaching a standing position. The timing of neck and trunk extension may need to be assisted. All the necessary automatic adjustments are impoverished in these patients and help may be needed. Sometimes verbal help is needed but more often actual assistance by simply adjusting the movements and waiting for the patient to react may be more helpful. This enables the patient to feel and perhaps see the successful activity. At all times the effect on the whole patient must be observed since it is quite possible to be gaining more normal tone in one part of the patient at the expense of another.

Movement of a normal nature does appear in itself to reduce excessive tone and consequently this should be encouraged in the patient. However, care must be taken if conscious volitional movement is demanded. Due to reflex release, some motoneurone pools are already in an excitatory state and any volitional effort is likely to act as a triggering mechanism to those motoneurone pools giving associated muscle contraction in the spastic pattern. Such patients should not be encouraged to make strong volitional effort since this is inclined to facilitate the production of spastic patterning. Conscious voluntary activity should be kept to a minimum until it is not accompanied by undesirable associated activity. Instead, appropriate stimuli should be given to encourage more normal responses which will automatically help to reduce the patterns of spasticity.

Other methods of reducing spasticity include the application of heat or cold for relatively prolonged periods of time. These can have dramatic effects on some patients provided a large enough area of the patient is included. Total immersion in ice cold water has been recommended for some cases of multiple sclerosis who show spasticity and the author has seen very impressive temporary results from this approach. The patient who responds to this shows a marked improvement in movement ability for several hours before the process has to be repeated again.

Deep rhythmical massage with pressure over the muscle insertions has proved effective in some cases and many authorities advocate slow, steady and prolonged stretching. This last method does have its dangers since, if the stretching is forced against severe spasticity, the hyperexcitable stretch reflex reacts even more strongly and damage to the periosteum of bone may occur where excessive tension has been applied by the tendons of the stretched muscles.

Rhythmical, slowly performed passive movements through normal patterns may also be helpful and in the more moderate cases the patient may subconsciously join in and by his own activity a reduction in spasticity may occur. Quick movements, abruptly performed, and noisy surroundings are most detrimental as are excitement, anxiety or any form of discomfort.

SENSATION OF NORMAL POSITION AND MOVEMENT

This is of vital importance. A patient who is dominated by reflex patterns never experiences the sensation of normal movement and position unless helped to do so. He is denied normal stimulation and either cannot know or soon forgets the normal. Very quickly the abnormal feels normal and vice versa.

A patient showing extensor spasticity of the lower limb will most often hold the limb in hip extension, adduction and medial rotation, knee extension and foot plantar flexion, i.e. mass extensor synergy of the lower limb. Such a patient when standing or sitting may never be able to experience weight-bearing through the heel. When weight is taken through the heel the stimulus encourages a true supporting reaction which gives co-contraction of hip, knee and ankle muscles, flexors as well as extensors, in a malleable co-contraction suitable for normal weight-bearing. Thus there is no hope for the patient who is in extensor synergy unless some method of applying the more appropriate stimulus is found.

If an abnormal position makes a starting point for a movement then an abnormal movement must occur. Because of their spasticity many patients are forced by circumstances to repeat abnormal movement patterns. By repetition the nervous pathways used to cause these movements are facilitated and the abnormal movements therefore occur more and more readily. When this has occurred correction is difficult, if not impossible. Because of this it is important to give early treatment to the whole patient so that, as far as possible, the sensation of normal movement is retained.

Praise for a movement should only be given if it really is good because, having received praise, the patient will try to repeat the same performance. If it was a good movement the second attempt is also likely to be good, but if it was unsatisfactory at first the repeated movement will also be poor and this faulty pathway has been facilitated.

FACILITATION OF NORMAL MOVEMENT PATTERNS

More normal movement patterns can be produced when domination by reflex mechanisms is minimised. Thus, when the patient appears to be relatively free, movement should be encouraged. Movement itself will reduce spasticity if it follows normal patterns. Often automatic adjustment of position is easier to produce than conscious volitional activities. Figures 7/6 and 7/7 illustrate some movements and positions which are helpful if encouraged and some which should be discouraged. Rotational movements of the trunk and limbs are important and spiral rolling patterns involving head, shoulder girdle, pelvis and limbs should be encouraged.

In most cases it is helpful to follow a neurodevelopmental approach with these patients. They often have a vocabulary of movement pattern less versatile than that of a newly born child. Thus they are more likely to learn movement control if they are encouraged to follow the sequence of events seen in the movement patterning of a child.

Basic functional movements are the ones to encourage at first. The child does not develop skilled hand movements until the hands are freed from being props for balance. The same holds good for adults showing spasticity. One does well if the upper limbs can be trained to support the patient. The ambition to train skilled hand movements should be deferred until this is achieved.

It is important to appreciate that points (1), (2) and (3) (p. 191) are best dealt with at one and the same time. In other words one does not arrange for the patient to fulfil the aim of reducing spasticity and then proceed to applying appropriate sensation and then re-educate movement. The patient should be placed in an area suitable for seizing the opportunity of moving as and when a reduction in tone is felt and as a suitable stimulus has had an effect.

The physiotherapist must constantly observe the effect of her efforts on the whole patient and if an opportunity arises to use a movement which is occurring in a normal manner she should use

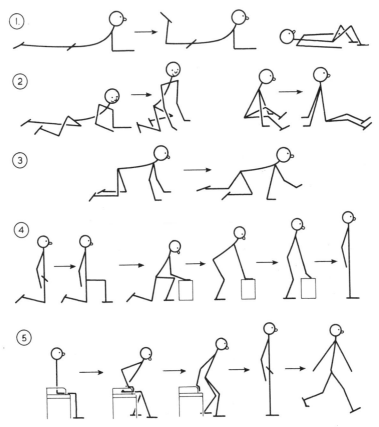

FIG. 7/6 Patterns of movement to be encouraged

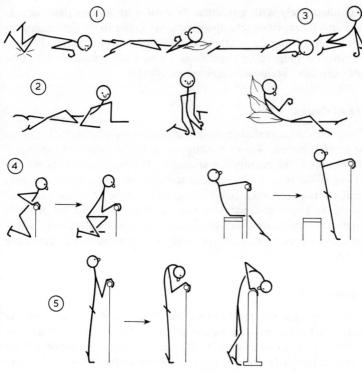

FIG. 7/7 Patterns of movement to be discouraged

it without delay. For this reason a sample list of activities is impossible to offer since fixed methods are not applicable.

Functional activities

It is in the field of spasticity that most controversy occurs regarding functions of daily living. If the aim is normal movement only those functions which do not produce pattern abnormalities should be encouraged and progress should be made relative to this. The physiotherapist should, in this case, be the person to decide which functions are suitable.

If, however, the aim is to gain functional independence at all costs, then movement abnormalities may have to be ignored or even encouraged in order to gain some sort of ambulation. Strictly speaking, the skill of a good physiotherapist should not be used for long if this is the aim, since well-trained aides could fulfil it

quite adequately with guidance. It is most important that consultants and therapists exchange views and come to an agreement on
which line of approach is to be followed and also when further
attempts to help the patients are to be abandoned. Conflicting
views can have seriously detrimental effects.

Use of drugs

There are drugs available which will have an inhibitory effect on
the stretch reflex. These mainly work by blocking the synaptic
functions of internuncial pathways. If they are effective the
patient is likely to be hypotonic with underlying movement patterns of the flexor/extensor synergies. Such patients are best
treated as hypotonic patients but great care should be given if
resisted exercises are used. Free active patterning with some automatic compression stimuli and gentle balance activities are more
suitable.

Rigidity

In this situation the patient tends to show excessive postural fixation, axial rotation is non-existent and normal balance reactions
do not appear to be available. The patient tends to adopt a fixed
head and shoulder positioning and movements which would normally be those of trunk rotation either do not occur at all or occur
by the patient moving round as a whole.

The face adopts a mask-like rigidity and the patient appears to
be unresponsive to stimuli. A tremor is often present when resting, which disappears when purposeful movement occurs. All
these symptoms are seen when the centres concerned with automatic reactions are the site of lesion, so that these reactions do
not occur.

Increase in tone causes opposition to all movements, which are
therefore slow in being produced and are not readily accompanied
by automatic postural adjustments.

As in the case of spasticity the abnormality effectively prevents
the patient from experiencing normal sensory information and he
quite rapidly 'forgets' the normal and accepts the abnormality as
normal.

The physiotherapist can help the patient in several ways, but
she must always have the following aims at the back of her mind:
1. To encourage a reduction in the overall sensitivity of the
   stretch reflex mechanism.

2. To help the patient to experience more normal reactions.
3. To encourage movements to follow normal patterns in as wide a range and as freely as possible.

REDUCTION IN OVERALL SENSITIVITY OF THE
STRETCH REFLEX MECHANISM

There are several methods available to achieve this aim and the sooner the patient is treated the more effective is treatment likely to be. Methods include: teaching general relaxation in a comfortable, well-supported, recumbent position; the application of rhythmical massage of a sedative nature; and the use of rhythmical passive and/or assisted active movements.

The most effective method is likely to be to give rhythmical passive to active movements with the patient recumbent or semi-recumbent.

The movements which are of most value to the patient are those which are not available to him. Trunk rotations are particularly useful, and may be carried out through a small range at first, gradually increasing the range and speeding up the rate of rhythm of the movement as the rigidity subsides. Such movements can be done passively by the physiotherapist, but she should not discourage the patient from helping if he can. It is not total relaxation that is wanted but only a sufficient reduction in tone to make movement more possible.

Probably the side lying position is a most convenient one for this purpose since trunk rotations can be most easily produced in this position and can also be easily converted into rolling activities when the patient has enough freedom to do so. In addition the patient's scapula is freely available and can be moved prior to encouraging greater range of activity in the whole body.

Since many patients showing rigidity are elderly, the fully recumbent position is not always suitable and rotations may have to be performed in other positions. It is quite possible to help a patient to rotate at the trunk in sitting by moving the upper trunk upon the lower and one can even involve the trunk diagonal patterns of flexion with rotation to one side, followed by extension with rotation to the other.

Limb movements can be encouraged in a similar way involving the diagonal patterns, if possible, and starting with a small range and progressing to a large range as the movement becomes more available. If the patient assists so much the better.

EXPERIENCING MORE NORMAL REACTIONS

Helping the patient experience the more normal reactions is very much linked with the methods suggested in the previous section. As the patient loosens up when the overall tone of the muscles is reduced, opportunities to react to situations should be given and help to reach and experience the reaction should be offered as needed. For instance if trunk rotation is being encouraged in side lying the patient will gradually loosen up and start to participate. The upper limb should then be encouraged to come forward to receive weight as the trunk comes forward ready for going into prone lying. If the limb does not react automatically the therapist can repeatedly encourage rotation and bring the patient's arm and hand forward into the supporting position. Gradually the patient will appreciate the sensation and will join in until all the physiotherapist need do is gently push the shoulder forward to initiate the reaction. A similar method of encouraging the appropriate lower limb reactions may also be used.

If the trunk rotations are being done in sitting, other balance reactions may be added. Such reactions as hand support forward or hand support sideways may be encouraged. Even the lifting reactions of the limbs on the side away from which the patient is shifted can be helped by the skilled physiotherapist in this way, so that the patient experiences the sensation of balance reactions.

By lifting reactions are meant the reactions of the body to displacement of weight sideways or backward. If the body-weight is displaced sideways the upper limb on that side moves sideways to receive some of the weight. The other upper limb lifts sideways to try to pull the body back to its original base. The lower limbs, if free, may also participate by rotating (see Fig. 6/3, p. 120).

Any sign of regression back into rigidity to an excessive degree should be countered by further rotations. Trunk rotations with rhythmic arm swinging can be very helpful and give the arm swing sensation required when walking. Many physiotherapists encourage this by having the patient sitting or standing holding one end of a pole in each hand. The physiotherapist is holding the other ends of the poles and using her arm swing she can encourage the arm swing of the patient.

ENCOURAGING MOVEMENTS TO FOLLOW NORMAL PATTERNS
IN AS WIDE A RANGE AND AS FREELY AS POSSIBLE

This automatically links with the previous two sections and has to some extent already been encouraged. Movement patterns may be encouraged with minimal resistance for guidance. The range should be small at first and slowly encouraged to larger range and faster movement. The patient has to be 'pumped up' to more rapid and fuller range of activity. This also applies to functions such as standing up and sitting down, rolling over and getting started with walking activities.

For the younger patient the author has found the following type of activities most successful:

1. Rhythmical rolling in a spiral manner, first helping the patient and later starting the movement for the patient and allowing him to react by following.
2. Encouraging the adoption of side sitting and moving on to all fours and then sitting on the opposite side. This is started on all fours and the patient sways rhythmically towards the side upon which he will eventually sit before rising back to all fours. At first he does not sit at all but gradually approaches the sitting position as a fuller range is available. This activity encourages trunk and limb rotation and if rhythmical it will help to keep the overall tone reduced.
3. Rhythmical crawling may also be encouraged by swaying the body-weight forward and backward and eventually encouraging a step forward reaction of the limbs.
4. Hand support forward half kneeling, changing legs rhythmically, may also help and eventually leads to the adoption of standing.
5. The standing activities should include rhythmical walking, which is best started by rotating the trunk at the shoulders so that an easy arm swing rhythm is started. The patient's body-weight is then pushed gently forward at hip level to encourage a stepping reaction in the lower limbs.
6. The customary stooping position should be avoided and the patient encouraged to maintain as upright a position as possible. As mentioned previously, many physiotherapists use poles to initiate walking and do so by encouraging the patient to step forward with the right leg as the left arm comes forward.
7. Gradually the walking should include turning and stepping backward and also across the other leg. These activities may be done as conscious volitional activities but, if possible, should eventually become an automatic response to disturbance of balance.

One cannot do quite such agile activities with the older patient and some of the following suggestions may prove helpful:

1. Sitting: assisted active trunk rotations to encourage a hand support sideways sitting position.
2. Hands supporting to one side: encourage standing up by leaning back to leaning forward and standing up. Rhythmical swaying may be more suitable at first and then gradually changed to standing up.
3. Standing up to sitting down as before, progressing to standing up again with the hands supporting to alternate sides. This also involves trunk rotations which are so easily lost in these patients.
4. Arm swinging and walking can be encouraged as in the younger person.

In both types of patients limb patterns through full range should be encouraged in addition to functional mat type activities.

Patients' relatives can be taught to help reduce the rigidity at home by encouraging rotational movement and perhaps helping to give the necessary 'pumping up' procedures prior to achieving a particular function. It is most important to keep these patients as functionally independent as possible and relatives must be encouraged to give minimum assistance of an 'educated' nature.

The patient can help himself to a tremendous degree once he receives adequate guidance and provided he receives appropriate encouragement from his relatives. It can be helpful to allow him to have a period of intensive physiotherapy at intervals and to encourage him to be responsible for his own welfare ('movement-wise') in the periods when he has no formal treatment. An early morning 'warm-up' exercise session involving trunk rotations and rhythmical swinging movements of arms and legs can be very valuable when he is otherwise receiving no treatment.

Odd jobs about the house which require movement are more suitable than those which can be done sitting down. They may take a longer time for the patient to perform but they are a treatment in themselves.

Static activities are undesirable and rhythmical stabilisations do not usually help these patients and so should be avoided if possible.

Drugs are available to reduce rigidity and some surgical procedures have given a measure of relief. The patient may then show variable movement problems and has to be dealt with according to individual peculiarities.

It cannot be emphasised too much that the earlier the patient receives treatment the more effective it will be. When a patient is first suspected of showing rigidity symptoms he is unlikely to show gross abnormality and will not have so much underlying joint stiffness or have 'forgotten' normality to such a degree. He is therefore more able to be receptive to help. This is directed at helping him to help himself. He may then well be able to minimise his symptoms more effectively for longer.

If the patient is very rigid when he first receives help he may also have painful joint stiffness and have mechanical difficulty in addition to physiological problems. Normal movement will be very unusual to him and the likelihood of his being able to help himself adequately is considerably more remote.

THE PROBLEMS OF ATHETOSIS, CHOREA AND BALLISMUS

These three movement abnormalities are grouped together since all show the presence of involuntary activity and fluctuations of tone. The physiotherapist has to meet problems with these patients when they appear. At one time she may be required to encourage stability in the same way as she would a hypotonic patient and at another time she may have to help in the inhibition of abnormal activities while encouraging normal purposeful movement patterns.

Excitement should be avoided at all costs since this increases the symptoms.

Athetoid patients frequently have problems with body image and steps must be taken to improve this by experiences of normal activities and stimuli.

Many athetoids are helped in stability by compression forces being applied through weight-bearing joints. Some children benefit by wearing little leaded caps which add to the weight of the head and give compression force to the vertebral column. This helps to stimulate stabilisation. Much of the action advised in preceding sections is useful for these patients and the physiotherapist must use her ingenuity in selecting those activities which help and discarding those which do not. She must receive a constant 'feedback' from the patient and adjust her stimuli accordingly.

Drugs and surgery have been used to control the symptoms of these disorders and have met with varying success. In such circumstances the patient is still left with movement abnormalities which have to be assessed and treated accordingly.

Biofeedback equipment as mentioned at the end of Chapter 6 may also be of value to the therapist treating problems discussed in this chapter. The signal of muscle activity can be used to indicate successful patterning to the patient or, more negatively, it can be used to indicate unwanted activity.

PROBLEMS OF DEFORMITY

Adaptive shortening of soft tissues is likely to occur when habitual posturing is adopted by patients who have any disease or injury problem. In neurological problems it is particularly likely to occur when no movement is available to the patient and when there is imbalance of muscle pull.

There are many methods of preventing the onset of deformities of this nature. These include:

Passive movements

These were already suggested in an earlier section as being helpful in the maintenance of a knowledge of body image. When used to prevent deformity the physiotherapist must bear two facts in mind:

1. She must maintain the biological length of the muscles which work over the joints she is moving. This means that her passive movements must involve elongating the muscle over all its movement components. For example, to maintain the length of gastrocnemius she must dorsiflex the foot and extend the knee and her return movements should be plantar flexion of the foot and flexion of the knee. In that way she has fully lengthened gastrocnemius which pulls over the back of the knee and ankle and she has also put it into its most shortened position.

2. She must maintain the biological pliability of the ligaments of the joints she is moving. This means that she must be cautious when moving a joint over which a 'two-joint' muscle works since it could restrict the range of movement available before the ligaments are fully elongated. For example, ankle dorsiflexion is limited by gastrocnemius if the knee is held extended as the ankle is dorsiflexed. Therefore the ligaments of the joint are not fully elongated by the time movement has stopped. Thus in this case the tension should be taken off gastrocnemius

by flexing the knee before dorsiflexing the foot. A greater range will then be found to be available.

Careful positioning of the severely disabled patient

This should be done in such a way that constant adoption of one position is avoided. Limbs and trunk should be supported in a variety of positions throughout the day. Extreme positioning of any joint should be avoided.

Splintage

This is most helpful in patients with peripheral problems as it prevents the flaccid muscle groups from being constantly stretched by normal opposing muscle action. Splints should never be left on permanently but should be used as resting splints when the patient is likely to adopt a prolonged poor position of the joints concerned. Lively splints are very useful since they allow movement to occur and simply return the limbs to a normal position at the end of the movement. They are more functional than the simple rest splints.

Many people use splintage with central nervous system problems but it should only be used in certain well-considered circumstances. Splints applied to such cases effectively prevent normal movement patterns and pressure from the splint may actually increase the spastic patterning. For example a plaster cast applied to the lower leg and foot to keep the foot in dorsiflexion may effectively stimulate (by pressure on the ball of the foot) an extensor response which will take the form of mass extensor synergy. This could be undesirable and worse than no splintage at all. Only in some circumstances is splintage helpful in these disorders.

Use of bed cradles

These are very helpful. They lift the weight of bedclothes off the limbs, which may be paralysed, and therefore the bedclothes do not force the feet into plantar flexion.

The cradle is also useful when hypertonicity is a problem since the constant irritation of bedclothes can stimulate withdrawal reflexes which encourage flexion deformities.

If deformity is already present by the time the patient comes for help, the problem is much greater. The patient may require more help to counter the problem such as traction, manipulation, and surgery. In the latter case tendons may be divided and lengthened or muscles are disattached and left to re-attach in a more suitable position.

The physiotherapist may be able to help in some cases by the application of serial plasters designed to correct deformities gradually.

Some patients, particularly those with lower motoneurone problems, develop adaptive shortening of the muscles antagonistic to those which are paralysed. The physiotherapist can help considerably here to encourage a new resting length for these muscles by using any or all of the following methods:

1. The application of prolonged (about 10–20 minutes) cold packs to the adaptively shortened muscle. The packs must extend over the whole length of the muscle. This method encourages inhibition of the muscle which will relax more, making it possible to lengthen it more easily.

2. The use of 'hold, relax' techniques in which the adaptively shortened muscle is put into as elongated a position as is comfortable and then made to contract statically – hence the term 'hold'. As the contraction is held for a prolonged time it begins to weaken. When this occurs the patient is instructed to relax while the physiotherapist supports the joint or joints involved. When relaxation has occurred the physiotherapist further elongates the muscle passively. If successful she will find that the muscle will allow itself to be elongated more as it has relaxed sufficiently to allow an increase in length.

   There are various theories as to why this should work. Some authorities say that the muscle relaxes more because of fatigue and others consider that the Golgi tendon organs which lie at the musculotendinous junction are stimulated by the contracting muscle pulling on the tendon. As was stated earlier these organs have an inhibitory influence on the motoneurone pools of their own muscle and may therefore help to induce this excessive relaxation (autogenic inhibition).

   Cold packs may be applied at the same time as 'hold, relax' techniques.

   'Hold, relax' is most suitable for use when the adaptively shortened group are opposed by completely flail antagonists.

3. A modification of the above is the 'slow reversal, hold, relax' technique. In this case the procedure is as for 'hold, relax' but after the relaxation stage has occurred the patient is stimulated

to use the antagonist to the adaptively shortened muscle concentrically. In other words the adaptively shortened muscle is
made to contract statically by a 'hold'. It is then commanded
to relax and the reverse movement is brought about by active
concentric activity of its antagonist. This technique is most
useful when there is some activity available in the antagonist.
The phenomenon of reciprocal inhibition is added to the phenomenon of autogenic inhibition in this case.

The above techniques are only of value when movement limitation is due to changes in length of muscle. They do not help if
the limitation is due to ligamentous or bony changes.

Some workers claim to have used the above techniques to relax
spastic muscle groups. The author does not use this particular
technique for fear of facilitating spastic patterning. The student
should, however, keep an open mind in all such matters and
decide for herself which methods she will use, noting the results
and accepting those which give good results while rejecting those
which do not.

PREVENTION OF INJURY

This has been largely dealt with on page 148, since much of the
damage which can occur in these cases is due to sensory loss.

The patient must be made aware of the dangers, if possible,
and if he cannot change his position himself he must be frequently
turned. He must be kept scrupulously clean and have his skin
toughened and protected against the possibility of pressure sores.

If any area shows signs of breaking down it may be stimulated
by ice massage to improve the local circulation, or by heat or mild
doses of ultraviolet light. The use of heat has its dangers since
sensory loss may make the patient endure a temperature that is
too hot for safety. Cold is, therefore, the method of choice.

The use of ripple mattresses, sheepskins, protective rings and
constant changes of position should effectively prevent the onset
of pressure sores. If they do develop they are very detrimental to
the patient's general condition and must be treated as a serious
problem.

CIRCULATORY PROBLEMS

Many patients show disturbances of circulation. Some of these are due to lack of movement and some are due to disturbance in some part of the autonomic system.

In the lower motoneurone problem the loss of 'muscle pump' activity will cause slowing of the circulation through the affected area and, in addition, the peripheral autonomic nerve fibres may also be involved.

These problems can be helped by encouraging activity in other parts of the body. This will speed up circulation generally.

Whirlpool baths for the affected areas may also be used. These will promote circulation to the skin over the affected muscle groups. Contrast baths may also prove valuable. They may stimulate such blood vessel activity as is available.

The central autonomic problem is described in Chapter 14. Essentially the patient has to adapt gradually to change of position which puts greater demands upon the problem of maintenance of blood pressure.

In cases of causalgia, in which there is disuse due to pain, similar methods may be used to those advocated for the lower motoneurone problem. Wax baths may also help here, but on the other hand they may cause onset of pain and so should be used with reservation.

Many patients who have hemiplegic symptoms have problems in the posturing of the shoulder girdle. This can cause pressure and kinking of the axillary vessels giving rise to oedema which is further encouraged by lack of use and the dependent position. In this case the weight of the limb may have to be relieved by sling support to reduce pressure on the axillary vessels. This is unfortunate since it discourages movement of the limb. However, the sling need not be retained all the time and other treatments for oedema may be given which involve movement. As soon as the posturing of the patient improves the sling should be discarded.

RESPIRATORY PROBLEMS

Many patients show respiratory problems. These range from those which are due to paralysis of the muscles of respiration to those which are due to restriction of exercise because of the patient's disability.

Patients who have paralysis of the respiratory muscles will obviously need the help of a ventilator and will be in an intensive therapy unit. They may also require to have assisted coughing or may even need suction to help to remove secretions.

Only the local peripheral problems will totally escape from respiratory difficulties. The head injury case may well require tracheostomy, suction and to be ventilated (IPPV).

The patient with a central nervous system disorder of the progressive variety will be inclined to develop respiratory distress as the disease progresses. The muscles supporting the thoracic inlet may be hypotonic and will allow respiratory movements to have a suction effect on the chest wall in this area, thus diminishing the amount of air the thorax can house. Such patients may also have deglutition problems and it is possible for food to be inhaled.

Even the less handicapped patient may show weakness of respiratory movements and will need some help.

Breathing exercises should be incorporated into the treatment of all the heavily handicapped patients. They may be facilitated in lower motoneurone cases by using appropriate arm patterns and by giving repeated contractions to the muscles of inspiration. Both inspiratory and expiratory phases should be emphasised to get maximum respiratory excursion.

The central problem requires a more relaxed approach but respiration must not be forgotten. It is particularly important for patients with rigidity and to those with numerous problems as in multiple sclerosis.

The advanced case of multiple sclerosis and also the patient with weakness in the thoracic inlet and deglutition group (omohyoid, mylohyoid, digastricus, thyrohyoid and sternothyroid) may be helped by giving head and neck patterns of a resisted nature, stabilisation of the head and neck and combining these with respiration.

PROBLEMS OF SPEECH

These problems are properly left to the speech therapist who is the specialist. The physiotherapist may be able to endorse the work of the speech therapist if the two team members can discuss matters with each other.

It is possible to stimulate movement of the tongue by using a spatula and moving the tongue with it, encouraging the patient to participate. Ice frozen on to the spatula may also help as the cold is a stimulus. As the water forms from the melting ice it acts as a lubricant to the tongue and mouth.

Activity of buccinator can also be encouraged by pressure from the spatula against the inside of the cheek. This may help to train the patient to keep the cheek against the teeth and therefore prevent collection of saliva. This can be very useful when treating facial palsy as the stretch stimulus can be used by pressing the cheek outwards while commanding the patient to pull in.

Speech in the severely handicapped is not easily available unless there is control of head position and the physiotherapist may be required to help in this way.

Deglutition is also difficult without head control and may be impossible if the patient is recumbent. The patient who has swallowing difficulties should be fed, if possible, in an upright position.

To speak, we also have to be able to swallow as otherwise we spit as we speak. The swallowing muscles may be stimulated by stroking or brushing over the anterior aspect of the under-surface of the chin and neck and by icing the tongue and lips.

EXERCISE TOLERANCE

This becomes lost if respiration and circulation are impaired but it may also be lost due to disuse. The wheelchair patient never fully uses himself unless encouraged to do so. If possible he should be encouraged to indulge in as active a type of exercise as possible to maintain good exercise tolerance.

Other patients should be given activities in their programme which tax them to their limits so that they maintain good general health. The only exception to this would be, perhaps, the patient who has had a cerebrovascular accident or one with cardiac complications.

Care must be taken to see that the patient and relatives understand that to be overweight is detrimental. The less exercise the patient is able to indulge in, the lighter should be the diet. Over-eating is a common problem to the handicapped patient.

PAIN

This, as has been stated before, is a problem most associated with irritative lesions. Relief of the irritation leads to relief of the pain. Pain may also be the result of faulty posturing or of faulty muscle synergy leading to inflamed bursae, etc.

Pain relieving methods include: gentle heat to encourage relaxation; prolonged cold, which often helps when heat fails; transcutaneous nerve stimulation which uses an electrical impulse to deflect the conduction of pain impulses by influencing the 'pain gate'; soothing massage techniques associated with correction of malposturing and the use of movement activities which help to reduce the discomforts of constant joint positioning.

Many patients who have loss of synergy in the shoulder have severe shoulder pain which spreads down the arm. The hemiplegic patient is particularly prone to this. The pain can often be relieved by the application of a cold pack over the shoulder area incorporating pectoralis major, deltoid and the scapula. If this is followed by rhythmical traction versus compression stimuli the patient frequently reports relief of pain. The explanation for this is obscure but it may be that the cold helps to relax the painful muscle spasm which will be superimposed upon the patient's other symptoms and the compression alternately with traction may stimulate more normal muscle synergy and therefore joint protection.

If the pain is part of a neuritis the position of the vertebral column and shoulder girdle is important.

Cervical traction may be advised as a measure to relieve pressure on the nerve roots and therefore act as a relief to irritation.

The pain of causalgia is another difficult problem and all pain relieving methods may be attempted. Heat is not always successful and may be dangerous if the patient's ability to appreciate degrees of heat is impaired.

Thalamic pain is not very responsive to physiotherapy and drugs may be the only thing to help the patient.

Drug therapy is used widely in the relief of pain which cannot otherwise be helped and even surgical interference may be attempted as a method of blocking sensory input of a painful nature.

LOSS OF CONSCIOUSNESS

Patients showing loss of consciousness require special care in an intensive therapy unit. Attention must be paid to the accompanying respiratory problems and the physiotherapist may be called in to help in these matters.

As was indicated in Chapter 4 there are various levels of unconsciousness and much care must be taken to talk *to* the patient and not about him in case he is receptive to some stimuli.

EPILEPSY

Seizures of this nature are usually held in check by the administration of phenobarbitone and allied drugs. The physiotherapist must know whether her patient is prone to these attacks so that she is not completely unprepared should one occur during a treatment session.

If the seizure is of a minor nature it may pass almost unnoticed, but if it is of a more major type then care must be taken to prevent the patient from injuring himself and other people. Such patients should not be left unattended nor should they be treated in areas where they could come to any severe injury should they have an attack. Pool therapy may well be unwise for these patients on two counts. First, there is a danger of inhalation of water and possible drowning. Second, the shimmering effect of light on the water may well trigger off an attack.

Epilepsy can be triggered off by light wave bands giving visual stimulation and for this reason some patients show the onset of an attack if they sit watching television for long. This is particularly likely to happen if they are too close to it and in a darkened room.

The flickering light coming through trees and from the road upon which there are multiple areas of shade and light may also be a contributory factor and patients who are travelling as passengers are advised to close their eyes when the light fluctuates in this way. Short wave diathermy has been known to have a similar effect and care should be taken if such treatment is contemplated for any patient known to have epilepsy.

It is as well for the physiotherapist to know this since patients often complain of feeling unwell or of having a mild attack when watching television. The physiotherapist may be able to help by explaining the cause.

INCONTINENCE OF URINE AND BACK PRESSURE

As was explained in Chapter 4 many of the more severely handicapped patients show these symptoms. Catheterisation is the standard method of dealing with this, but unfortunately it often leads to urinary infections which have to be controlled by antibiotics.

Back pressure into the kidneys can be relieved periodically by allowing the patient to adopt the upright position for periods during the day. If the patient is unable to stand he may be supported on a tilting couch which can be wound up into the upright position. The patient may have to be secured by strapping into position, but provided adequate padding is given, there is no danger of skin pressure.

This method of procedure can be useful for the patient suffering from multiple sclerosis who has reached the bedfast stage, and who is in danger not only of having urinary problems but also of going into a flexion position. The weight-bearing stimulus through the feet encourages extension and counteracts the flexion, while the urinary complications are minimised.

The patient may be held in this position in the gymnasium (which is a change from the ward) where he may have free use of any movements available in the arms and where he can make social contact with other patients. This may seem to be of small value but values must be related to the situation of the patient. If left, he would be curled up into flexion at this stage, have kidney failure, pressure sores and be unable to make any social contacts; the remaining weeks would be spent in more discomfort than necessary.

FUNCTIONAL INDEPENDENCE

At some stage in his rehabilitation the patient will require help towards functional independence. Exactly when this is encouraged will depend upon the type of condition and the method of management being used.

To be manageable at home the patient should be able to move himself up and down and about his own bed. He should be able to transfer himself from his bed to a chair of any kind and if he is a wheelchair patient, he should be able to manoeuvre the wheelchair about the house and transfer from wheelchair to toilet seat and into the bath, etc. All these things should be possible with minimal assistance from relatives. In some cases special hoists have to be supplied to patients to help them to be independent and aids have to be given to make some functions possible. It is, however, most important that aids are only supplied as a last resort or as an intermediate measure from which the patient will progress.

The physiotherapist and occupational therapist are involved in functional independence and should work in close conjunction with each other.

Such activities as dressing and washing must be related to the patient's ability to balance in various positions and to carry out fine movements of the hands. Although the occupational therapist is very involved with this aspect the physiotherapist must also take an interest since she is probably responsible for the balance training and will know when the patient can be expected to use hand skills.

For the housewife kitchen training is dealt with as a rule by the occupational therapist who is concerned with any adaptation required for the patient's own kitchen. However, the physiotherapist may well be able to help by giving the patient the necessary skills of movement so that she may use her kitchen either as it is or with its adaptations.

Home visits may be necessary and should be made ideally by the occupational therapist and the physiotherapist together. Much of the patient's treatment programme can be adjusted to suit the particular home problems and the physiotherapist gains much by seeing the difficulties likely to be faced by the patient.

In some cases functional independence cannot be achieved without some kind of aid such as a weight-relieving or weight-bearing orthosis, a pair of sticks, elbow crutches, or a wheelchair. The patient must be correctly assessed for these appliances and must also be adequately instructed in their use.

The education of relatives is important. When the patient is sent home the relatives have an all-powerful position and can make or break the patient's progress. They need help to understand the problems faced by the patient and to know how best they can help him. If they smother him with help they may make him relinquish his independence and then he will be wholly dependent and become a burden. If they offer too little help life may become too difficult for the patient and he will give up trying. Thus the relatives have a considerable responsibility when the patient finally goes home.

Finally, the need to get out and to see other people is very great and relatives and patient alike must appreciate that confinement to four walls eventually imprisons the mind. Herein lies a great problem. Handicapped people often rely upon others to help them to get out and if they do not get away from home they become fractious and difficult since their horizons become narrowed. The opening of day centres for severely handicapped patients helps a great deal. Patients who have been away from home for a day meet their relatives in the evening with refreshed minds and have something to offer as a social contact. Naturally it is hoped that most patients will be able to work but those who cannot must not be forgotten and it is for these patients that day centres are of most value.

PROGRESSIVE DISORDERS – THE USE OF EARLY PHYSIOTHERAPY

The most commonly seen progressive neurological disorder in the physiotherapy department is multiple sclerosis. Unfortunately such patients are most usually referred to the physiotherapist when their motor disability has reached quite an advanced stage and their body image has already become quite abnormal. The reasons for delaying their referral are most usually:

(a) The reluctance to admit to the patient that he may have a progressive neurological disorder – particularly if there is any doubt in the diagnosis.

(b) The lack of appreciation that a physiotherapist can be of any help to a patient during the early stages of the development of the symptoms.

(c) The inability of the physiotherapist to analyse the patient's early movement difficulties and to appreciate what is needed to help the patient to exploit his own nervous system to its maximum capacity.

It is not generally understood that movement therapy really starts by helping the patient to improve his body image and that even 'normal' people have very little knowledge about their bodily movements. The ability to move and achieve normal functional skills is taken for granted and little or no interest is taken in 'how' this is done unless a particular and new skill is required for a special reason. It is not, therefore, surprising that patients with a slowly progressive disorder are not aware of how much they are affected by the change in their nervous system. They may feel unsteady and a little bit clumsy but may put it down to an 'off' day or the fact that they are getting a little bit older or to some other possible cause. They will even then only be aware of the limb activity and are unlikely to realise that the important equilibrium reactions of the trunk are deteriorating and are possibly creating the difficulty. Such patients often present with such minimal symptoms that the non-specialist is unable to detect anything amiss. However, if such patients are carefully tested for equilibrium reactions and are put into reflexogenic postures the movement difficulties become much more apparent.

While accepting that the disease process cannot be delayed, the reduction in functional ability can be alleviated if, at this early stage, the patient is helped to find a way of producing the appropriate balance reactions and rebuilding them into his repertoire of movement. In other words, a 'revision' course of equilibrium reactions, rolling in a spiral manner, lateral reactions of the trunk to weight transference in sitting and standing, can often reinstate these reactions so that the patient functions with more confidence and maintains the more normal body image for longer. Additionally, such patients can be given advice regarding the importance of rest/activity programmes, the dangers of over-fatigue, of habitually adopting reflexogenic resting postures, the hazards of prolonged bed rest (which can lead to a much more profound loss of postural reaction than is experienced by the neurologically 'normal' patient) and the need to maintain a healthy respiratory and circulatory system. Such patients do not need more than a few intensive sessions to set them on the right road to caring for themselves. It is not desirable to interfere with a patient's lifestyle in the interests of physiotherapy at this stage. The role of the physiotherapist should be that of educator and adviser and, after the few intensive sessions to teach the patient appropriate maintenance activities, the patient should be left alone to take care of himself, but given a 'life-line' to the therapist who can be contacted if further help is needed, or who will contact the patient for assessment at appropriate intervals. Physiotherapists should welcome the opportunity to have patients at this stage because many problems can be delayed if this opportunity is seized.

A similar approach is needed for the patient with early Parkinson's disease and also, if the patient is receiving medication to replace the dopamine balance, a short burst of intensive physiotherapy can be very valuable. Such a patient may well have had quite severe symptoms prior to medication and it is, unfortunately, assumed that medication will restore him to normal. Instead, patients often feel very disorientated and lacking in confidence because the body image he had in response to rigidity is no longer appropriate or, he may retain 'rigidity type' movement patterns because he has 'forgotten' the normal reactions. A little help from a therapist may make all the difference and this, again, should take the form of a 'revision' course on balance reactions and re-education of the body image for functional activities.

When either of these conditions has progressed to a more advanced level, whether or not the patient was seen in the early stages, the principles outlined earlier in this chapter still hold good but the therapist and the patient must take a realistic approach and appreciate that progress to a higher functional level will be limited by the extent of the damage and that the nervous system can only be exploited to its individual limits. Much help is needed to enable the patient to adapt to the changing situation and, at each stage of the disease, the important factor is the quality of the patient's existence. Therapists must try to remember that the therapy is given to help the patient to live his life as best he can and that therapy sessions should not themselves become the patient's life. However, in the very advanced stages, the therapist must try to help the relatives to understand the patient's difficulties, offer help and advice over specific problems, particularly in relationship to appropriate posturing of the patient for feeding activities, the avoidance of pressure sores and the need for mental stimulation.

REFERENCES

Cotton, E. and Kinsman, R. (1983). *Conductive Education for Adult Hemiplegia*. Churchill Livingstone, Edinburgh.

Dunkin, E. (1981). Motor skill training. In *Psychology for Physiotherapists*. The British Psychological Society, London.

Turnbull, G. (1982). Motor learning theory. *Physiotherapy*, **68**, 2.

BIBLIOGRAPHY

Basmajian, J. V. (1980). *Therapeutic Exercise*, 3rd edition. Williams and Wilkins, Baltimore.

Bobath, B. (1978). *Adult Hemiplegia: Evaluation and Treatment*, 2nd edition. William Heinemann Medical Books Limited, London.

Brunnstrom, M. (1970). *Movement Therapy in Hemiplegia: A Neurophysical Approach*. Harper and Row, New York.

Carr, J. H. and Shepherd, R. B. (1979). *Early Care of the Stroke Patient*. William Heinemann Medical Books Limited, London.

Carr, J. H. and Shepherd, R. B. (1980). *Physiotherapy in Disorders of the Brain*. William Heinemann Medical Books Limited, London.

Carr, J. H. and Shepherd, R. B. (1984). *A Motor Re-learning Programme for Stroke*. William Heinemann Medical Books Limited, London.

Cohen, J. and Clark, J. (1979). *Medicine, Mind and Man.* W. H. Freeman and Company, Reading and San Francisco.

Farber, S. (1982). *Neurorehabilitation, a Multisensory Approach.* W. B. Saunders Co, Philadelphia.

Knott, M. and Voss, D. (1969). *Proprioceptive Neuromuscular Facilitation Patterns and Techniques*, 2nd edition. Harper and Row, New York.

Lee, J. M. and Warren, M. P. (1978). *Cold Therapy in Rehabilitation.* Bell and Hyman, London.

Lubbock, G. (ed.) (1983). *Stroke Care: An Interdisciplinary Approach.* Faber and Faber, London.

Sullivan, P., Markos, P. and Minor, M. (1982). *An Integrated Approach to Therapeutic Exercise.* Reston Publishing Company Inc., Reston, Virginia.

PAPERS

Atkinson, H. W. (1973). The limitations of facilitation techniques. *Physiotherapy*, **59**, 1, 6–8.

Basmajian, J. V. (1976). Electromyographic investigation of spasticity and muscle spasm. *Physiotherapy*, **62**, 10, 319–23.

Bishop, B. (1974). Vibratory stimulation: Part I – Neurophysiology of motor responses evoked by vibratory stimulation. *Physical Therapy*, **54**, 12.

Bishop, B. (1975). Vibratory stimulation: Part II – Vibratory stimulation as an evaluation tool. *Physical Therapy*, **55**, 1.

Bishop, B. (1975). Vibratory stimulation: Part III – Possible applications of vibration in treatment of motor dysfunctions. *Physical Therapy*, **55**, 2.

Bryce, J. (1976). The management of spasticity in children. *Physiotherapy*, **62**, 11, 353–7.

Davies, P. M. (1972). Practical neurological assessment. *Physiotherapy*, **58**, 12, 398–402.

De Souza, L. H. (1984). A different approach to physiotherapy for multiple sclerosis patients. *Physiotherapy*, **70**, 11, 429–32.

Gautier-Smith, P. C. (1976). Clinical management of spastic states. *Physiotherapy*, **62**, 10, 326–8.

Goff, B. (1969). Appropriate afferent stimulation. *Physiotherapy*, **55**, 1, 9–17.

Goff, B. (1972). The application of recent advances in neurophysiology to Miss M. Rood's concept of neuromuscular facilitation. *Physiotherapy*, **58**, 12, 409–15.

Goff, B. (1976). Grading of spasticity and its effect on voluntary movement. *Physiotherapy*, **62**, 11, 358–61.

Huberman, G. (1976). Organised sports activities with cerebral palsied adolescents. *Physiotherapy*, **62**, 11, 362–4.

Hudgson, P. (1976). Clinical features of spastic states. *Physiotherapy*, **62**, 10, 323–5.

Illingworth, R. S. (1965). Sequence of development in the child. *Physiotherapy*, **51**, 6, 176–8.

Lane, R. J. (1969). Physiotherapy in the treatment of balance problems. *Physiotherapy*, **55**, 10, 415–20.

Manning, J. (1972). Facilitation of movement – the Bobath approach. *Physiotherapy*, **58**, 12, 403–8.

Piercy, J. M. (1973). The place of facilitation in non-neurological problems. *Physiotherapy*, **59**, 1, 2–6.

Todd, J. M. (1972). Facilitation of movement as taught at Vallejo. *Physiotherapy*, **59**, 12, 415–19.

Wilson, J. (1976). Spastic states in childhood. *Physiotherapy*, **62**, 11, 350–3.

Wyke, B. (1976). Neurological mechanisms in spasticity: a brief review of some current concepts. *Physiotherapy*, **62**, 10, 316–19.

ACKNOWLEDGEMENTS

The author expresses her thanks to everyone who has helped her in the preparation of these chapters. She is particularly grateful to the late Margaret Knott of Vallejo, California, and Dr and Mrs K. Bobath of the Western Cerebral Palsy Centre, London, who originally stimulated her interest in this work; to Julia McGuinness-Scott for her advice and help with the notation; and to her patient and forbearing staff, all of whom have helped in a variety of ways. Finally, she thanks the patients she has treated and her students – they are the best teachers of all.

Chapter 8

The Rood Approach

by B. GOFF MCSP, ONC, DipTP

The Rood approach is based on the known physiological facts that skeletomotor units with different enzyme profiles play a distinct role in control of movement and posture, and how afferent input can influence different controls on these in the central nervous system (CNS).

The techniques that will be described are used for patients with neurological conditions, but they are also effective in conditions such as rheumatoid arthritis, osteoarthritis, soft tissue injury and post-fractures. In these conditions the techniques are used to reduce the protective muscle spasm, increase soft tissue range and to elicit normal postural reactions.

The technique takes its name from the late Margaret Rood, an American physical therapist who, in 1956, stated that 'muscles have different duties. Most of them are a combination, but some predominate, in "light work", others in "heavy work"' (Tables 8/1 and 8/2).

The essential features of this technique may be summarised as follows:

1. Identification of goals.
2. Identification of factors contributing to poor function.
3. Following a sequence of positions and activities of normal motor development and selecting those most relevant to individual needs.
4. Selection of appropriate afferent stimuli to exploit potentiality of tissues to change at molecular level. This facilitates attainment of motor goals and helps to prevent perpetuation of abnormal influences imposed by pathological changes.
5. Pertinent timing of stimuli.
6. Ensuring repetition in association with the environs, and thus managed without therapy so that a lasting effect is obtained.

TABLE 8/1 Muscle work patterns

Light work	Heavy work
Phasic movement	Tonic co-contraction
Fast glycolytic (FG) motor units	Slow oxidative (SO) motor units
Superficial, usually multiarthrodial	Deep one joint
Fusiform or strap; small area of attachment	Pennate; large area of attachment
Great increase in blood supply if active	Rich blood supply at all times
High metabolic cost; rapidly fatigue	Low metabolic cost; slow to fatigue
Flexors and adductors	Extensors and abductors

TABLE 8/2 Facilitation and inhibition of patterns of muscle work

Light work patterns	Heavy work patterns
Facilitated by:	*Facilitated by:*
Quick stretch	Quick stretch
Unpleasant stimuli	Joint compression in correct alignment
Potentially harmful stimuli; pain (nocioceptors)	Pressure on weight-bearing surfaces, distal end fixed
Specific receptor sites on lips, tongue, soles of feet, palms of hand	Resistance distally to extension or abduction of proximal limb joint
	Extensor aspect uppermost
Input from semicircular canals, e.g. movement of head in space	Input from utricle and saccule; static position of head in space

Objective activities

Inhibited by:	*Inhibited by:*
All stimuli for heavy work (see above), e.g. compression of the long axis of body segments	All stimuli for light work (see above), e.g. pain
	Movement of head

Trophic changes occur by axoplasmic flow in nerve processes over periods of time as well as immediate effects by transmission of nerve impulses.

Goals: These may be communication; manipulative skills; or gross motor function.

Clinical examination for defects: This will include assessment of sensation; perception; postural reactions; quality of movement; muscle tone; and noting if there are any local circulatory defects.

TABLE 8/3   Sequences in gross motor development

A. *Total movement patterns*	*Description*	*Remarks*
A1	Supine Withdrawal pattern Total flexion, tonic posture pattern Heavy work, trunk, neck and proximal extremity joints Reciprocal innervation Bilateral Centred at 10th thoracic vertebra	Miss out in very young except those with extensor spasticity
A2	Roll over Flexion top arm and leg Phasic movement pattern	Use first for young child CVA Hemiplegia
A3	Pivot pattern Total extension Reciprocal innervation bilateral Centred at 10th thoracic vertebra	Avoid if extensor spasticity predominates

B. *Fixed distal segments*	*Description*	*Remarks*
B1	Co-contraction neck, vertebral extension	Use for hyperkinesia of head and neck Use to stabilise eyes if nystagmus
B2	Forearm support Alignment must be correct to avoid trauma to glenohumeral joint	
B3	All fours	
B4	Sitting Auto-facilitation by pressure on knees through to heels	

	Examples	
C. Movements over fixed distal segments to gain mobile stability	For example: Rock side to side, backward and forward Turning movements	
D. Skilled movements Distal end of limbs free	Objective activities, e.g. reaching, crawling, walking	

SEQUENCES (Table 8/3)

Total body position and activity should be considered with special regard to the head in relation to gravity and to the rest of the body.

1. Total movement is facilitated in the normal early patterns of curl up, stretch out and rolling, omitting undesirable ones, for example, total extension if extensor spasticity predominates. This will secure any component, muscle activity or movement, if the necessary muscles are innervated and appropriate stimuli are used.
2. Postural stability is facilitated by using positions with the distal segment fixed, and compression is given through correctly aligned head, trunk or limbs.
3. Movement, active or passive, over the fixed distal segment(s) prepares for dynamic stability.
4. Lastly, movement is facilitated with the distal end of the part free. Objective and functional activities are used.

In the above sequences head control is obtained before that of arms and upper trunk, and lastly control of lower trunk and legs, thus the principle of cephalocaudal development is observed. Movement control follows the sequence of flexion, extension, adduction, abduction and, lastly, rotation as in ontogenetic development.

RECEPTORS

Cutaneous

Cutaneous stimulation by quick light brushing: This is used as a preparatory facilitation to increase excitability of motor neurones which supply inhibited muscles. The area to be brushed is specific in terms of the nerve root supply to skin and muscle; these must be the same and the skin must lie on the same aspect of the part as does the muscle. In most cases the skin overlying a muscle shares its root supply. A changing stimulus is needed and is continued only for a short time in one place. A soft artist's or decorator's brush is used, or, if available, an electrically-powered brush.

For skin supplied by anterior primary rami the excitatory effect is local and mainly to superficial muscles.

For skin supplied by posterior primary rami the effect is excitatory to deep back muscles.

On the face the effect is to muscles of mastication and possibly also of expression through the intersegmental connections of cranial nerves V and VII.

A delay of up to 20 minutes occurs before the maximal effect if the nerve pathways to the inhibited muscles have not been used recently. Rapid skin stimulation is useful for an area with poor circulation, for example, if brushing is given to the entire surface of a hand or foot. If reflex pathways to and from the spinal cord are intact, loss of cutaneous sensation does not negate the effectiveness of skin stimulation. Loeb and Hoffer (1981) noted that 'new data are presented demonstrating that cutaneous stimulation causes rapid and large modulation of muscle spindle sensitivity presumably through complex gamma motoneurone reflexes'.

Brief application of cold: In the form of a quick wipe with an ice cube this also has an excitatory effect which is immediate and most effective when applied to skin overlying the extensors of limbs and when the part is warm. Brushing or ice application to the palmar surface of the finger tips alerts mental processes but should be avoided if spasticity is present. Ice applied to the lips or tongue facilitates sucking, swallowing and speech.

Slow stroking: If this is carried out from neck to sacrum over the centre of the back it will reduce choreo-athetosis or excessive muscle tone. It should be applied rhythmically for 3 minutes.

PRECAUTIONS

Use of brushing: Brushing is the most powerful tool physiotherapists have, so they must use it with discretion and in the full knowledge of its potential.

1. The area brushed is very specific so therapists must be aware of the effect likely on dermatomes and myotomes.
2. It should be used only for up to 3 seconds in one place at one time, longer may inhibit rather than facilitate. The stimulation can be repeated in bursts at intervals; the maximum effect is delayed for 20 to 30 minutes where nerve pathways have not been active through disuse or inhibition.
3. Do not use mechanical tools with revolutions of 360 or higher to operate a brush as this can completely inhibit nerve pathways.

4. In cases of flaccidity, especially in an infant or young child with no mechanism for response, brushing may cause a seizure; should this occur slow rhythmical stroking should be used over the posterior primary rami dermatomes for 3 minutes.
5. Brushing the skin of the ear and the outer thirds of the forehead has a central inhibitory effect and should be avoided when treating a low energy individual. It should also be avoided if brainstem injury exists as it may result in a coma. The same applies to slow stroking of the back. (Revive by the application of ice to the lips and the tongue.)

Use of ice: Great care must be observed when applying ice:
1. Ice used behind the ear can lead to a sudden lowering of the blood pressure.
2. Ice applied to special receptor areas in the sole of the foot or the palm of the hand is potentially nocioceptive so its use should be avoided in very young children, the highly strung patient or in anyone who is emotionally unstable.

   Ice can be safely applied to the specific receptor areas on the lips and tongue as this is pleasant; contact with the teeth should be avoided as this may be painful.
3. Ice applied over the skin supplied by the posterior primary rami may set up a chain of effects on viscera over which one has no control. For example, the blood supply to viscera may be affected by the application of ice to a dermatome sharing the same segmental nerve supply.
4. Ice used in the region of the left shoulder may be dangerous if there is known cardiac disease.

Muscle spindles

Quick, unexpected stretch: On any muscle this has a facilitatory effect via the spindle afferents from a primary ending (Ia) and must therefore be avoided if spasticity prevails.

Slow full stretch: If this is applied to deep muscle components passing over one joint only it will be inhibitory to the muscle stretched, and excitatory to the antagonist(s). Full length is gradually obtained and should be held for 5 minutes.

Other stimuli then follow to elicit correct postural use of the part. The inhibitory effect is mediated via secondary spindle endings (II). The therapist should avoid stretching synergic multiarthrodial muscles. As long ago as 1960 Hunt and Perl found that group II afferents produce reflex inhibition in extensors and excitation in flexors; and Boyd (1981) noted that 'present work confirms the long-accepted view that the secondary ending (II) is a length-measuring device which derives most of its input from nuclear chain fibres'.

A chain reaction can be gained – for example, if slow stretch is

TABLE 8/4   Muscles and their responses

Multiarthrodial muscles; flexors and adductors (FG motor units)	Stimulus	One-joint muscles; extensors and abductors (SO motor units)
Excitation via primary ending activates muscle stretched and inhibits antagonists	Stretch Quick part-stretch	
	Full stretch maintained for 5 minutes or more	Inhibition via secondary ending to homonymous and synergic muscles and activation of antagonistic flexors or adductors
Many contraction receptors (Golgi) which inhibit muscle contracting. Difficult to maintain in contraction voluntarily if *no* facilitation is given	Contraction without resistance even of gravity	Few contraction receptors (Golgi). Less effect on antagonist and not as difficult to maintain in contraction voluntarily

Multiarthrodial muscles; flexors and adductors (FG motor units)	Stimulus	One-joint muscles; extensors and abductors (SO motor units)
Major facilitation to muscle being resisted	Contraction plus stretch or outside resistance, i.e. against a load	Contraction of a resisted muscle, if resisted near the joint, gains major facilitation to agonists. If a long lever is used, by resisting at distal end of limb, it will result in co-contraction of agonists and antagonists including those at proximal joints
Inhibition Use to inhibit spasticity in flexors and adductors	Joint compression, i.e. in long axis of the body segments in correct weight-bearing alignment	Gains co-contraction with greatest facilitation to one-joint extensors and lengthening of antagonistic flexors
Reduces tone, e.g. relaxes the long flexors of the fingers and thumb	Pressure over distal attachment of superficial muscles	
Releases the long flexors of the fingers and thumb	Firm pressure over palmar aspect of metacarpals	Reduces palmar grip, facilitates normal grasp

applied to the soleus muscle, with the knee flexed, reciprocal activation of dorsiflexion is obtained which in turn inhibits the gastrocnemius muscle; the extensor thrust is prevented and a normal stance facilitated. Other groups of deep muscles which respond well to this technique to reduce spasticity are the vastus medialis and lateralis of the quadriceps muscle, the hip abductors, the lumbar and cervical deep extensors, the posterior muscles of the glenohumeral joint and the shoulder girdle retractors (Table 8/4).

VIBRATION

Muscle spindles can be stimulated by vibration applied by a mechanical vibrator at the musculotendinous junction with the muscle on stretch. The facilitation gained increases the strength of a contraction and may overcome inhibition in a muscle. This reflex is known as the tonic vibratory reflex (TVR). Burke et al (1976a and b) have shown that some fusimotor drive to a muscle is essential for production of the TVR. Cutaneous brushing prior to the use of a vibrator should enhance its effect.

Golgi tendon organs (Ib)

These receptors which lie in series with contractile muscle fibres at the musculotendinous junction are known as contraction receptors and are auto-inhibitory to a non-resisted repeated contraction of a muscle. Their inhibitory effect can be cancelled by concurrent facilitatory influences, so to exploit the inhibition no resistance is given even by the force of gravity and a small range repeated contraction is requested. This applies mainly to multiarthrodial muscles with fast glycolytic motor units, for example, superficial flexors and to adductor muscles. If the patient has some control of movement, spasticity in flexor or adductor muscles can be reduced by stimulating the Golgi tendon organs. The patient is taught to produce, repeatedly, very small range contractions of the spastic muscle and its antagonist. There must be no resistance from gravity or other forces; the part should be supported, effort avoided and no facilitation given. After many repetitions in a very small range, stimuli can be given to elicit strong isotonic contraction of the antagonistic extensor or abductor groups.

The spastic group of muscles is thus lengthened and the process can be repeated using a starting position in which the spastic muscles are longer than previously. Gradually, by several series of repetitions, considerable relaxation can be obtained. The technique is particularly useful for the adductor muscles of the hip or the shoulder joints.

Note: The effect of inhibition is on the flexor and adductor groups of muscles in which the Golgi tendon organs are numerous, and no inhibition occurs on the extensor or abductor muscles in which there are few or no Golgi tendon organs. (For further reading see Houk and Henneman (1967), p. 239.)

Mechanoreceptors in dermis and joints

Receptors found in the ligaments and capsules of joints are known to play a vital role in the control of posture and movement. A classification of these receptors is given by Wyke (1972).

Maintained or intermittent pressure on normal weight-bearing areas increases activity in slow-acting motor units which stabilise the part and have maximal effect on the muscles on the opposite surface to the part stimulated. For example, pressure under the medial side of the heel activates the dorsiflexor muscles which evert the foot, facilitates dorsiflexion in eversion and corrects the tendency to plantar flexion and inversion in a spastic leg.

In the upper limb spasticity and protective muscle spasm are reduced and deep postural tone is increased by pressure on the heel of the hand, firm rubbing along the posterior border of the ulna, and compression through the long axis of the upper, or whole, arm with the head of humerus in its correct contact position with the scapula. Alignment must be correct so that the part could, or does, take weight painlessly. In cases of spasticity with ulnar flexion of the wrist, pressure should be given through the pisiform bone, and the wrist gradually taken into radial extension; the radial extensor muscles are then activated and spasticity reduced.

When pressure from the top of the skull to the ischial tuberosities is given through a correctly aligned head and trunk, the deep postural muscles are activated and the head and trunk stabilised. In sitting, aided if necessary by corrective seating appliances, a weighted cap worn on the head will stabilise the head and trunk. In cases of hemi-athetosis a weighted shoulder bag worn over the lower shoulder will help to gain a symmetrical posture.

When the head, trunk or a limb is held in an unsupported position so that the extensor aspect is uppermost, the part is automatically held steady with little or no conscious effort. This contrasts with the difficulty in maintaining an unsupported position with the flexors uppermost. Prone positions, with the head or trunk unsupported, facilitate stability by an increase in postural tone. An asymmetrical posture of head and/or trunk is corrected by placing the patient in side lying over pillows, so that the convex side is uppermost while the head and legs are not supported. Skin stimulation is given near the centre of the back on the convex side only. As active correction occurs light resistance is given at the head and pelvis to increase the strength of contraction in deep muscles on the convex side. The patient then sits and, if necessary, compression is given over the shoulder on the concave side; a weighted shoulder bag can be worn to maintain correction.

Resistance to muscle action which is applied near a proximal limb joint gains major facilitation to the agonist, but if resistance is given with a long lever, that is, applied at the distal end of a limb, co-contraction will occur of all the muscles at the proximal joint.

Once stability of a weight-bearing part is obtained, movement should be added keeping the distal segment fixed on a supporting surface so gaining dynamic stability in preparation for control of movement with the distal end free. This sequence follows that of the infant who gains dynamic stability of the shoulder girdle and arm in forearm-support prone lying, rocks backwards and forwards and eventually achieves the ability to lift one arm and correctly reach out to grasp a toy.

Pressure on the distal attachment of the superficial muscles and on the palmar surfaces of the metacarpals allows the long flexor muscles to be released (see techniques for spasticity, p. 237).

Labyrinthine system

The position or movement of the head in space stimulates the receptors in the utricle and saccule and in the semicircular canals. Static positions will stimulate the utricle and saccule and influence postural tone; the tonic labyrinthine reflexes of the neonate are modified as righting and equilibrium reactions develop. The influence of retained or released tonic reflexes must be observed and positions must be selected to reduce these.

Movement of the head stimulates the semicircular canals and elicits movement, reducing excessive postural tone and aiding the initiation of movement in cases of bradykinaesia. This is most effective with the head in a vertical position and is easy to achieve by seating the patient in a revolving chair.

To elicit total extension of head, trunk and extension and abduction of the limbs the patient is placed prone on a tilting plinth or large ball and rocked head up and down alternately. This is the pivot pattern shown in Table 8/3. It has been suggested 'that other input from neck and labyrinthine reflexes at times produce greater activation of the fast-twitch than slow-twitch muscles, indicating the possible existence of alternative control mechanisms for fast and slow twitch units' (Burke, 1980).

Receptors in special sense organs

Use should be made of stimulation of receptors in the nose and mouth to mobilise the face or to elicit tongue movements. Examples include using a drop of a dilute solution of quinine placed on the back of the tongue to overcome tongue thrust, and solutions of ammonia held under the nose to release a parkinsonian mask. Dilute unsweetened lemon juice stimulates thin saliva flow and aids swallowing and clearing secretions from the throat.

Optical righting reactions can be elicited and motivation is gained either by looking at objects or following their movement.

Muscle response to stimuli is summarised in Table 8/4.

In the intact nervous system many afferent nerve impulses do not reach the sensorium, and even in patients who lack sensation input has an effect on the autonomic and somatic motor systems without reaching the sensorium. Rood techniques have been used to facilitate the respiratory muscles in unconscious patients (Bethune, 1975).

TIMING

A selection of body positions and activities can be made so that the sequences followed are timed for maximum facilitation. For example, head control is ensured by selecting the first positions in Table 8/3 before using techniques to facilitate swallowing or speech. Correct timing of stimulation is vital, for example, skin brushing precedes all other stimuli to allow for the delay in its facilitatory effect. Verbal commands for activity, or to hold a position, should coincide with the application of stimuli which gain an immediate effect, as, for example, does the application of a wipe of ice to skin over extensor muscles.

REPETITION

Axoplasmic flow along nerve processes produces changes in the molecules of nerve and muscle tissue. Repetition of regimes of activity over sufficient periods of time are needed to effect changes in muscle-unit type so that they are more suited to the demands made upon them. Regimes of activity must be planned and ways found which will enable patients to follow them in their daily routine at home for sufficient periods regularly and over a long enough span to ensure lasting beneficial effects.

TREATMENT PLANNING

No treatment follows a set pattern but should be planned to meet individual needs and will be adjusted as evaluation of its effectiveness indicates. The following is a selection of stimuli and activities for common syndromes.

Hypokinaesia

Causes of hypokinaesia include lower motor neurone lesions, dense sensory loss, and the flaccid stage of hemiplegia.
1. Skin brushing can be used to facilitate key muscles.
2. Total movement will facilitate any weak components.
3. Stimuli from bone taps, quick ice, and vibration should be used as appropriate.
4. Deep muscles can be activated by choosing positions with the distal end of segments fixed, and then applying compression and resistance distally to gain co-contraction.
5. Rocking movements prepare for subsequent activity with the distal part free.

Bradykinaesia

The semicircular canals are stimulated by using a revolving chair; passive or active head and shoulder rotation; or activities, such as alternately punching a suspended target placed so that the patient must reach up and forward to reach it.

As a preparation for walking, the rhythm of arm and leg movements can be facilitated by the use of poles held by the patient and by the therapist who is standing behind him. Alternate arm swinging can thus be assisted and cadence maintained; marking time with the legs can be added to arm swinging, progressing from standing to walking.

It is possible to modify a rigid walking frame to provide a

tactile and auditory stimulus as each step is taken (Lubbock and Robson, 1981).

Hyperkinaesia

Syndromes which are classified as hyperkinetic include those with low or fluctuating postural tone, involuntary movements and inco-ordination.

Ontogenetic sequences are used with emphasis on positions and stimuli to increase postural tone. A selection of positions is shown in Figure 8/1. In all positions, support must be given while using stimulation of mechanoreceptors until the deep muscles are able to contract and hold the position. If correct positions are obtained weights or weighted garments can then be used to improve stability. Heavy work patterns are used and activities with facilitation (see Tables 8/1, 8/2 and 8/4).

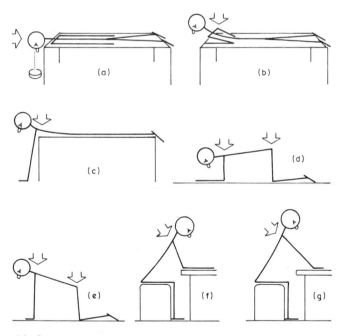

FIG. 8/1 Sequences of positions to gain stability: arrows indicate resistance. (a) Prone lying, head unsupported, eyes focused on object below; (b) Forearm prone lying; (c) Arm support prone lying; (d) Forearm support prone kneeling; (e) Prone kneeling; (f) Forearm support stoop stride sitting; (g) Arm support stoop stride sitting

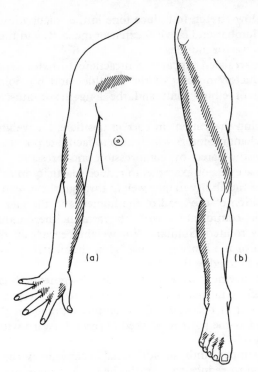

FIG. 8/2 Areas to brush to (a) inhibit spasticity in the finger and thumb flexors and adductors, wrist ulnar flexion, elbow flexion and retraction at shoulder; and (b) to inhibit extensor thrust of a spastic leg. Inhibits toe flexion and adduction, plantar flexion and inversion of foot and hyperextension of knee. Also by brushing lateral side (L2 dermatome) inhibits adductors of hip (L2 root supply but on medial side of thigh)

Spasticity

Spasticity varies so much in type, distribution and severity that it requires careful selection of suitable techniques followed by an evaluation of their effectiveness. Some of these are discussed under the following headings:

SPASTICITY WITH SOME VOLUNTARY MOVEMENT CONTROL

1. Light brushing to facilitate key muscles which oppose spastic groups (Fig. 8/2).
2. Follow the sequences described above, and adapt them according to needs, for example, omit total extension and pivot patterns if extensor tone is strong.

3. Use a slow stretch to reduce tone in the soleus muscle, quad-riceps, lumbar and cervical extensor muscles, and the shoulder girdle retractor muscles.

4. Use non-resisted repeated contractions to reduce spasticity in the adductor muscles of the shoulder and hip joints, flexor muscles of elbow joint and the long flexor muscles of the fingers.

5. By placing the patient in correct positions for weight-bearing the mechanoreceptors which help to facilitate postural stability can be stimulated by compression and pressure on weight-bearing areas. For example, to reduce spasticity in the arm and facilitate the ability to take weight through the forearm or hand the position of the head of the humerus in the glenoid cavity must be comfortable, with the arm neither adducted nor medially rotated. Similarly, for weight-bearing on the leg the position of the hip joint must be in the neutral position, that is, not adducted or flexed.

6. Teach movement over the fixed distal segments, finally elicit-ing selective normal movements for function. Repeat facilitat-ing stimuli as necessary, for example, tapping on the heel of the hand as the patient is asked to reach forward with an open hand.

For the upper limb an additional technique is the use of a hollow cone to reduce tone in the hand. A cone is placed in the

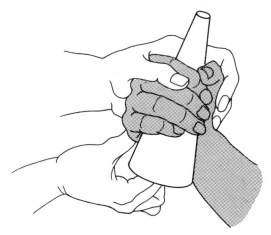

FIG. 8/3 Inhibition of spasticity of hand and wrist. Patient's spastic right hand (shaded) is firmly pressed around a hollow cone by the therapist's hands whose right fingers give pressure through the inside of cone on to the ulnar aspect of the patient's wrist, i.e. on the pisiform bone

hand with its base to the ulnar side, and the digits are moulded around it giving pressure through the cone on to the tendons of the superficial flexors and the palmar surface of the metacarpals (Fig. 8/3). The flexors will relax so that the patient can grasp the cone without a palmar grip, the tips of the digits being lifted off the cone.

Note: If a release of grasp reflex obtains (see below) this technique should not be used.

A sequence to reduce tone in the leg is described on page 228.

SPASTICITY IN COMPLETE CORD LESIONS

All the above techniques can be used except the non-resisted repeated contractions as these require volitional control. Selective free movements are impossible, but by placing the patient in normal weight-bearing positions (see pp. 352 and 376), and by using compression through the long axis of the limb, or the trunk, it is possible to reduce spasticity. Functional activities such as transfers and dressing are then facilitated, reinforcement of spasticity is avoided and the risk of contractures and pressure sores is reduced.

It is a known fact that some input to spinal neuronal sets originates at other levels in the spinal cord and are transmitted by intersegmental and commissural systems. These extend the range of intrinsic spinal control and add to the repertoire of movement allowed by spinal organisation alone (Kidd, 1980).

Released grasp reflex

Firm slow massage, using the heel of the hand applied to the non-weight-bearing areas of the patient's palm or the medial side of the sole of the foot, will inhibit a retained grasp reflex in an infant or a released grasp reflex in an adult. The operator must avoid contact with the finger tips or the ball of the foot.

Facilitation of swallowing and speech

A stable head position should be facilitated as described on page 230. Other techniques which can be used include (1) light brushing to the upper lip, face and throat avoiding the undersurface of the floor of the mouth, (2) the application of ice to the lips and tongue, (3) resisted sucking and (4) the application of a wipe of ice to the lower neck anteriorly.

Sucking or sipping a drink of dilute unsweetened lemon juice helps to clear secretions in the throat by stimulating flow of thin saliva.

REFERENCES

Bethune, D. A. (1975). Neurological facilitation of respiration in the unconscious adult patient. *Physiotherapy* (Canada), **27**, 5, 241-5.

Boyd, I. A. (1981). The action of three types of intrafusal muscle. In *Muscle Receptors in Movement Control*, p. 17, (eds. Taylor, A. and Prochazka, A.). Macmillan, London.

Burke, D., Hagbarth, K., Wallin, G. and Lofstedt, L. (1976a). The responses of human muscle spindle endings to vibration of non-contracting muscles. *Journal of Physiology*, **261**, 673-93.

Burke, D., Hagbarth, K., Wallin, G. and Lofstedt, L. (1976b). The responses of human muscle spindle endings to vibration during isometric contraction. *Journal of Physiology*, **261**, 695-711.

Burke, R. E. (1980). Motor unit types: functional specializations in motor control. *Trends in Neurosciences*, **3**, 11, 255-8.

Hunt, C. C. and Perl, E. R. (1960). Spindle reflex mechanisms concerned with skeletal muscle. *Physiology Review*, **40**, 538-79.

Kidd, G. (1980). Neuromuscular control of the skeleton. In *Scientific Foundations of Orthopaedics and Traumatology*, pp. 122-3, (eds. Owen, R., Goodfellow, J. W. and Bullock, P.). William Heinemann Medical Books Limited, London.

Loeb, G. E. and Hoffer, J. A. (1981). Muscle spindle function. In *Muscle Receptors in Movement Control*, p. 219, (eds. Taylor, A. and Prochazka, A.). Macmillan, London.

Lubbock, G. and Robson, P. (1981). Walking frames. *Physiotherapy*, **67**, 2, 45.

Rood, M. S. (1956). Neurophysiological mechanisms utilized in the treatment of neuromuscular dysfunction. *American Journal of Occupational Therapy*, **4** (Part II), 220-5.

Wyke, B. D. (1972). Articular neurology: a review. *Physiotherapy*, **58**, 3, 94-9.

BIBLIOGRAPHY

Burke, D. (1980). Muscle spindle function during movement. *Trends in Neurosciences*, **3**, 11, 251-3.

de Domenico, G. (1979). Tonic vibratory reflex. *Physiotherapy*, **65**, 2, 44-8.

Haase, J., Cleveland, S. and Ross, H. G. (1975). Problems of postsynaptic autogenous and recurrent inhibition in mammalian spinal cord. *Review Physiology Biochemistry and Pharmacology*, **73**, 73-129.

Houk, J. and Henneman, E. (1967). Responses of Golgi tendon organs. *Journal of Neurophysiology*, **30,** 466–89.

Kidd, G. and Brodie, P. (1980). The motor unit: a review. *Physiotherapy*, **66,** 5, 146–52.

Pennow, B. and Saltin, B. (1971). *Muscle Metabolism During Exercise. Adaptive Changes in the Morphology and Enzymes of Skeletal Muscle.* Plenum Press, New York.

Valbo, Å. B., Habarth, K. E., Troebjork, H. E. and Wallin, B. G. (1979). Somatosensory proprioceptive and sympathetic activity in human peripheral nerves. *Physiology Reviews,* **59,** 4, 944.

Chapter 9

Clinical Aspects of Stroke

by J. P. H. WADE BA, MD, MRCP

Strokes are by far the most common cause of neurological disability in the adult population. They are responsible for about a quarter of all deaths in the developed countries and account for much disability in the elderly. Of patients who suffer a stroke, about a third will die, a third will survive but with severe disability and the remainder will make a good recovery with functional independence. The onset is usually sudden with maximum deficit at the outset, so the shock to patients and relatives is extreme.

DEFINITION

The term 'stroke' is synonymous with cerebrovascular accident or CVA, and is a purely clinical definition which, according to the World Health Organisation, can be defined as a 'rapidly developed clinical sign of a focal disturbance of cerebral function of presumed vascular origin and of more than 24-hours' duration'. Included within this definition are most cases of cerebral infarction, cerebral haemorrhage and subarachnoid haemorrhage but deliberately excluded are those cases in which recovery occurs within 24 hours. These latter cases are designated 'transient ischaemic attacks' (TIA) and because they are often a harbinger of completed stroke, they have received considerable attention over the past two decades.

ANATOMY AND PHYSIOLOGY

The brain is a unique organ in that the neurones depend on a continuous blood supply because metabolism is almost exclusively aerobic. This means that the production of energy (and energy is required to maintain both neuronal structure and function) necessitates a continuous supply of oxygen and glucose delivered to the neurones by the arterial blood. If the brain is deprived of blood, consciousness is lost within seconds and permanent damage occurs within minutes. Other tissues, such as muscle, are not only able to metabolise glucose without oxygen (anaerobic respiration) but they also contain limited amounts of glucose stored in the form of glycogen, so they are relatively immune to transient failures of blood supply.

Perhaps because of the brain's unique vulnerability, evolution has seen to it that its blood supply is copious and anatomically diverse. The brain receives about a quarter of the cardiac output and this ensures that the amounts of oxygen and glucose exceed baseline requirements by a considerable margin. Thus blood returning to the heart (via the jugular veins) is still three-quarters saturated with oxygen and little depleted of glucose. The supply of nutrients can be considered as luxurious and the cerebral circulation responds rapidly to fluctuating local metabolic requirements by focal dilatation and constriction. Overall, a complex physiological mechanism ensures that the blood supply remains stable over a wide range of arterial blood pressure, a phenomenon termed 'autoregulation'.

Blood arrives at the brain via four major vessels (Fig. 9/1). The right carotid artery arises from the innominate artery, and the left carotid artery directly from the aorta; they pass up the front of the neck, through the skull floor to the base of the brain where each artery divides into two and the branches (anterior and middle cerebral arteries) supply the frontal, parietal and temporal lobes. The two anterior cerebral arteries join anteriorly through the anterior communicating artery and this forms the front of the circle of Willis. This safeguard means that severe stenosis, or even occlusion, of one of the internal carotid arteries does not usually lead to stroke, since blood can pass from right to left (or vice versa) via the anterior communicating artery. There are two other arteries, known as the vertebrals, which are smaller than the internal carotids and are branches of the subclavian vessels. These run up the neck within the transverse processes of the cervical vertebrae and enter the posterior fossa through the foramen magnum. They anastomose in front of the brainstem to form the basilar artery and branches of that artery supply the medulla, pons, cerebellum and mid-brain. At the top of the mid-brain, the basilar artery divides into two posterior cerebral arteries which

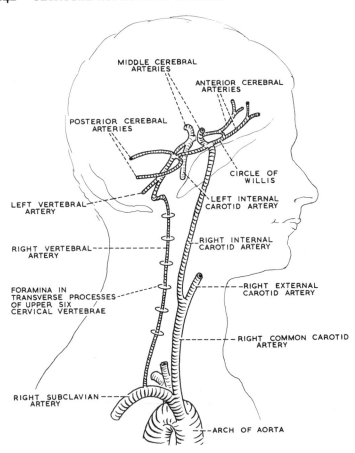

FIG. 9/1 Blood supply to the brain showing the circle of Willis

turn backwards to supply the occipital lobes. These two arteries are also joined to the back of the circle of Willis by small posterior communicating arteries and so an anastomosis occurs between the internal carotids and the vertebral circulation. This offers a further safeguard, and it is not uncommon to see patients who are well despite having bilaterally occluded internal carotid arteries.

The branches of the major cerebral vessels (anterior, middle and posterior cerebral arteries) do not, however, anastomose with each other and they are therefore termed *end arteries*. The parts of the brain they supply are relatively well designated and distinct although anastomoses do occur at the periphery of each region.

If one of these vessels is occluded, then relatively stereotyped brain damage occurs in the area which it supplies.

TYPES OF STROKE

Ischaemic

The most common cause of stroke is due to obstruction to one of the major cerebral arteries (middle, posterior and anterior, in that order) or their smaller perforating branches to deeper parts of the brain. Brainstem strokes, arising from disease in the vertebral and basilar arteries, are less common. Some 70 to 75 per cent of all strokes are due to occlusion, either as a result of atheroma in the artery itself or secondary to emboli (small clots of blood) being washed up from the heart or diseased neck vessels. The patient does not usually lose consciousness but may complain of headache, and symptoms of hemiparesis and/or dysphasia develop rapidly. The hemiplegia is initially flaccid but within a few days this gives way to the typical spastic type. The middle cerebral artery supplies most of the convexity of the cerebral hemisphere and important deeper structures, so there is a dense contralateral hemiplegia affecting the arm, face and leg. The optic radiation is often affected leading to a contralateral homonymous hemianopia and there may be a cortical type of sensory loss. Aphasia can be severe in left hemisphere lesions and there may be neglect of the contralateral side. In right hemisphere lesions, parietal damage can lead to visuo-spatial disturbances. If the main part of the middle cerebral artery is not affected, but one of its distal branches is, then the symptoms will be less extreme.

The most prominent symptoms following posterior cerebral artery occlusion are visual and usually comprise a contralateral homonymous field defect. More complicated disturbances of visual interpretation or complete blindness can follow bilateral infarcts. The posterior cerebral artery also supplies much of the medial aspect of the temporal lobe and the thalamus, so strokes may involve memory and contralateral sensory modalities. The anterior cerebral artery supplies the medial aspect of the frontal lobe and a parasagittal strip of cortex extending back as far as the occipital lobe. Occlusion of this artery may therefore give rise to a contralateral monoplegia affecting the leg, cortical sensory loss and sometimes the behavioural abnormalities associated with frontal lobe damage.

Occlusion of the vertebral arteries, or the basilar and its branches, is potentially much more damaging since the brainstem contains centres which control such vital functions as respiration and blood pressure. The nuclei of the cranial nerves are clustered in the brainstem and the pyramidal and sensory tracts course through it. Thus, ischaemic brain damage may itself be life-threatening and if the patient survives, he may be severely incapacitated by cranial nerve palsies, spastic quadriplegia and sensory loss. Having said that, however, recovery after brainstem stroke is often gratifyingly complete.

Haemorrhagic

About 5 to 10 per cent of strokes are caused by haemorrhage into the deeper parts of the brain. The patient is usually hypertensive, a condition which leads to a particular type of degeneration known as lipohyalinosis in the small penetrating arteries of the brain. The arterial walls weaken and as a result small herniations or micro-aneurysms develop. These may rupture and the resultant haematoma may spread by splitting along planes of white matter to form a substantial mass lesion. Haematomas usually occur in the deeper parts of the brain, often involving the thalamus, lentiform nucleus and external capsule, less often the cerebellum and the pons. They may rupture into the ventricular system and this is often rapidly fatal. The onset is usually dramatic with severe headache, vomiting and, in about 50 per cent of cases, loss of consciousness. The normal vascular autoregulation is lost in the vicinity of the haematoma and since the lesion itself may have considerable mass, intracranial pressure often rises abruptly. If the patient survives the initial ictus, then profound hemiplegic and hemisensory signs may be elicited. A homonymous visual field defect may also be apparent. The initial prognosis is grave but those who do begin to recover often do surprisingly well as the haematoma reabsorbs, presumably because fewer neurones are destroyed than in severe ischaemic strokes. Occasionally, early surgical drainage can be remarkably successful, particularly when the haematoma is in the cerebellum.

Younger, normotensive patients sometimes suffer from spontaneous intracerebral haematoma from an underlying congenital defect of the blood vessels. Such abnormalities are commonly arteriovenous malformations (AVMs); circumscribed areas of dilated and thin-walled vessels which can be demonstrated angiographically. Patients with AVMs are liable to subsequent re-bleeding and surgical excision is undertaken when possible.

Subarachnoid haemorrhage (SAH)

Between 5 and 10 per cent of strokes are due to subarachnoid haemorrhage with bleeding into the subarachnoid space usually arising from a berry aneurysm situated at or near the circle of Willis. The most common site is in the region of the anterior communicating artery with posterior and middle cerebral artery lesions almost as frequent. Congenital factors play some part in the aetiology of berry aneurysms but it is not predominantly a disease of the young since hypertension and vascular disease lead to an increase in aneurysm size and subsequent rupture.

The patient complains of sudden intense headache often associated with vomiting and neck stiffness. Consciousness may be lost and about 10 per cent will die in the first hour or two. Of those that remain, 40 per cent will die within the first 2 weeks and the survivors have a substantially increased risk from re-bleeding for the next 6 weeks or so. A hemiplegia may be evident at the outset if the blood erupts into the deep parts of the brain, and other focal neurological signs may evolve over the first 2 weeks because there is a tendency for blood vessels, tracking through the bloody subarachnoid space, to go into spasm leading to secondary ischaemic brain damage.

Early investigation by angiography, followed by a competent neurosurgical procedure to clip the aneurysm and prevent re-bleeding offers the best hope for recovery.

Less frequent causes of stroke

Stroke may occasionally occur in the context of a generalised medical disorder which either affects the arteries or the blood going through them. An arteritis, or inflammation of the arteries, may complicate meningitis, particularly tuberculous, and strokes were relatively common in tertiary syphilis. The collagen vascular diseases, particularly systemic lupus erythematosus (SLE) and polyarteritis nodosa, may affect medium and small cranial arteries. Temporal arteritis, an inflammatory condition predominantly affecting the extracranial and retinal arteries in the elderly, may also give rise to stroke by intracranial involvement. Bacterial infection of damaged heart valves (bacterial endocarditis) is sometimes complicated by stroke, either as a result of an immune-mediated arteritis or as a consequence of septic emboli impacting in the cranial arteries. Emboli may also arise from the left atrium in patients with atrial fibrillation, particularly if there is coincidental mitral stenosis. More recently, an association between mitral valve prolapse (floppy valve), which is a fairly common congenital abnormality, and ischaemic stroke has been demonstrated. Haematological diseases such as polycythaemia rubra vera, thrombocythaemia and sickle cell disease can provoke stasis in the intracranial arteries, thus leading to ischaemic brain damage. Completed stroke occasionally complicates severe migraine if the vessel spasm which normally produces only temporary symptoms is of such intensity and such duration that ischaemic damage occurs. Finally, there is some evidence that women taking the contraceptive pill, particularly if it has a high oestrogen content, suffer slightly higher incidence of stroke than those not on the pill. The absolute risk is small but enhanced by cigarette smoking.

THE STROKE-PRONE POPULATION

Once a stroke has occurred, neurones are irreparably damaged but there is a border zone around the infarct where non-functioning neurones may still be viable if an adequate blood supply can be restored. There is no certain way of doing this at present and so much attention has concentrated on trying to define those subjects in the normal population who are at risk from having a stroke before they show signs of a compromised cerebral circulation. The risk factors might then be amenable to treatment in the hope that the stroke could be prevented from occurring (Table 9/1). The most comprehensive epidemiological study to date has been conducted in Framingham, Massachusetts (Kannel and Wolf, 1983) and the first point to emerge is that while the chance of having a stroke increases with age, it should not be considered as a natural concomitant of increasing age. The most significant risk factor to emerge is hypertension, either systolic ($>$160mmHg) or diastolic ($>$90mmHg). The risk of stroke increases dramatically with increasing blood pressure and there is good evidence that prophylactic hypotensive therapy alleviates this susceptibility. Patients with diabetes are also much more likely to suffer a stroke than subjects with normal blood glucose. Abnormal blood lipids, smoking and a positive family history are independent risk factors but their effect is relatively minor. The 'final common pathway' for all these risk factors is the arterial disease atherosclerosis, a disease of the larger and medium-sized arteries characterised by the deposition of cholesterol and other substances in the arterial wall. The irregular vessel wall provokes clot formation in the lumen of the artery, which may completely occlude the vessel or may dislodge to form emboli. Hypertension and other risk factors therefore predispose to ischaemic strokes, but it will be recalled that the most usual cause for intracerebral haematoma is also hypertension and the associated small vessel disease (lipohyalinosis).

TABLE 9/1   Risk factors for stroke

Hypertension	Heredity
Diabetes mellitus	TIA
Cardiac abnormalities	Carotid bruit
Hyperlipidaemia	Oestrogen contraceptive pill
Cigarette smoking	Elevated haematocrit

Atherosclerosis is a generalised disease so if the stroke-prone patient is studied he may also have evidence of ischaemic heart disease (angina or previous myocardial infarction) and peripheral vascular disease (claudication). Atrial fibrillation is often a manifestation of ischaemic heart disease and may itself predispose to stroke because blood clots tend to form in the left atrium and these can subsequently dislodge and embolise to the brain. Prolapsed mitral valve has also been mentioned as a potential source of emboli.

Less important risk factors include an elevated haematocrit and the oestrogen-containing contraceptive pill (see above).

THREATENED STROKE

Transient ischaemic attacks (TIA)

A transient ischaemic attack refers to a stroke-like syndrome in which recovery is complete within 24 hours. They are important to recognise because some patients (about 10 per cent per year) will go on to have a complete stroke. The symptoms depend on which part of the brain has been temporarily deprived of blood. Thus, if the left middle cerebral artery has been briefly occluded, then symptoms may comprise weakness and clumsiness of the right side and difficulty making oneself understood (dysphasia). The symptoms evolve rapidly, and resolve more gradually, but it is unusual for the whole episode to last more than an hour and there are no permanent sequelae. Sometimes the retinal artery is involved and here the patient complains of a unilateral visual field disturbance, or blindness, often descending like a curtain across the vision. Within half-an-hour or so (often much more rapidly) the veil lifts and vision is restored. This syndrome is known as amaurosis fugax and it is particularly important because observations have been made on patients during the attacks which have thrown light on the mechanism of TIA in general.

By the use of the ophthalmoscope, the observer can see the retinal vessels and several authors have reported small platelet and cholesterol plugs, blocking the retinal arteries during an attack of amaurosis fugax (Fisher, 1959). These plugs subsequently disperse, blood flow is re-established and vision recovers. The emboli may come from atherosclerotic plaques in the internal carotid artery, sometimes the heart acts as the source, and it is argued that TIAs characterised by hemispheric disturbances are due to the same process, with emboli ascending to the cerebral arteries rather than the ophthalmic and retinal vessels. Brainstem TIAs also occur with symptoms ranging from transient vertigo to sudden loss of consciousness, and here emboli are thought to arise from the vertebral arteries, aorta and heart. The importance of TIA is that if a source of emboli can be defined, then it is sometimes amenable to surgery (e.g. carotid endarterectomy) or medical treatment with anti-platelet drugs such as aspirin.

Leaking aneurysm

About 40 per cent of patients who develop a subarachnoid haemorrhage due to rupture of an aneurysm have preceding symptoms which suggest minor leaks. These usually occur within a month of the major bleed and often go unrecognised by patient and doctor alike. Symptoms which suggest a minor subarachnoid bleed are sudden headache accompanied by nausea, photophobia and sometimes neck stiffness. The symptoms can resolve rapidly and may be incorrectly attributed to migraine. If a bleed is suspected then it should be confirmed by CT scan and/or lumbar puncture because most of these patients will go on to a major bleed with devastating consequences. The operative risk in a healthy subject who has had a minor bleed is much less than in the patient who has suffered a major subarachnoid haemorrhage.

Asymptomatic carotid bruit

A noise (or bruit) is sometimes heard over the carotid artery during the routine medical examination. The bruit suggests turbulent blood flow due to underlying atherosclerosis and it is referred to as an asymptomatic carotid bruit if present in an otherwise healthy individual. Some 5 per cent per year of patients who have a bruit will go on to have a stroke, though not always in the distribution of the diseased artery. However, this group is receiving considerable attention at present in the hope that a sub-group particularly at risk can be identified. These subjects could then be offered prophylactic treatment with aspirin and/or carotid endarterectomy.

INVESTIGATION OF THE PATIENT WITH STROKE

The first objective is to decide which of the three main types of stroke (ischaemic, haemorrhagic or SAH) the patient has had. The history and clinical examination are, of course, helpful and may give the answer. It is important to check the pulse for irregularities of cardiac rhythm, auscultation of the heart may suggest valvular disease and the carotids should always be checked for bruits which, when present, suggest turbulent blood flow due to underlying atherosclerosis. The CT scan will differentiate between ischaemia and haemorrhage since blood shows up as a hyper dense mass lesion whereas ischaemic lesions are less dense than normal brain.

When the history suggests subarachnoid haemorrhage, confirmation can be obtained by examining the cerebrospinal fluid at lumbar puncture. If this is bloodstained, then angiography should be undertaken in an attempt to define the source of bleeding.

Patients with small ischaemic strokes, who have made a good recovery, are investigated along the same lines as those with TIA. The rationale for this is an attempt to prevent further and more devastating strokes. The cause may be immediately apparent such as severe hypertension, in which case investigations will be limited to those indicated in the evaluation of hypertension. Assuming the patient is normotensive, then routine blood tests, which should include haematocrit, ESR, VDRL and blood sugar may be helpful. An ECG and echocardiogram should certainly be performed if there is any chance that the heart is acting as a source of emboli. A carotid bruit would suggest that emboli might be arising from diseased neck vessels, in which case a carotid angiogram may be performed.

MANAGEMENT

Patients with subarachnoid haemorrhage are treated surgically provided they are considered fit enough to withstand surgery. If they are not, then treatment is conservative with prolonged bed rest (4 to 6 weeks) and some authorities favour medication designed to prevent clot lysis. Some patients with haematomas are also treated surgically, but for the most part the treatment of patients suffering stroke is conservative and undertaken by general physicians. The neurological deficit is usually maximal at the outset and, if not severe, the patient can be satisfactorily managed at home. In practice, many patients are admitted to hospital for a short period of treatment and investigation. Patients with more severe stroke will require admission because they and their relatives will be unable to cope at home. At present, there are no drugs which convincingly reduce infarct size and therefore initial treatment is essentially conservative. In some cases a secondary deterioration occurs 2 or 3 days after a stroke usually due to evolving oedema around the infarct. This may respond to dexamethasone or intravenous mannitol although these agents are not very effective in treating the oedema which accompanies stroke. Severe hypertension should be cautiously treated and biochemical abnormalities corrected. The patient must be nursed carefully, his airway may need protecting, bulbar function may be compromised and he is at risk from secondary pneumonia. Most recovery occurs within the first 8 weeks, but about 10 per cent will show some improvement in their walking beyond that and almost 30 per cent will show improvement on their activities of daily living score over the initial 6 months.

All the data suggest that further recovery after 6 months is much slower, so it is during the first few months that the energies of the rehabilitation are likely to be the most fruitful (Brocklehurst et al, 1978). For a classical account of the course of motor recovery following stroke, the reader should consult the excellent paper by Twitchell (1951). Most stroke survivors have a hemiplegia but this is not necessarily the chief barrier to recovery of the ability to walk and an independent life. Cognitive defects are common and may impair the patient's ability to learn new strategies (Adams and Hurwitz, 1963). Patients with receptive dysphasia or defective memory, for instance, will find it difficult to co-operate with the rehabilitation programme. Other barriers include the neglect and denial of paralysed limbs sometimes seen after parietal lobe lesions, and disturbances of emotional behaviour, which may be directly attributed to the cerebral lesion or be part of a depressive reaction in response to a devastating illness. If depression is considered severe, then it is certainly worth a therapeutic trial of an antidepressant drug.

If the stroke is restricted and recovery good, or if the patient has only suffered from TIA and by definition has no residual deficit, then treatment aimed at obviating recurrence may be much more aggressive, depending on the results of the investigations. If the heart is considered a likely source of emboli, then long-term treatment with anticoagulants may be indicated. Atherosclerosis, leading to tight stenosis of the internal carotid artery can be confirmed angiographically and treated surgically by carotid endarterectomy. The surgeon opens the artery and scrapes the lumen, a procedure which when done well is relatively safe and which may reduce subsequent embolic events. If the artery is completely occluded, some surgeons will consider a transcranial by-pass operation in which a branch of the superficial temporal artery is anastomosed to the middle cerebral artery on the surface of the brain. This appears to be an extremely safe undertaking but the indications for doing it remain rather obscure. In cases where the arterial disease is not considered surgically remedial, or when the general condition of the patient precludes anaesthesia, then drugs like aspirin, which reduce platelet aggregation may prevent further episodes by stopping platelets accumulating at sites of vessel disease.

THE FUTURE

There seems no doubt that the incidence of stroke is declining in the Western world at a rate of about 5 per cent per year. The explanation of this is uncertain but it seems probable that the recognition and effective treatment of hypertension is playing an important role. If this is so, then the reduction may be expected to continue as doctors and patients become increasingly aware of the dangers of sustained hypertension. The recognition that TIA often precedes completed stroke may also be contributory since medical and/or surgical treatment at that stage is probably effective in reducing the incidence of subsequent stroke. The main hope rests on preventive measures because it seems unlikely that one will be able to dramatically change the outcome of completed stroke once it has occurred. Once stroke has occurred, much requires to be done in terms of the organisation of rehabilitation facilities. Whether the arrival of the 'stroke unit' facilitates this remains to be seen; hopefully it will encourage greater collaboration between members of the health team.

REFERENCES

Adams, G. F. and Hurwitz, L. J. (1963). Mental barriers to recovery from strokes. *Lancet*, **ii**, 533-7.
Brocklehurst, J. C., Andrews, K., Richards, B. and Laycock, P. J. (1978) How much physical therapy for patients with stroke? *British Medical Journal*, **1**, 1307-10.
Fisher, C. M. (1959). Observations of the fundus oculi in transient monocular blindness. *Neurology*, **9**, 333-47.
Kannel, W. B. and Wolf, P. A. (1983). Epidemiology of cerebrovascular disease. In *Vascular Disease of the Central Nervous System*, pp. 1-24, (ed. Ross Russell, R. W.). Churchill Livingstone, Edinburgh.
Twitchell, T. E. (1951). The restoration of motor function following hemiplegia in man. *Brain*, **47**, 443-80.

BIBLIOGRAPHY

Barnett, H. J. M. (ed.) (1983). *Symposium on Cerebrovascular Disease. Neurological Clinics*. 1. W. B. Saunders Company, Philadelphia.
Ross Russell, R. W. (ed.) (1983). *Vascular Disease of the Central Nervous System*. Churchill Livingstone, Edinburgh.

Chapter 10

Hemiplegia - Assessment and Approach

by J. M. TODD BSc, MCSP *and* P. M. DAVIES MCSP, Dip Phys Ed

Lesions which result in hemiplegia occur in the brain or upper segments of the spinal cord and can affect any age group. The characteristic feature of hemiplegia is the loss of voluntary movement with alteration of muscle tone and sensation throughout one side of the body.

ASSESSMENT

A thorough assessment of each patient's problems is essential if the treatment is to be successful. The therapist needs to observe the patient closely while he moves against gravity and performs activities. She should watch him not only in the treatment area, but also in other instances which occur during his daily life. At first, these may be only in and around his bed, but later she will need to observe how he moves when he walks outside, is confronted by other people, climbs the stairs or sits down at the table to eat. Observation alone does not provide sufficient information as to why the patient has difficulties. The therapist needs to feel the difficulties as well. She must use her hands to feel muscle tone and the resistance it offers while the patient is moving. With her hands she can feel the ease with which he transfers his weight and maintains his balance. To understand what she observes and feels the therapist needs to remember that the inability to move normally is due to disturbed tone and reciprocal innervation, not to actual muscle weakness.

Assessment is a continuous process as even during one therapy session changes will occur and the treatment must be adjusted accordingly.

When assessing the problems the therapist is constantly comparing the way in which the patient moves to the way in which the same movement would normally be performed. In her treatment she will be trying to facilitate normal patterns of movement. It is essential, therefore, that she knows how each movement sequence should be carried out and how balance is maintained.

THE NORMAL POSTURAL REFLEX MECHANISM

To assess and treat the problems of the hemiplegic patient the factors underlying normal movement must be understood. The normal postural reflex mechanism which provides a background for movement has two types of automatic reaction: righting reactions and equilibrium reactions.

Righting reactions allow the normal position of the head in space and in relation to the body, and normal alignment of trunk and limbs (Bobath, 1978). They give the rotation within the body axis which is necessary for most activities (see Chapter 3).

Equilibrium reactions maintain and regain balance. More complex than the righting reactions, they may be either visible movements or invisible changes of tone against gravity. Basic patterns of movement evolve from the righting reactions of early childhood, which later become integrated with the equilibrium reactions (see Chapter 3) (Fiorentino, 1981).

The brain is continuously receiving sensory impulses from the periphery, informing it of the body's activities. All movement is in response to these sensory stimuli and is monitored by proprioceptors (in muscles and joints), extroceptors (in skin and subcutaneous tissue) and telereceptors (the eyes and ears). Without sensation human beings do not know how to move or how to react to various situations, but in the conscious state intention may govern these reactions.

Normal function of the body depends on the efficiency of the central nervous system as an organ of integration. Every skilled movement depends on:

NORMAL POSTURAL TONE

Postural tone, which is variable, provides the background on which movement is based, and is controlled at a subcortical level. It must be high enough to resist gravity yet still permit movement. Hypertonicity is loss of dynamic tone, giving stability without mobility. Hypotonicity precludes the stable posture necessary for movement. With each movement posture changes, and cannot be separated from it.

NORMAL RECIPROCAL INNERVATION

Reciprocal innervation allows graded action between agonists and antagonists (Bobath, 1974). Proximally the interaction results in a degree of co-contraction which provides fixation and stability. Distally, skilled movements are made possible by a greater degree of reciprocal inhibition.

NORMAL PATTERNS OF MOVEMENT

Movement takes place in patterns that are common to all although there are slight variations in the way different people perform the same activity. Normally, the brain is not aware of individual muscles, only of patterns of movement produced by the interaction of groups of muscles.

DIFFICULTIES ASSOCIATED WITH HEMIPLEGIA

When treating the hemiplegic patient it must be remembered that the problem is loss not only of voluntary control but also of normal movement patterns, with abnormal tone, abnormal sensation and the presence of stereotyped associated reactions.

Alteration in tone

It is important to note the distribution of abnormal tone and to observe factors which contribute to its increase or decrease.

After the onset of hemiplegia the abnormal quality of postural tone appears initially as hypotonus, but at a very early stage increased tone may become apparent in certain groups, e.g. finger flexors or retractors of the scapula, so that a mixture of flaccidity and spasticity is present. Tone usually changes and increases as the patient becomes more active. The basic tone may change gradually for 18 months or longer. When hypotonicity is present the tone is too low to initiate movement. There is a lack of resistance to passive movement and the patient is unable to hold a limb in any position. When hypertonus develops there is resistance to passive movement and active movement is difficult or impossible. The increase in tone is usually more marked in certain patterns involving the anti-gravity groups of muscles, i.e. the flexor groups in the arm and the extensor groups in the leg.

Reflex activity and alterations in posture may also affect the distribution of tone, e.g. there may be resistance to extension of the arm when it is held by the side but resistance to flexion if held above the head. If marked co-contraction is present, resistance to all passive movement may be felt (see Chapter 7). Effort, stress, fear and pain increase tone.

Associated reactions

Associated movements occur in the normal person during strenuous activity, but with hypertonicity they appear as associated reactions in abnormal stereotyped patterns which inhibit function.

Sensory disturbance

It is important to be aware of any reduction in sensory input although accurate testing is frequently difficult. Proprioception and stereognosis is noted in addition to superficial and deep sensation and temperature. Information about disturbance of body image and unilateral neglect is also recorded.

There may be disturbance of awareness of parts of the body in relation to each other or their position in space. Loss of sensation impairs the patient's ability to move and balance normally. In many cases, the deficit can be attributed to inattention towards the affected side rather than actual loss of feeling. Impairment of sensation can be improved with treatment, and there would seem to be many exceptions to the traditional belief that impaired sensation precludes functional recovery and that the loss is greater in the arm than the leg (see Chapter 6).

Loss of selective movement

The degree and quality of voluntary control is recorded carefully. Although many patients with hemiplegia appear able to move all parts of their bodies, they may be unable to move one part in isolation without other muscles acting simultaneously in a stereotyped mass pattern of movement. These synergies are stereotyped because the muscles that participate in the patterned motion and the strength of their responses are the same for every effort, regardless of demand. This primitive pattern response is a voluntary act, initiated when the patient wishes to perform a task (Perry, 1969). For example, he may be able to grip only while the elbow flexes and the shoulder adducts, or stand up with the hip and knee extended and the foot plantar flexed. Similarly, dorsiflexion of the foot may only be possible when the hip and knee are flexed.

The therapist must remember that not only are the arm and leg affected but the whole side, and therefore the trunk will be similarly affected. Movement does not become effective unless and until the undesired components of movements in these reflex patterns can be inhibited at the same time that the desired components are excited (Kottke, 1980).

Loss of balance reactions

Normally, with every movement, posture must be adjusted to maintain balance, but with altered tone the required reactions are impaired or absent. The presence or absence of such reactions and also their quality are noted during all the basic functional activities.

Communication

If speech is affected it is important to understand the deficit in order to modify instructions and suitably adapt the approach. There may be an actual language problem where there is difficulty expressing ideas or interpreting the written or spoken word, or there may be a purely sensory motor problem where correct articulation is hampered by loss of voluntary control. Often a combination of factors contributes to the difficulty.

Non-verbal communication in the form of head posture and movement as well as facial expression is often hampered by altered tone and sensation. All sensorimotor difficulties affecting movements of the tongue, lips, jaw and facial expression should be assessed and then treated by the physiotherapist. Difficulty with eating may arise because any movement problem which occurs throughout the body can be present inside the mouth.

APPROACH TO TREATMENT

The unilateral approach

It is generally accepted today that patients who have suffered a stroke need not spend the rest of their lives in bed, but most traditional methods of treatment are directed towards gaining independence by strengthening and training the sound side to compensate for the affected side. Many disadvantages are inherent in such methods:

1. The resultant one-sidedness accentuates the lack of sensation and awareness.

2. Relying on a tetrapod or stick for balance not only increases spasticity and abnormal associated reactions, but prevents use of the unaffected hand for functional tasks (the hand being solely involved in maintaining the patient in an upright position).

3. One-sidedness requires increased effort to perform any function, making movement tiring and difficult. Consequently, spasticity increases and movement becomes more abnormal in a self-perpetuating manner.

4. Progressive spasticity in the lower limb demands increasingly complex appliances which are difficult, if not impossible, for the patient to apply himself, and which may ultimately fail to control the position of the foot.

5. Increased tone in the upper limb leads to a distressingly obvious deformity which hinders mobility and everyday activities including washing and dressing.

6. The patient has no means of maintaining his balance or saving himself when he falls toward the hemiplegic side or backward as the stick or tetrapod would leave the floor. He is, therefore, very afraid of walking or moving while standing.

The bilateral or symmetrical approach

Preferable methods stress the need to re-educate movement throughout the body, realising that as the quality of movement improves function will automatically improve. They aim to normalise tone and to facilitate normal movement, thus providing the sensorimotor experience on which all learning is based. If the patient is allowed to move in an abnormal manner with abnormal muscle tone, such experience of movement will be all he knows and correction afterwards will be more difficult. Everyone, regardless of age, should be treated in a way which gives the opportunity to develop maximum potential (Adler et al, 1980). Even if dramatic motor recovery is not achieved each patient will be able to function better and live more normally. For those who have not reached complete independence at least they will feel safer and move more freely, and therefore will be easier to help.

All treatment should be directed towards obtaining symmetry with normal balance reactions throughout the body. The affected side should be bombarded with every form of stimulation possible to make the patient aware of himself as a whole person again. Re-education of bilateral righting and equilibrium reactions in the head and trunk are vital if independent balance is to be regained.

From the beginning, the patient must be discouraged from using the good arm to assist every movement as this reduces stimulation of the normal postural reflex mechanism and could prevent return of control on the affected side.

The patient should never struggle to perform an activity which is too advanced for him. Any movement he is unable to manage himself should be assisted to make the action smooth and easy without being passive. Excess effort induces abnormal tone and unwanted associated reactions (Brunnstrom, 1970). Assistance should be gradually lessened until he performs the movement unaided. Repetition re-establishes a memory of the feeling of normal movement.

When and if movement returns to the limbs it will be in abnormal patterns. It is most important to make the patient very aware of unwanted abnormal movements or associated reactions; such stereotyped patterns must be firmly corrected at once to prevent them becoming established habits (Kottke, 1980). It is vital to teach him to inhibit such reactions himself, e.g. he must learn to stop the arm flexing up or the leg shooting into extension each time he does anything.

It is important that the fight against the hemiplegic posture be carried out on a *24-hour basis* and not only by the intermittent therapy session (Ruskin, 1982).

If everyone in contact with the patient reinforces the approach from the start, hours of physiotherapy time will be saved, easier and quicker learning is facilitated and the final result will be far more satisfactory. Because it is an overall management of the patient, he is never 'too ill to treat'.

INSTRUCTION FOR NURSES AND RELATIVES

Careful instruction and involvement of nurses and relatives are of paramount importance and will eliminate or minimise many of the complications associated with hemiplegia.

For the nurses

POSITION OF THE BED IN THE WARD (Fig. 10/1)

The patient benefits if the position of his bed in the ward or room makes him look *across* his affected side at general activity or items of interest, e.g. television (Fig. 10/1). Similarly, with the locker on his affected side, he has to reach across the midline for a glass of water, tissues, etc.

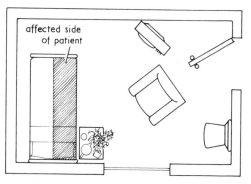

FIG. 10/1 Position of the bed in ward

NURSING PROCEDURES (Fig. 10/2)

Great therapeutic value can be incorporated in routine procedures by encouraging the patient's participation. While bathing him in bed, the nurse can focus his attention on each part of the body by naming it, and asking for his help to facilitate washing, e.g. rolling on to his side with her aid, and holding up the affected arm with

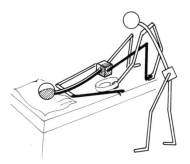

FIG. 10/2 Presentation of bedpan by nurse. (The right side of the patient is affected and is shown in black)

the sound hand; or rolling actively as she is making the bed. When a bedpan, medicine or food are brought to the patient, the approach should be from his affected side, thereby increasing his awareness of it (Fig. 10/2).

POSITIONING THE PATIENT IN BED

The bed must have a firm mattress on a solid base and the height should be adjustable. It will need to be lowered to enable easy and correct transfer of the patient into a chair. Five or six pillows will be required to maintain the correct alignment of the head, trunk and limbs. The patient's position should be changed frequently to avoid chest complications, pressure sores and discomfort. Two- to three-hourly turning is advisable in the early stages while the patient is confined to bed. Even when he is out of bed during the day and more active, correct positioning at night must continue.

POSITION LYING ON THE AFFECTED SIDE (Fig. 10/3)

1. The head is forward with the trunk straight and in line.
2. The underneath shoulder is protracted with the forearm supinated.
3. The underneath leg is extended at the hip and slightly flexed at the knee.
4. The upper leg is in front on one pillow.
5. Nothing should be placed in the hand or under the sole of the foot because this would stimulate undesirable reflex activity, i.e. flexion in the hand and extensor thrust in the leg.

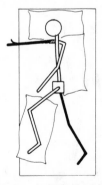 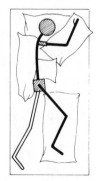

FIG. 10/3 (*left*) Position of patient lying on the affected side

FIG. 10/4 (*right*) Position of patient lying on sound side

POSITION LYING ON THE SOUND SIDE (Fig. 10/4)

1. Patient is in full side lying, not just a quarter turn.
2. The head is forward with the trunk straight and in line. If necessary a pillow under the waist will elongate the affected side further.
3. The affected shoulder should be protracted with the arm forward on a pillow.
4. The upper leg is in front on one pillow. (The foot must be fully supported by the pillow and not hang over the end in inversion.)
5. A pillow is behind the back.
6. Nothing should be placed in the hand or under the sole of the foot.

POSITION IN SUPINE (Fig. 10/5)

1. The head is rotated towards the affected side and flexed to the good side.
2. The trunk is elongated on the affected side.
3. The affected shoulder is protracted on a pillow with the arm elevated or straight by the side.
4. A pillow is placed under the hip to prevent retraction of the pelvis and lateral rotation of the leg.
5. Nothing should be placed in the hand or under the sole of the foot.

In the supine position there will be the greatest increase in abnormal tone because of the influence of reflex activity, and this position should be avoided whenever possible.

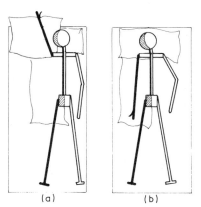

FIG. 10/5 (a) Position in supine with the arm elevated. (b) Position in supine with the arm at the side on a pillow

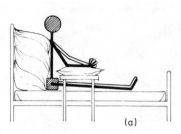 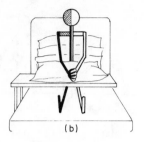

FIG. 10/6 Sitting in bed: (a) side view and (b) front view

SITTING IN BED (Fig. 10/6)

Sitting in bed for meals is not desirable, but may be necessary to fit in with staffing and ward routine. The half-lying position should never be used, as there is increased flexion of the trunk with extension in the legs and greater risk of pressure sores.

1. The patient should be as upright as possible with the head and trunk in line and his weight evenly distributed on both buttocks.
2. The affected arm is protracted at the shoulder, both hands are clasped together and placed forward on a bed-table.
3. The legs are straight and not laterally rotated.

TRANSFERRING FROM BED TO CHAIR (Fig. 10/7)

Much damage can be done to the patient's shoulder as well as to the nurse's or therapist's back during this manoeuvre if it is performed incorrectly. It can also be a very frightening time for the patient if he is suddenly transferred without any explanation or chance to move himself. The following is an easy, safe, therapeutic way of transferring a patient from bed to chair.

The chair is placed in position on the affected side and the patient is rolled or assisted on to his affected side. The helper places one hand under the patient's affected shoulder, swings his legs over the edge of the bed with her other hand, and brings the patient to the sitting position. During this phase elongation of the trunk occurs, and if a pause is needed to rearrange clothes, etc., the patient can be propped on the affected elbow and take weight through it (Fig. 10/7a).

The patient, with his hands clasped together in front of him, is helped to move to the edge of the bed. He transfers his weight over to one side and then to the other and moves the opposite hip forward each time as if he was walking on his buttocks. The assistant's arms are placed under the patient's shoulders with her

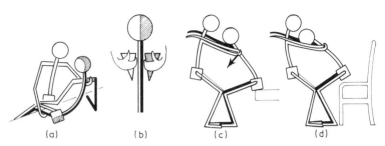

FIG. 10/7 Transferring from bed to chair. (a) Bringing the patient from lying to sitting over the side of the bed. (b) Starting position for transfer, from behind patient. (c) Starting position for transfer from side. (d) Pivot round to chair – seat well back in chair

hands over the scapulae while her legs wedge the patient's feet and knees (Fig. 10/7b and c). The patient's arms are placed round the helper's waist or on her shoulders, but he must not grip his hands together. If he does he will pull on the assistant's neck so that she takes his weight instead of him bearing weight through his legs. His trunk is then pulled well forward and he is brought to standing by pressure forward and down on the shoulders, so that his weight goes equally through both legs. No attempt is made to lift him up at all. The assistant's weight counter-balances the patient's, and with shoulders and knees fixed he is pivoted round to sit on the chair (Fig. 10/7c and d).

Transferring in such a way emphasises the hemiplegic side and encourages weight-bearing and weight transference to that side.

TRANSFERRING MORE ACTIVELY

A stool or chair placed well in front of the patient will enable him to come forward more easily, until, with his clasped hands on the chair, his head is over his feet. The assistant holds his trochanters and helps him to lift his buttocks and turn them to sit well back in the chair, on the bed or toilet (Fig. 10/8).

Once he has learned to transfer in this way he can progress to transferring on his own. The same movement sequence is used, only now without the support of the stool. His clasped hands are stretched out in front of him (Fig. 10/9).

Transferring will then be a preparation for standing up from sitting, i.e. the patient will have learned to bring his weight sufficiently far forward over his feet to enable him to come to standing without pushing back into extension.

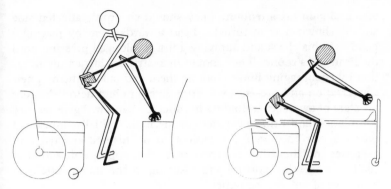

FIG. 10/8 (*left*) Transferring more actively with assistance

FIG. 10/9 (*right*) Transferring more actively on his own

SITTING IN A CHAIR (Fig. 10/10)

A better sitting posture can be obtained in an upright chair.

1. The chair should be of sufficient height to allow the patient's hips, knees and ankles to be at approximately right angles when he sits well back in the chair.
2. His head and trunk are in line with the body-weight evenly distributed over both buttocks. His hands are clasped and placed well forward on a table in front of him.

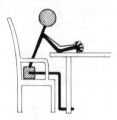

FIG. 10/10 Sitting in a chair

For the relatives

Within the first few days the physiotherapist should meet the patient's relatives and explain his difficulties and how they can help to overcome them. They will appreciate being involved, and having something concrete to do while visiting; they often have more time to spend with the patient than either nurses or therapists.

When visiting a hemiplegic patient, relatives tend to sit on his unaffected side as his head is usually looking that way, and it is easier to gain his attention. They should sit on his affected side and be shown how to turn his head towards them by placing a hand over his cheek and applying a firm prolonged pressure until the head stays round. They should then strive to attract his attention by encouraging him to look at them and talk to them. Their conversation and presence will stimulate him and help to restore his state of awareness. Holding his affected hand will give sensory stimulation and bring awareness of the limb. Initially, interested relatives can encourage the patient to do his self-assisted arm exercises and later, they can encourage other appropriate activities such as correcting posture and assisting in the therapeutic performance of self-care activities.

REFERENCES

Adler, M. K., Brown, C. C. and Action, P. (1980). Stroke rehabilitation – is age a determinant? *Journal of the American Geriatric Society*, 28(11), 499–503.

Bobath, B. (ed.) (1978). *Adult Hemiplegia: Evaluation and Treatment.* William Heinemann Medical Books Limited, London.

Bobath, K. (1974). *The Motor Deficit in Patients with Cerebral Palsy.* (Medical education and information unit of the Spastics Society.) William Heinemann Medical Books Limited, London.

Brunnstrom, S. (1970). *Movement Therapy in Hemiplegia. A Neurophysiological Approach.* Harper and Row, Hagerstown, USA.

Fiorentino, M. R. (1981). *A Basis for Sensorimotor Development – Normal and Abnormal.* Thomas, Springfield.

Kottke, F. J. (1980). From reflex to skill: the training of co-ordination. *Archives of Physical Medicine and Rehabilitation*, 61, 551–61.

Perry, J. (1969). The mechanics of walking in hemiplegia. *Clinical Orthopaedics*, 63, 23–31.

Ruskin, A. P. (1982). Understanding stroke and its rehabilitation. Current concepts of cerebrovascular disease. *Stroke*, 17(6), 27–32.

Chapter 11

Hemiplegia – Physiotherapy

by J. M. TODD BSc, MCSP *and* P. M. DAVIES MCSP, Dip Phys Ed

Treatment must commence immediately after the onset of hemiplegia. Progress will be more rapid if the patient is treated two or three times a day in the early stages, even if only for 10 minutes at a time.

The patient's ability and tolerance are directly related to the site and severity of the lesion and his physical condition prior to the illness rather than to the length of time since the incident. Treatment must progress accordingly.

Most patients are able to sit out of bed within a few days and it is important for them to move from the ward or bedroom so that they are stimulated by the change of surroundings. Shaving, wearing make-up and dressing in everyday clothes all help to overcome the feeling of being an invalid.

Rehabilitation in a hospital department has the advantage of invaluable contact with other people and patients with similar problems as well as the stimulation of leaving home and dealing independently with new situations. Many stroke patients never attend hospital and are treated in their homes. The physiotherapist in attendance must use all her ingenuity to provide a similar rehabilitation without special apparatus and to overcome the limitations of space. However, adequately instructed relatives and friends can provide a very effective learning environment and are often able to give more reinforcement to the concept.

The following outline of physiotherapy is not a fixed regime or programme for all patients but provides suggestions for activities which will be of benefit to many. Careful and continuous assessment must be made as the problems arising from hemiplegia will be different for each individual and may alter from day to day. Treatment must be carefully selected and progressed.

For simplicity the activities have been divided into sections but the therapist must be aware that one part of the body cannot be treated in isolation, e.g. working on the leg in sitting or standing may adversely affect the trunk and arm if they are flexing and retracting with effort. Similarly, attention must always be given to the trunk before normal movement of the limbs can be achieved.

ACTIVITIES IN LYING

Mobilising the arm

Although most hemiplegics with severe paralysis will never regain full functional use of the affected arm, it is important that it should remain fully mobile. A stiff painful arm impedes balance and movement of the whole body, limits treatment and interferes with daily living. If full passive elevation of the arm is performed every day the complication need never arise. The movement should be performed in such a way that no pain is elicited. Pain around the shoulder would indicate that sensitive structures around the joint were being compromised (Davies, 1985).

ELONGATION OF THE TRUNK (Fig. 11/1)

The patient lies in half crook lying with his affected leg flexed and adducted. Place one hand on his pelvis, the other hand over his shoulder and elongate his trunk until his hip remains forward off the bed.

MOVEMENT OF THE SCAPULA (Fig. 11/2)

One hand is placed over his scapula, the other supporting his arm. With the shoulder protracted, the scapula is elevated and

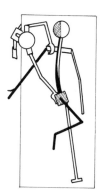

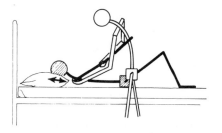

FIG. 11/1 (*left*) Elongation of the trunk

FIG. 11/2 (*below*) Mobilisation of the scapula

depressed until spasticity is released and it moves freely. While the scapula is being moved, the arm is eased into lateral rotation.

ELEVATION OF THE ARM (Fig. 11/3)

Maintaining lateral rotation at the shoulder, the elbow is extended, and the arm lifted into full elevation with supination of the forearm, extension of the wrist and fingers and wide abduction of the thumb. The arm is moved until it will stay in elevation without pulling down into flexion.

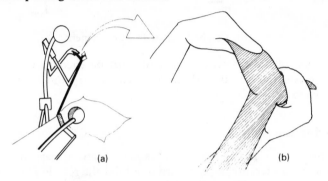

(a)   (b)

FIG. 11/3 (a) Elevation of the arm. (b) Close-up of hand grip

ABDUCTION OF THE ARM (Fig. 11/4)

From full elevation the arm is taken out to the side in abduction and up again maintaining the extension at the elbow, fingers and wrist with supination of the forearm.

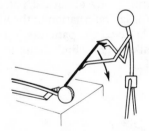

FIG. 11/4 Arm out to abduction

SELF-ASSISTED ARM MOVEMENTS (Fig. 11/5)

The patient is taught at an early stage to clasp his hands together, interlacing the fingers, and to lift them up into full elevation. The movement should begin with protraction of the shoulders and

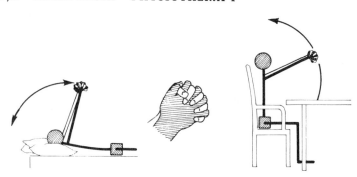

FIG. 11/5 Self-assisted arm movement

extension of the elbow. The patient must be encouraged to perform this activity frequently throughout the day and to continue this when he is sitting in a chair.

Moving the leg

To prevent associated reactions his hands can be clasped in elevation or, preferably, he can learn to inhibit the reaction by letting the arm remain relaxed at his side.

HIP AND KNEE FLEXION OVER THE SIDE OF THE BED (Fig. 11/6)
Place his leg over the side of the bed with his hip extended and hold his knee in flexion and his foot in full dorsiflexion until there is no resistance. Maintain the position of the foot and knee and guide the leg up on to the bed while he actively assists. Repeat the movement preventing any abnormal pattern occurring, e.g. extension of the knee or lateral rotation of the hip.

If the exercise is perfected the patient will be able to bring his leg forward when walking and climb stairs in a normal manner, one foot after the other.

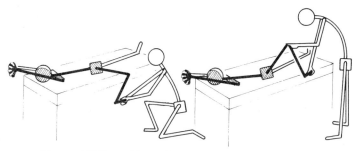

FIG. 11/6 Hip and knee flexion over the side of the bed

KNEE EXTENSION WITH DORSIFLEXION (Fig. 11/7)

His foot is held in dorsiflexion, and his leg is moved from full flexion into extension without his toes pushing down and without rotation at the hip. The patient takes the weight of his limb, making it feel light throughout.

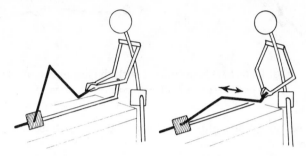

FIG. 11/7 Control of knee extension through range

HIP CONTROL WITH THE FOOT ON THE BED (Fig. 11/8)

In crook lying, the patient moves alternate knees smoothly into medial and lateral rotation without his other leg moving and without tilting his pelvis.

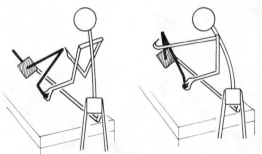

FIG. 11/8 Hip control with the foot on the bed

HIP CONTROL WITH THE HIP IN EXTENSION (Fig. 11/9)

In half crook lying with his affected leg flexed and adducted the patient lifts his affected hip forward off the bed and, maintaining hip extension, moves his knee out and in.

ISOLATED KNEE EXTENSION (Fig. 11/10)

Place the patient's foot against your thigh to maintain dorsiflexion

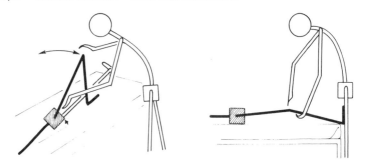

FIG. 11/9 (*left*) Hip control with the hip in extension
FIG. 11/10 (*right*) Isolated knee extension

and ask him to straighten his knee without pushing down with his foot.

Bridging

BRIDGING WITH ROTATION OF THE PELVIS (Fig. 11/11)

Maintaining good extension at the hips the patient rotates his pelvis equally to either side while preventing any associated movement in his affected leg.

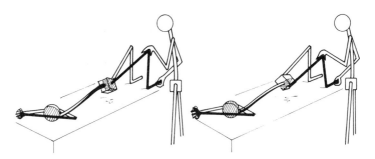

FIG. 11/11 Bridging with rotation of the pelvis

BRIDGING ON THE AFFECTED LEG (Fig. 11/12)

The patient bridges on both legs and lifts his sound foot off the bed while maintaining the same position of the pelvis and affected leg.

Progress to raising and lowering his hips several times.

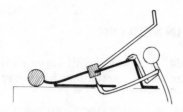

FIG. 11/12 Bridging on the affected leg

Rolling

Correct rolling brings awareness of the affected side, release of spasticity by rotation between the shoulder girdle and pelvis and facilitates active movement in the trunk and limbs.

TO THE AFFECTED SIDE (Fig. 11/13)

With his affected arm in abduction, the patient is asked to lift his head and bring his sound arm across to touch his other hand. Instruct him to lift his sound leg across his affected leg without pushing off from the bed.

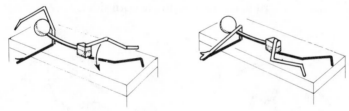

FIG. 11/13 Rolling to the affected side

TO THE SOUND SIDE (Fig. 11/14)

The patient's affected leg is guided over his other leg with less and less assistance until he can perform the action himself. He can clasp both hands together and rotate his upper trunk by moving both arms to the sound side.

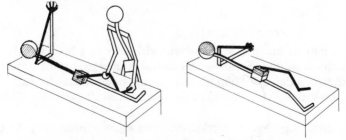

FIG. 11/14 Rolling to the sound side

ACTIVITIES IN SITTING

The patient should be moved into sitting as soon as possible even if he is not fully conscious, to stimulate balance reactions.

WEIGHT TRANSFERENCE FROM SIDE TO SIDE; FEET UNSUPPORTED (Figs. 11/15 and 11/16)

The therapist sits on the patient's affected side and draws his body toward her so that his body-weight passes through one buttock only. Elongate his trunk on that side and inhibit any flexion in his arm. His good leg is then free to be raised in the air. His body-weight is shifted over his sound side, and his head is placed in position if it does not right automatically. Side flexion of his trunk on the affected side is facilitated by giving pressure at his waist with one hand and encouraging him to lift his buttock clear of the bed.

The movement is repeated in a rhythmic manner until automatic head and trunk righting occurs to both sides.

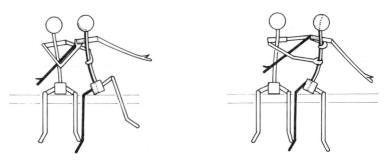

FIG. 11/15 (*left*) Weight transference in sitting to the affected side

FIG. 11/16 (*right*) Weight transference in sitting to the sound side

MOVING IN SITTING (Fig. 11/17)

The patient must move in sitting without using his hand. He is taught to shuffle or walk on his buttocks forwards and backwards and later sideways. Help him by placing one hand under each hip or thigh and then rock and move him from side to side.

WEIGHT TRANSFERENCE THROUGH THE ARMS BEHIND (Fig. 11/18)

Both arms are taken carefully behind the patient with his hands

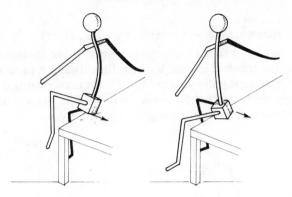

FIG. 11/17 Moving in sitting

being supported on the therapist's hands. Extension is facilitated by using a sharp push-pull action up through his arms until they support his weight. Progress by shifting his weight from one side to the other without his elbow bending.

WEIGHT TRANSFERENCE THROUGH THE ARM SIDEWAYS (Fig. 11/19)

A similar activity is practised with his affected arm at the side. His hand is placed flat on the bed or plinth and with one hand under his axilla and the other supporting his elbow, the therapist draws the patient toward her elongating his trunk at the same time.

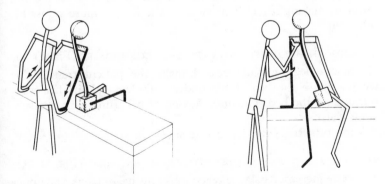

FIG. 11/18 (*left*) Weight transference through the arms behind

FIG. 11/19 (*right*) Weight transference through the arm sideways

INDEPENDENT MOVEMENT OF THE LEGS (Fig. 11/20)

To prepare for walking teach the patient to move his legs without moving his trunk. Lift one leg at a time asking him to make it feel light by taking the weight himself. He must maintain control while his leg is lowered on to the bed. Ask him to keep his trunk still and not to lean back throughout the activity.

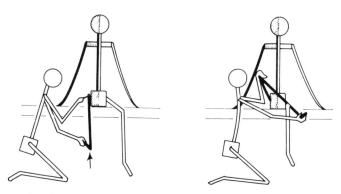

FIG. 11/20 (*left*) Lifting one leg at a time in sitting

FIG. 11/21 (*right*) Sitting with affected leg crossed, inhibiting extensor thrust

INHIBITION OF EXTENSOR THRUST (Fig. 11/21)

The patient's affected leg is crossed over the sound one and is held in full flexion and lateral rotation with the foot and toes in full dorsiflexion until it will stay in position on its own. Maintain inhibition at his foot and ask the patient to uncross his leg and lower it, making it feel light and to raise it once more across his other leg.

RAISING THE HIP IN SITTING WITH THE LEGS CROSSED (Fig. 11/22)

While one leg remains crossed make the patient transfer his weight on to the hip of his underneath leg and lift his other buttock off the bed. Facilitate flexion of his trunk with pressure at his waist.

Repeat the same activity to both sides.

BALANCE REACTIONS OF THE UPPER TRUNK AND HEAD (Fig. 11/23)

Facilitate increased balance reactions of his head, trunk and upper limbs by lifting both legs together and rotating them to either side. Alter the speed and position to obtain the required reactions

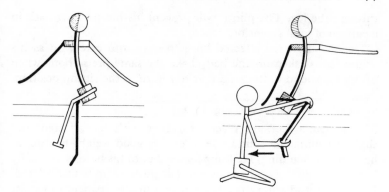

FIG. 11/22 (*left*) Sitting with crossed legs raising alternate hip off the bed

FIG. 11/23 (*right*) Lift both legs together and rotate them

in the rest of the body. The affected arm should assist balance in a similar way to the sound arm and not pull into flexion.

STANDING FROM A HIGH BED OR PLINTH TO THE GROUND (Fig. 11/24)

The patient wriggles to the edge of the bed and puts his affected leg to the floor without his foot pushing down. If necessary mobilise his foot by pressing down over the front of his ankle to ensure that his heel is on the ground and that dorsiflexion is possible.

When his affected foot is on the floor practise isolated knee extension before bringing his hip forward to take full weight

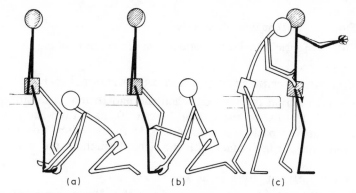

(a)   (b)   (c)

FIG. 11/24 Standing from sitting. (a) Affected leg on the ground with foot dorsiflexed. (b) Isolated knee extension. (c) Coming off on to the affected leg

through the leg. The plinth will prevent his hip pushing back in a pattern of total extension.

Do not allow his affected knee to snap into extension as his sound leg is taken off the bed. Take the same precautions when lifting his sound buttock up first to return to the sitting position.

STANDING FROM A CHAIR (Fig. 11/25)

The patient's feet are placed together with his affected foot slightly behind the sound one to ensure good weight-bearing as he comes to standing. He leans forward until his head is vertically in front of his feet and stands without pushing up with his hand. If his trunk and arm retract too much at first the patient can assist standing by pushing his arms out in front of him with hands clasped together. When returning to sitting his affected foot remains behind and his head is kept well forward while his bottom is placed far back in the chair. He must not put a hand down on the chair as this spoils the symmetry and alters the weight-bearing. Instead he should look behind and back up until he is correctly aligned with the chair.

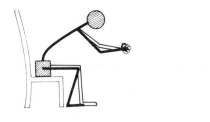 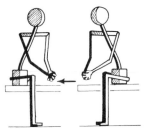

FIG. 11/25 (*left*) Standing from a chair

FIG. 11/26 (*right*) Moving the bottom from side to side in sitting

MOVING IN SITTING WITH THE FEET ON THE FLOOR (Fig. 11/26)

A similar action is practised when the patient moves in sitting. With his feet flat on the ground he can lift his bottom and place it forward or back and from one side to the other. His heels should remain in contact with the floor throughout the activity.

TRUNK CONTROL (Figs. 11/27 and 11/28)

With his hands clasped in front of him, and elbows extended, he can practise reaching out to either side, well forward and down to his feet.

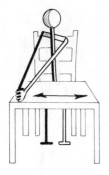 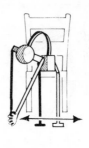

FIG. 11/27 (*left*) Reaching sideways and forward

FIG. 11/28 (*right*) Reaching down to feet

ACTIVITIES IN STANDING

Correct weight-bearing at an early stage provides good afferent stimulation and is a most effective way of normalising tone. Preparation for walking can be carried out adequately in an area of one square metre. It is of no benefit to practise walking with a patient who is unable either to take weight on his affected leg or bring it forward in a reasonably normal manner unless these can be facilitated. The same applies to someone who already walks with a poor gait pattern because repetition merely reinforces the experience of incorrect movements which in time may actually contribute to a reduction in ability. It is better to assess the difficulty carefully and practise relevant activities.

Weight-bearing on the affected leg
(Preparation for the stance phase of gait)

1. Standing on the patient's affected side draw his weight towards you, giving as much support as he requires. Ask him to take steps forward with his sound leg. Prevent his knee from snapping back into extension by keeping his hip well forward.
2. In the same position ask the patient to place his sound foot lightly on and off a step in front of him (Fig. 11/29).
3. Repeat the activity with the step placed well out to the side. Encourage the patient to keep his affected hip against your hip (Fig. 11/30).
4. Still preventing his knee from locking back ask the patient to

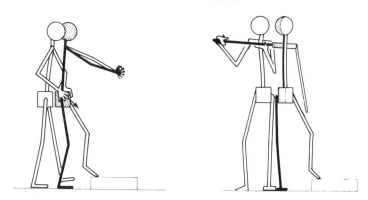

FIG. 11/29 (*left*) Placing the sound leg on a step

FIG. 11/30 (*right*) Stepping out to the side with the sound leg

draw large letters on the floor with his sound foot, ensuring weight-bearing on a mobile leg (Fig. 11/31).

5. Make the patient stand on his affected leg and lightly place his sound foot at a right angle in front or behind the other foot, without transferring his weight on to it (Fig. 11/32). If the activity is performed accurately it helps him to gain control of the hip abductors and extensors.

6. Place the patient's affected leg on a 15cm (6in) step in front of him. With your hand pushing down on his knee and keeping his weight well forward, he steps up on to the step (Fig. 11/33).

7. Practise stepping down with his sound leg placing it further

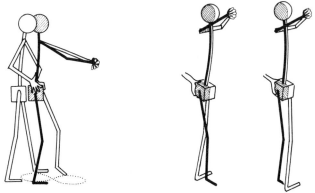

FIG. 11/31 (*left*) Making a figure-of-eight with the sound leg

FIG. 11/32 (*right*) Placing the sound foot at right angles to the hemiplegic foot

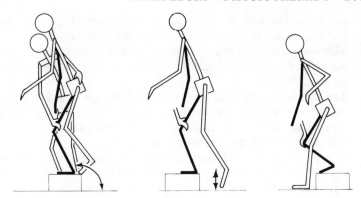

FIG. 11/33 (*left*) Stepping up with the affected leg on the step

FIG. 11/34 (*centre*) Putting the sound leg further and further back (Eros)

FIG. 11/35 (*right*) With the affected leg on the step, step up and over

and further back, and tapping it on the floor behind keeping the weight forward on his affected leg (Fig. 11/34).

8. Put his affected leg on the step and help the patient to push up and step right over and back again (Fig. 11/35).

Releasing the knee and moving the hemiplegic leg
(Preparation for the swing phase of gait)

1. The patient stands with his feet close together. Guide his pelvis forward and down to release his knee on the affected side. Instruct him to straighten it again without pushing his whole

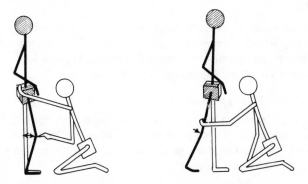

FIG. 11/36 (*left*) Releasing the hemiplegic leg in standing

FIG. 11/37 (*right*) Releasing the knee with hemiplegic leg behind side back. His heel must remain in contact with the floor, this is only possible if his pelvis drops forward (Fig. 11/36).

2. The same activity is practised in step standing with his affected leg behind, and the weight forward over his extended sound leg (Fig. 11/37).

3. The patient stands with the weight on his sound leg. Facilitate small steps backward with the other foot by holding his toes dorsiflexed and instructing him not to push down. Do not allow him to hitch his hip back (Fig. 11/38).

4. The patient walks sideways along a line crossing one foot in front of the other. When his sound leg takes a step, his affected hip must be kept well forward so that his knee does not snap back into extension (Fig. 11/39).

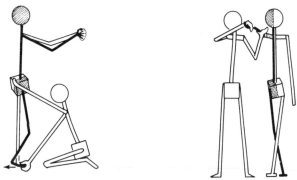

FIG. 11/38 (*left*) Taking small steps backward with affected leg

FIG. 11/39 (*right*) Walking sideways behind a line

Stairs

Climbing stairs at an early stage, even before independent gait is achieved, is both therapeutic and functional. The patient is taught to perform the activity in a normal manner, i.e. one foot on each step and without the support of the hand-rail.

ASCENDING (Figs. 11/40 and 11/41)

In the early stages it may be necessary for the therapist to lift his affected leg on to the step rather than allowing him to struggle. Support his affected knee as he steps up with his sound leg and keep his weight well forward.

DESCENDING (Fig. 11/42)

Guide the pelvis well forward on his affected side as he puts the

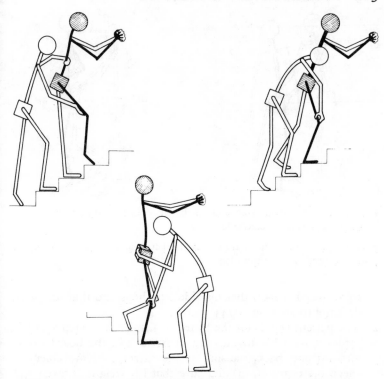

FIG. 11/40 (*above left*) Climbing stairs assisting the affected leg up

FIG. 11/41 (*above right*) Climbing stairs supporting the affected knee to step up

FIG. 11/42 (*below*) Descending stairs – hand supporting the affected knee

foot down, preventing the leg pulling into adduction. The therapist's hand on his knee will give support as he steps down with his sound leg.

Activities on the tilt board (Figs. 11/43 and 11/44)

The tilt board is not essential for treatment but is most helpful when re-educating correct transference of weight.

1. Stand on the floor behind the patient and help him to step on to the tilt board with one foot on either side. His feet should be parallel to one another throughout the exercise. Tilt the board slowly from side to side, pausing at each extreme to correct the patient's position and make sure that his hip comes

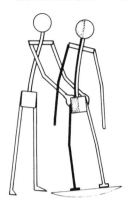 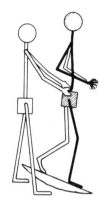

FIG. 11/43 (*left*) Stride standing on the tilt board – side lengthening as weight comes over affected side

FIG. 11/44 (*right*) Step standing on the tilt board – hemiplegic leg in front – weight over the front leg

    right over his foot, that his side lengthens and that his pelvis does not rotate (Fig. 11/43).

2. The patient stands on the board so that he is in step standing across it with his affected leg in front. Tilt the board slowly forward and back, pausing at the extreme of movement to check his position, making sure that his weight is taken well forward over the front foot without the pelvis rotating. His feet must remain parallel (Fig. 11/44).

3. The same activity is performed with his affected leg behind.

Facilitation of gait

Once the patient has sufficient tone and movement in his leg, walking can be assisted providing the therapist or relative is able to prevent abnormal patterns of movement and a reasonably normal gait can be facilitated. His pelvis is held on either side from behind and the action is made as smooth and rhythmic as possible. It is important to keep the affected hip well forward during the stance phase on that side so that the knee does not snap back into extension (Fig. 11/45). Downward pressure on the pelvis during the swing phase helps him to release the knee instead of hitching the hip to bring the leg forward.

The arms may be held forward to help overcome any flexion and retraction on the affected side or remain at his side without any associated increase of tone.

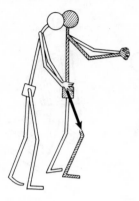

FIG. 11/45 Preventing the knee 'snapping back' into extension. The arrow shows the direction of the assistant's pressure (downwards and forwards)

As walking improves less assistance is required and a normal reciprocal arm swing can be facilitated by lightly rotating the trunk from the pelvis or shoulders.

To be confident when walking the patient needs to be able to turn his head, to talk, and to step to one side to avoid obstacles which means he can regain his balance and save himself automatically.

USE OF A STICK

If balance and weight transference are properly trained the patient should not need to lean on a stick. Avoid the use of a tetrapod at all costs as it is clumsy, unsightly and prevents the patient from using his sound hand for more skilled tasks.

Activities on the mat

To assist the patient getting down on to the mat stand behind him and ask him to step forward with the sound leg and kneel down on his affected leg. The affected hip is supported from behind by the therapist's knee to prevent him from collapsing as he brings the other knee down (Fig. 11/46).

1. In kneel standing support him from behind, with your arms over the front of his shoulders and your hands behind each side of his pelvis. Move his weight sideways over his affected leg, with his trunk lengthening on that side and his hip kept

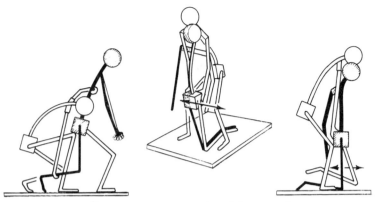

FIG. 11/46 (*left*) Ässisting the patient to kneel down on the mat

FIG. 11/47 (*centre*) Kneel standing – transfer weight over affected leg – hip forward

FIG. 11/48 (*right*) Stepping forward with sound knee – affected hip stable

well forward. Repeat the movement to the sound side. The patient should practise holding the position with the weight fully over each side, with less and less assistance (Fig. 11/47).

2. Also in kneel standing the patient takes steps forward and back with his sound knee, while keeping his affected hip stable (Fig. 11/48).

3. With assistance the patient sits down to either side, and learns to balance in side sitting without using his hands to support him (Fig. 11/49).

4. The patient steps forward with his sound foot and practises activities balancing in half kneel standing, for example tapping lightly on the floor with his foot (Fig. 11/50).

5. The patient can get up from the floor by kneeling up on both

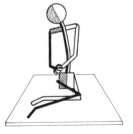
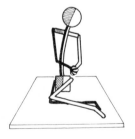

FIG. 11/49 Side sitting from kneeling

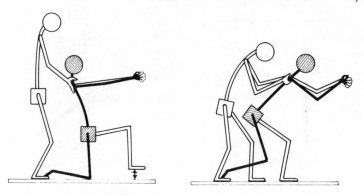

FIG. 11/50 (*left*) Half kneel standing – tapping with sound foot

FIG. 11/51 (*right*) Assisting the patient to stand from kneeling

knees, stepping forward with his sound foot, and standing up. Assistance is given by the therapist placing her hands under his shoulders to guide him well forward as he pushes up to standing (Fig. 11/51).

It is worth mastering these activities as they will also enable the patient to get in and out of the bath without using aids and, even if complete independence is not attained, the assistance required will be much less strenuous.

ACTIVITIES FOR THE RECOVERING ARM

When the hemiplegic arm shows signs of recovery every effort must be made to encourage movement and restore function as much as possible.

There is usually difficulty in isolating movement to one part of the limb, and in stabilising proximal joints while the hand performs more skilled actions. Total patterns of movement tend to dominate.

In lying

1. After inhibiting the arm fully in elevation ask the patient to let it stay there, and then move it slightly in all directions with the elbow extended. Gradually increase the range until he can lower it slowly to his side and lift it again, and take it out sideways to full abduction and up to vertical again (Fig. 11/52).

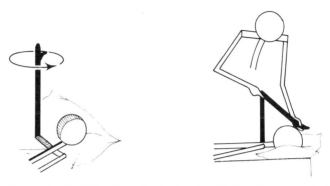

FIG. 11/52 (*left*) Small circles in the air with the elbow extended

FIG. 11/53 (*right*) Touching the head and up again

2. Ask the patient to touch his head (and lift his hand up again) without his elbow pulling down to his side. He can also place his hand on the opposite shoulder and lift it again. The therapist can assist by maintaining extension of his fingers and thumb as he does so and by reminding him that his elbow must remain in the same position (Fig. 11/53).

3. While the therapist holds his hand in extension and his forearm supinated, ask him to extend and flex his elbow; small movements without the shoulder participating (Fig. 11/54).

4. (a) Holding a pole with both hands let him lower it and raise it slowly while maintaining elbow extension (Fig. 11/55).
   (b) Practise walking his hands along the pole, while it is held in elevation.

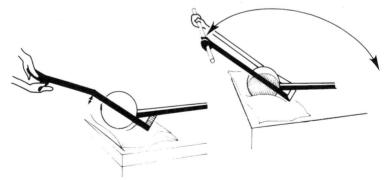

FIG. 11/54 (*left*) Flexion and extension of the elbow with the hand in dorsiflexion

FIG. 11/55 (*right*) Holding a pole in both hands, lowering and raising it

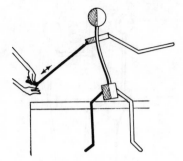

FIG. 11/56 Protective extension sideways – hand outstretched

In sitting

1. Practise protective extension sideways with his hand on the therapist's hand, giving small quick pushing movements up through the extended arm, until the arm can remain straight even when the therapist lets it go and the outstretched hand lands on the plinth (Fig. 11/56).
2. The patient holds a towel in his affected hand and allows the therapist to swing it round freely without him letting go, or pulling into total flexion to maintain his grip (Fig. 11/57).
3. Hold the rolled towel vertically in front of him and ask him to grip and release it, while walking his hand upwards. He must maintain elbow extension and shoulder protraction (Fig. 11/58).

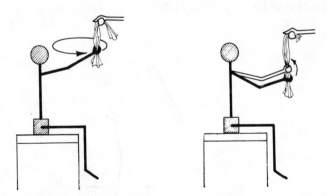

FIG. 11/57 (*left*) Holding a towel in the affected hand

FIG. 11/58 (*right*) Holding rolled towel, vertically walk hand upward

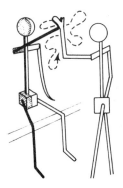

FIG. 11/59 Place hand flat against the therapist's hand and move without resistance

4. Place his hand flat against yours and ask him to follow your hand wherever it moves without resistance (Fig. 11/59).

In standing

1. Lift the patient's arm into elevation and ask him to leave it there when it feels light. The movement will be easier if his weight is on his affected leg.
2. The patient places both his hands flat on a table in front of him. Assist him to extend his elbows and maintain the elbow extension by keeping his shoulders forward. He then walks his feet away from the table and back again without changing the position of his arms (Fig. 11/60).

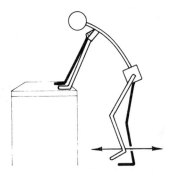

FIG. 11/60 Weight-bearing through the extended arms

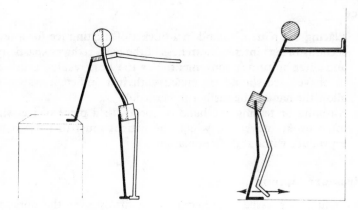

FIG. 11/61 (*left*) Weight-bearing on the affected arm while rotating the trunk away

FIG. 11/62 (*right*) Hands flat on the wall – lift sound leg

Ask him to turn his feet until he is sideways on to the table and reach out with his sound arm while his affected arm remains in position (Fig. 11/61).

3. The same activities can be practised with his arms outstretched and hands flat on a wall or mirror in front of him. He can also bend and straighten his elbows slightly without his hands sliding down (Fig. 11/62).

ADDITIONAL METHODS OF STIMULATION

Stimulation improves sensation and facilitates movement. Spasticity must be inhibited before any extra stimulation is given, and excitatory techniques should be graded very carefully because overstimulation will cause undesirable abnormal movements.

Weight-bearing is one of the most effective ways of bringing awareness and activity to the affected limbs.

Voice and use of words

The way in which the voice is used and the choice of words can help the patient to move correctly without excessive effort. The volume, inflection and speed of instructions can increase or decrease tone. Choose words which give the patient the feeling of the movement required, and change the words until the one which evokes the required response from the individual is found.

Ice

1. Placing the patient's hand in a bucket of melting ice for a few seconds brings intense awareness of the part, reduces spasticity and often improves movement. For the best results, crushed or shaved ice should be mixed with just sufficient water to allow the hand to be easily submerged.
2. Stroking or teasing the hand or foot with a piece of ice will often evoke movement which the patient must then learn to reproduce without the stimulation.

Pressure tapping

With fingers pressed together, tapping firmly over the dorsum and lateral aspect of the patient's foot encourages dorsiflexion. Elbow and hip extension can also be facilitated by tapping.

Heel banging

The patient sits in a chair or stool and his foot is held in full dorsiflexion with toes extended. With one hand on his knee bang his heel on the floor to facilitate active dorsiflexion. In the same position rub his heel firmly backwards and forwards on the floor to make him aware of the heel.

Tickle or flick his toes upwards to gain isolated dorsiflexion and extension of the toes. A bottle brush can be used in the same way to excite movement.

MANAGEMENT OF SOME COMPLICATIONS

If the methods of treatment described are carefully followed many complications and failures will be avoided.

Shoulder problems

THE SUBLUXED SHOULDER

Because of its extreme mobility the shoulder joint is commonly subluxed when the arm is significantly paralysed. The subluxation is not painful, but the shoulder can be traumatised easily if it is not carefully handled and positioned at all times (Davies, 1985). By correcting the downward rotation of the scapula, the natural passive locking mechanism of the shoulder is re-established (Basmajian, 1981).

When muscle tone or active movement in the rotator cuff muscles returns the correct alignment of the joint can be maintained. Physiotherapy therefore aims at correcting the posture of the shoulder girdle and stimulating activity in the stabilising muscles around the shoulder.

THE PAINFUL SHOULDER

If the scapula fails to rotate simultaneously when the arm is elevated or abducted, sensitive structures can easily be pinched between the head of the humerus and the acromion process, causing pain. The pain becomes increasingly severe if the trauma occurs often during the 24 hours.

Careful mobilisation of the shoulder after full release of spasticity around the scapula and in the trunk will soon free the shoulder and relieve pain.

A sling should never be worn as it reinforces the pattern of flexor spasticity and enforces immobility (Semans, 1965) both of which contribute to the condition in the first place. In any event a sling neither prevents subluxation nor reduces pain (Friedland, 1975).

The swollen hand

If the patient's hand suddenly becomes swollen and painful the therapist must take immediate steps to relieve the condition (Davis et al, 1977). If the oedema consolidates, the untreated hand will become permanently contracted and even if active movement returns can never be fully functional (Cailliet, 1980).

The contractures prevent supination of the forearm and dorsiflexion of the wrist. No flexion or abduction of the metacarpophalangeal joints is possible and the interphalangeal joints stiffen in slight flexion and can be neither fully extended nor flexed.

A small cock-up splint made of plaster of Paris and firmly bandaged with a crêpe bandage should be worn continuously till the swelling subsides. The hand should be placed in the ice bucket twice daily, the arm positioned in elevation at all times and the patient encouraged to do his self-assisted arm movements. If treated in this way the swelling should subside within a few days.

Splinting

Splinting reduces sensory stimulation and diminishes the need for activity and consequently inhibits the return of voluntary control as well as preventing normal movement. It is far better to retrain dorsiflexion and correct weight-bearing than resort to early bracing of the foot. An orthosis should only be used when all other methods of re-education have failed or when there is a risk of trauma to the ankle joint.

Foam rubber spreaders may help to inhibit flexion and adduction of the toes and fingers.

Hand splints should not be used as they tend to increase rather than decrease flexor spasticity (Mathiowetz et al, 1983).

INTEGRATION OF THERAPIES

As well as the involvement of relatives and nursing staff, close co-operation with all therapists is necessary to avoid confusing the patient and to ensure that all preparation for function proceeds along similar lines.

Reinforcement of principles and repetition of specific movement sequences can take place in actual situations in combination with re-education of speech or perceptual abilities and during the activities concerned with daily living. Affolter (1981) stresses the importance of using real-life events in the therapy to facilitate learning, and as Moore (1980) writes – 'the central nervous system learns by doing'.

One of the advantages of this method of management is the ease with which the level of function is maintained because of the manner in which daily activities are performed, serving as a continuous 'treatment'. The way the patient moves in sitting, dresses himself, stands from sitting, walks and climbs stairs will help to reduce spasticity and maintain or even improve the standard he has reached.

REFERENCES

Affolter, F. (1981). Perceptual processes as prerequisites for complex human behaviour. *International Rehabilitation Medicine*, 3(1), 3–9.
Basmajian, J.V. (1981). Biofeedback in rehabilitation: a review of principles and practices. *Archives of Physical Medicine and Rehabilitation*, 62, 469–75.

Cailliet, R. (1980). *The Shoulder in Hemiplegia*. Davis, Philadelphia.

Davies, P. M. (1985). *Steps to Follow*. Springer-Verlag, Berlin.

Davis, S. W., Petrillo, C. R., Eichberg, R. D. and Chu, D. S. (1977). Shoulder-hand syndrome in a hemiplegic population: a 5-year retrospective study. *Archives of Physical Medicine and Rehabilitation*, **58**, 353–6.

Friedland, F. (1975). Physical therapy. In *Stroke and Its Rehabilitation*, pp. 246–8, (ed. Licht, S.). Williams and Williams, Baltimore.

Mathiowetz, V., Bolding, D. J. and Trombly, C. A. (1983). Immediate effects of positioning devices on the normal and spastic hand measured by electromyography. *American Journal of Occupational Therapy*, **37(4)**, 247–54.

Moore, J. (1980). Neuroanatomical considerations relating to recovery of function following brain injury. In *Recovery of Function: Theoretical Considerations for Brain Injury Rehabilitation* (ed. Bach-y-Rita, P.). Huber, Bern.

Semans, S. (1965). Treatment of neurological disorders, concept and systems. *Journal of the American Physical Therapy Association*, **45(1)**, 11–16.

BIBLIOGRAPHY

In addition to the books which are listed in the references, and those in the Bibliographies on pages 217, 252 and 312 the following titles are helpful.

Affolter, F. and Stricker, E. (eds.) (1980). *Perceptual Processes as Prerequisites for Complex Human Behaviour*. Hans Huber Publishers, Bern.

Basmajian, J. V. (1979). *Muscles Alive. Their Functions Revealed by Electromyography*, 4th edition. Williams and Wilkins, Baltimore.

Blakeslee, T. R. (1980). *The Right Brain*. Macmillan, London.

Carr, J. H. and Shepherd, R. B. (1982). *A Motor Relearning Programme for Stroke*. William Heinemann Medical Books Limited, London.

Jay, P. E. (1979). *Help Yourselves: A Handbook for Hemiplegics and Their Families*, 3rd edition. Henry (Ian) Publications Limited, Hornchurch.

Johnstone, M. (1976). *The Stroke Patient: Principles of Rehabilitation*. Churchill Livingstone, Edinburgh.

Johnstone, M. (1978). *Restoration of Motor Function in the Stroke Patient: A Physiotherapist's Approach*. Churchill Livingstone, Edinburgh.

Luria, A. R. (1975). *The Man with a Shattered World*. Penguin Books, Harmondsworth.

Luria, A. R. (1975). *The Working Brain: An Introduction to Neuropsychology*. Penguin Books, Harmondsworth.

Chapter 12

Stroke Care in the Home

by F. W. FRAZER MCSP, BA(Hons), PhD

Stroke patients account for almost a twentieth of NHS resources, much of which is attributable to the admission to hospital of patients with acute strokes (Wade and Langton-Hewer, 1983). It is estimated that stroke is the third commonest single cause of admission (Garraway, 1976).

Various studies, including Waters and Perkins (1982) and Brocklehurst et al (1978), have demonstrated that the ratio of stroke patients treated at home as opposed to being admitted to hospital is roughly 3:2. Brocklehurst suggested that social factors are the most significant elements which influence the doctor in his decision to treat the stroke patient at home. It has been claimed, however, that many doctors lose interest in the stroke patient once the acute phase of the illness has passed and that most patients in the community receive very little, if any, long-term rehabilitation (Mulley and Arie, 1978).

A three-year study in the South Birmingham Health District showed that domiciliary physiotherapy is cost-effective, as well as achieving results which compare favourably with the hospital service (Frazer, 1980). During the study it was found that of a sample of 500 patients treated by the domiciliary service, one-third had suffered a stroke. The study demonstrated that severely handicapped stroke patients treated at home recovered equally as well as those admitted to hospital, and at a lower cost to the NHS. In a typical domiciliary case the mean cost of physiotherapy (based on a sample of 62 patients) was £72 (Isaacs and Evers, 1984).

There are a number of approaches to the treatment of the stroke patient, each with their enthusiastic advocates; this chapter borrows aspects of different techniques which are usually selected empirically and tailored to fit the needs of the individual patient and his family. The methods used are similar to those employed in hospital and the treatments in Chapters 10 and 11 can be applied equally well to the management of the stroke patient in the home. Within the home there are not the comprehensive facilities available in hospital; this factor along with problems of space, equipment, old and infirm relatives and unsuitable beds all create special challenges for the domiciliary physiotherapist when treating the stroke patient at home.

TREATMENT PLAN

Before treatment commences it is essential that a plan is prepared with a detailed assessment of the patient including physical dependency, communication problems, mental state, social background and medical diagnosis.

This initial record can be based on a number of different functional tests. No particular system of recording is wholly satisfactory and there is no general acceptance among physiotherapists as to which is most suitable. The ideal system needs to be easy to complete, simple, and reproducible by different physiotherapists on the same patient. The importance of accurate recording cannot be overstated.

As well as this initial assessment, there should be a continuous monitoring of progress, preferably by an independent physiotherapist, in order to obtain an unbiased assessment of the patient's achievement.

PROBLEMS ASSOCIATED WITH STROKE

These have been described in Chapters 10 and 11 and the same problems of hypotonia, spasticity, loss or disturbance of proprioception, perceptual and communication difficulties, visual and psychological problems will be present in the domiciliary stroke patient. In common with the hospital patient, many stroke victims suffer one or more of these problems in addition to the loss of motor function.

Although certain of these problems are regarded as the province of other specialties, the community physiotherapist needs to be capable of recognising *all* of the patient's problems and to be capable of providing basic advice and instruction on them.

PROBLEMS ASSOCIATED WITH DOMICILIARY TREATMENT

These can be considered under a number of headings which are not listed in any order of importance as the circumstances may alter from patient to patient: psychological, social, environment, equipment, communication, diagnosis, supporting services.

Psychological problems

Following a stroke, a major problem can be depression which may be severe, and long-standing. Lipsey et al (1984) estimated that depression can affect between 30 and 60 per cent of post-stroke patients. It is therefore essential that the domiciliary physiotherapist is aware of the signs and symptoms of depression so that she may alert the GP as appropriate.

It will be appreciated that an affective disorder such as depression involves an increase in intensity of normal emotions and that the boundary between normal and abnormal is imprecise. There are certain behaviours which are characteristic of the depressed state:

Depressed mood: The major complaint in most cases. This state is reflected in the posture, facial expression, speech and general appearance of the patient.

Difficulty in sleeping: Either difficult to get to sleep or early morning awakening.

Loss of energy: Patient feels tired and drained, may even imagine he has some serious disease.

Loss of interest: Patient loses interest in work, home, social activities, sex.

Loss of concentration: Patient is unable to concentrate, memory is unreliable. Pre-occupation with morbid self-doubt or guilt feelings.

Loss of appetite: Most patients lose their appetite, although younger people may over-eat as a compensation for feelings of inadequacy.

Transference is a term used to describe the development of an emotional attitude in a patient towards a therapist. It is not unusual for a patient to experience powerful feelings of love, hate and so on with regard to the physiotherapist. The patient may also have certain fantasies about the physiotherapist and it is important that she is able to appreciate that such events are a normal consequence of many therapeutic relationships.

Apart from the psychological problems experienced by some stroke patients, there are also psychological problems for the physiotherapist when faced with a large contingent of such patients in the community. The work is usually heavy and demanding both in terms of time and effort, with the likelihood of emotional demands on the physiotherapist which are, on occasions, more exhausting than their physical counterparts.

The fact that the majority of the stroke patients are aged 65 and over adds additional stress, as many patients of this age are suffering from more than one pathological condition or present with a serious social problem unconnected with the stroke.

As the domiciliary physiotherapist is working in comparative isolation, it is probable that she is faced by more difficulties and the need to accept more responsibility for her patient than her hospital counterpart. It is not unusual for her to have to decide whether a patient should be admitted to hospital and then to initiate the appropriate arrangements.

Social problems

In the hospital the patient is a part of a process which ensures that patients are fairly strongly regimented with regard to their treatment. If a physiotherapist shows the ward staff how to position the patient in a certain way this will usually be implemented whether the patient is able to agree or not. In the home the roles are reversed – the physiotherapist is a guest and if the patient does not wish to comply with her treatment procedures, he may refuse. It is vital that the domiciliary physiotherapist should gain the confidence and co-operation of the patient and his family as early as possible in the treatment course.

The physiotherapist will be teaching the family certain exercises and routines and she must rely on her own judgement as to the extent of family involvement for they are acting as unpaid helpers who will be providing care between visits. In such a situation it is not unusual for the physiotherapist to be seen as part of the family and she should retain her professional standing in order that role boundaries do not become unclear.

In dealing with any patient a friendly reserve should be adopted and it should be remembered that the dividing line between normal professional concern and friendship is easily misread. Making friends with a patient can lead to worry or even guilt; it is important to remember that some patients will misinterpret sympathy or similar attitudes which can lead him to develop unrealistic expectations about the clinical interaction. In this context 'friend' is taken to mean a person with whom a mutual need satisfaction can be realised. It is reasonable for the physiotherapist to express hopes, values and so on and to give support to the patient but she should not use the clinical interaction to support or satisfy her own needs or anxieties.

Problems with the environment

The treatment of the stroke patient will normally require very little equipment. The main item of equipment missing in the home is a set of parallel bars and a high mat. It is often difficult, if not impossible, to get an elderly person with a stroke down on to the floor and the appropriate treatment will, therefore, be given while the patient is on his bed. Tables or chairs can sometimes be substituted for the parallel bars unless there is a family handyman who can easily construct such an item with suitable lengths of scaffolding. Full length mirrors are not always available in the home but lengths of mirror which can be screwed to the wall can be obtained quite cheaply and are well worth the investment.

With an efficient community store there should be few problems with aids such as chairs, commodes, bath seats, transfer boards and so on and time spent in developing a good relationship with the clerical staff in this store is well rewarded.

Communication problems

As the physiotherapist is working single-handed within the community it is probable that she will experience problems arising from extended or non-existent lines of communication. To establish lines of communication is hard work and, initially, can be very time-consuming. These lines of communication are well established within the hospital but in many areas may be virtually unknown within the community. The general practitioner (GP), district nurse and health visitor may have an established communication procedure but often the physiotherapist can find herself having to contact these individuals separately which can prove both difficult and frustrating. Messages left with a third party are rarely delivered correctly and the domiciliary physiotherapist may have no option other than to spend several months establishing effective lines of communication with her colleagues in the community.

Diagnosis

Quite often the diagnosis which the domiciliary physiotherapist receives may be no more than a telephone message saying 'Mrs X, CVA, please treat'. There are always exceptions but sometimes it is difficult to contact the doctor on the day when he is needed. The establishment of group practices adds to this problem as some doctors may work only on certain days in the practice and cannot be contacted.

An additional task which, increasingly, is allotted to the domiciliary physiotherapist is the request from a consultant for her opinion as to whether the patient requires hospital admission for rehabilitation. She can also be asked whether she feels the patient requires surgery. This type of work is an example of the role extension possible within the community and adds greatly to the challenge presented by this type of work.

Supporting services

Often the physiotherapist is the first person to recognise a particular need in a family and then she is faced with how to arrange for certain supporting services for the patient and his family. In areas where there is no community occupational therapist the physiotherapist may have to request for alterations to be made within the home. Invariably there will be a delay before a rehabilitation officer calls from the local social services department with an even longer delay before the alteration is made. This is an area of responsibility which ought to be extended to the domiciliary physiotherapist who is trained to recognise such a need and, more important, is probably one of the first experts to visit the patient.

SUGGESTED SOLUTIONS

All the above problems can be alleviated, if not prevented, provided a number of basic steps are taken at the commencement of treatment. If the preparation of the treatment plan, following the initial visit, is based on the problem oriented assessment approach this will allow the various problems to be listed in order of importance and enable the physiotherapist to define her role with regard to each separate problem. In this way the total problem presented by any patient can be broken down into separate tasks, some of which are the province of other specialties, and this will prevent the physiotherapist from attempting to do too much for any patient. The domiciliary physiotherapist will often be faced with a 'problem patient' who is excessively demanding or difficult. It is probable that the same patient is just as much a problem for the doctor or the district nurse as he is for the physiotherapist.

The sense of isolation which is sometimes experienced by the domiciliary physiotherapist can be helped by regular attendance at the weekly ward meetings and by regular visits to the GP practices. Many GPs meet at intervals to hold clinical discussions and these meetings are often supported by drug companies. Such meetings are worth attending and the combination of business with pleasure can be recommended; the social atmosphere encourages a good working relationship between the disciplines. Many GPs welcome the physiotherapist's call at the surgery when they are more than willing to discuss the patient and compare notes.

It is recommended that the domiciliary physiotherapist participates in the hospital on-call and weekend rotas as this ensures frequent contact with her hospital colleagues as well as keeping her up-to-date with techniques. The domiciliary physiotherapist may be asked to visit luncheon and stroke clubs and such invitations should be accepted as they are a logical extension of her role in the community. She can enter a discussion about physical problems of patients and often performs a useful preventive role in this environment.

Frazer (1980) has suggested that the domiciliary treatment of the stroke patient is cost effective and it would therefore seem reasonable that the burden of car ownership and maintenance faced by the domiciliary physiotherapist might be eased by the provision of interest-free loans or alternatively by the provision of some form of sponsored transport within the community.

The social problems mentioned above require the physio-therapist to be adept at dealing with various social and ethnic groups. It is advisable that the domiciliary physiotherapist should have at least three years' experience since qualification, in order that she should have dealt with a wide range of people and con-ditions. Most university extra-mural departments organise courses on social behaviour or various aspects of sociology and it is recommended that intending domiciliary physiotherapists should attend such classes with the fees being refunded from the training budget.

The environmental problems are usually fairly easily solved. Many elderly people have their floors covered in rugs and carpets, laid one on top of the other, with a view to saving wear on the item underneath. Considerable tact is required to persuade them to remove these and it is often the case that they will be replaced as soon as the physiotherapist leaves. It has been found that clut-ter within the home is not a major cause of falls (Wild et al, 1981). When the patient is beginning walking practice, carpet can present a difficult surface; this can be overcome by laying a piece of plastic carpet protector over it. This can be bought in appro-priate lengths from most carpet shops at a reasonable price.

The patient's bed may need to be transferred downstairs and if no relatives are available the department porter might be willing to help. A commode will be required in the early stages of re-covery and a supply of disposable sheets and incontinence pads are useful, e.g. Kanga pants and Kylie sheets can be obtained from the community store.

The family who has a competent do-it-yourself member can avoid the long delays in having alterations to the home; provided the physiotherapist can give advice and instructions, many can do their own alterations.

The height of the bed can be adjusted either by using bed blocks or having the legs sawn off. The too soft mattress can be transformed by the use of a sheet of half-inch plywood of the appropriate size placed under it. If this should prove too expen-sive for the patient an old door, which often can be bought cheap-ly, is as effective.

If the family have insufficient pillows, paper pillow cases can be used to cover cushions or can be filled with foam off-cuts. While it is not suggested that the domiciliary physiotherapist should spend her time scrambling around junk yards, it is some-times the case that she is the only person available and it is a measure of her resourcefulness that such tasks get completed.

The remaining problems mentioned above can be avoided by establishing effective communication and it is essential that this is carried out as a separate exercise before any domiciliary service is commenced. When the service is established it is important to remember that good communication demands constant effort. This task is facilitated by the fact that most GPs and district nurses welcome the presence of a domiciliary physiotherapy service, and are receptive to positive suggestions from the physiotherapy staff. It is a simple matter to circulate information sheets which can be followed up with talks and demonstrations in postgraduate medical centres or district nurse education centres.

PHYSIOTHERAPY

The routine which is adopted for the patient nursed at home is broadly similar to that used in hospital. The extension of physiotherapy into the community has enabled many stroke patients to remain at home and there is evidence to suggest that patients receiving their rehabilitation at home recover equally well as those treated in the hospital.

In hospitals which do not have a stroke unit, there can be differences of expertise within the different wards and it is sometimes difficult to engage the co-operation equally of all ward staff. In this respect the domiciliary stroke patient is at an advantage as the provision of care is directed and monitored by the domiciliary physiotherapist.

It has been found that the improvement in patients discharged from a stroke unit had disappeared within one year (Garraway et al, 1980).

Early stages

Treatment will begin as soon as possible following the stroke and will include positioning, passive movements and care of the chest. The domiciliary physiotherapist will have access to intermittent positive pressure breathing (IPPB) machines, ultrasonic nebulisers and chest suction equipment; if required she can also arrange the supply of a tipping frame. If there is a chest infection present it is possible for her to visit the patient frequently during the early stages of recovery.

A full range of passive movements should be given each day

and the relatives will be shown these routines. Positioning of limbs should be taught and it is helpful to fix diagrams or pictures of the correct positioning above the patient's bed. Relatives are usually most anxious to be of assistance at this stage of rehabilitation and time spent in careful teaching is well rewarded.

It is important to remember that oedema of the hand is found in 16 per cent of all stroke patients; it is due to insufficient drainage from the lymphatics and the tendency for patients to forget the arm, allowing it to hang over the side of a chair. Passive movement and ultrasound can be used to eliminate this oedema which, if left, can rapidly become organised due to its high protein content (Howell, 1984).

POSITIONING

Co-operation between the physiotherapist and the district nurse is essential to ensure that the patient is placed in the correct position following routine nursing procedures. It is also important that the relatives receive consistent advice from both professions as there is nothing so detrimental as conflicting instructions.

It is usual for the district nursing officer to arrange study days when the domiciliary physiotherapist attends and demonstrates such techniques as positioning of limbs, bridging and handling the stroke patient. It is essential that the nurse and the relatives are shown how to lift the patient up and down and in and out of the bed. It must be repeatedly stressed that they should not support him underneath his affected arm as this can lead to the painful shoulder syndrome commonly found in the stroke patient. Provided the nurse, physiotherapist and family work closely together, it is possible to give a consistent service to the patient in the home.

BRIDGING

This simple procedure, which is taught to the patient and to his relatives from the earliest possible time following his stroke, makes it much easier to manage the patient in bed and facilitates such nursing procedures as sheet changing, care of pressure areas and use of the bedpan.

ROLLING

The ability to turn over in bed independently provides considerable stimulus to the patient and will contribute to an improvement in his morale. When it is appreciated that many stroke victims suffer depression which is often linked with the inability

to move without help it can be seen that any independent movement will be important to the patient.

Bridging and rolling can be taught easily to the relatives and
their use will make nursing considerably easier in the early stages
of recovery.

Exercise routine

The programme of exercise will closely follow that outlined in
Chapters 10 and 11 although there may be occasional modifications depending upon the time available to the physiotherapist.
Many of the procedures can be broken down into sections and
then taught to the relative, for example re-education of balance
can be taught in sequence starting with head control and progressing to the other elements described. It is possible for most
relatives to cope with this 'sectionalised' approach and it ensures
that the patient will be given a continuous and consistent treatment, even if it should be spread over a longer period with less
direct professional input.

The programme of exercises assumes a bilateral approach to
the restoration of function which constantly reinforces the awareness of the affected side. In the community where the patient is
either too old or too frail or his relative(s) is/are incapable of co-
operating in the rehabilitation, the method adopted may have to
concentrate on making the patient mobile by using the support of
a walking aid, perhaps utilising some form of knee brace, such as
the Swedish knee cage, or an ankle support.

The resulting pattern of walking is cumbersome and effectively
prevents a return to independence as the patient can never carry
anything or, while standing, manipulate any utensil. There may
be occasions when the use of a below knee leg iron is justified,
especially in cases where the patient is unaware that the ankle is
inverted and suffering repeated minor trauma.

Walking

When the patient has achieved reasonable standing balance, walking can be attempted even before he has mastered the ability to
swing his affected leg. The timing of this event will depend upon
a number of factors including the morale of the patient and his
family, his walking pattern and the space available within the
home. The re-education of walking will be along the lines of that
described in the preceding chapter.

ADVICE

It is recognised that the patient and his relatives will seek advice from the physiotherapists at all stages of his recovery. It is probable that the domiciliary physiotherapist is the person with whom the patient most readily relates and from whom advice most often will be sought. The advice which the physiotherapist is expected to provide is wide-ranging and she should beware of offering advice which is contradictory to that of the other professionals calling on the patient.

As far as advice on physical exercise is concerned it is probable that the physiotherapist is the person most suitable to provide it. In cases where advice on medication, social or psychological matters is required, the doctor or the social worker can be approached by the physiotherapist and asked for their opinions. It has been found that the patient is more likely to talk with the physiotherapist than most other professionals, possibly because of the special bond which develops during the course of the treatment.

A delicate area is that of sexual activity. There have been a number of instances where a stroke patient has suffered a second one following such activity. Physiotherapists are often asked for their advice on whether such normal pursuits should be attempted. The fact that the patient should ask for advice of this nature suggests that he should be encouraged to follow his desires, as the object of treatment is the restoration of function where possible. It is helpful to be reminded that doctors, when faced with similar questions, are no more experienced than most physiotherapists. Domiciliary staff would benefit by attending a counselling course organised by the Association to Aid Sexual and Personal Relationships (SPOD) (see page 636 for address).

FACTORS WHICH INFLUENCE RECOVERY

Patients who recover their muscle function within the first 2–3 weeks can be considered to have a good prognosis for rehabilitation. Neurological recovery is thought to begin at some point between the first and seventh week following the onset of the stroke, with little further neurological improvement following the 14th week. Functional recovery is closely linked with neurological recovery; it has been suggested that much of the early recovery, including that of the upper limb, may be due to the restoration of circulation to ischaemic areas of the brain with late recovery attributable to the transfer of function to undamaged neurones (Tallis, 1984; Thomas, 1984). One finding suggests that improvement can occur in performance 2 years after the stroke (Langton-Hewer, 1979). Factors which militate against recovery include severe spasticity, loss of sensation and mental confusion with inability to co-operate with the rehabilitation exercises.

The attitude of the relatives within the home is most important. Patients with many of the problems listed above can be maintained at home provided there is good family support. Such families will require long-term support from the domiciliary physiotherapist and it is common practice to keep such patients on the list of regular visits for periods of three or more years. There may not be any physical improvement in such cases but the weekly or fortnightly visit by the physiotherapist has been shown to be a significant factor in keeping the seriously impaired stroke patient at home. Any claim that the recovery of the stroke patient can be attributed mainly to circulatory and neurological factors can be questioned by examining a stroke patient who has been neglected for some reason. His limbs will be fixed in abnormal positions; contractures, pressure sores and incontinence will complete the picture and will all contribute to a severe nursing problem. The psychological state of the patient is an important factor in recovery and the sudden change in physical circumstances will, depending on his personality type, lead to depression or anxiety. The patient will worry about his future, especially with regard to his work and finances, and married patients may be concerned about a possible loss of attractiveness where their partner is concerned. All of these worries will depend upon the ability of the patient to be aware of his condition and are absent in a patient suffering from anosognosia. When these worries are superimposed upon either a speech defect or a perceptual difficulty, the physiotherapist needs constant patience and the ability to give continual reassurance.

Most physiotherapists will have had experience of a stroke patient who has been excessively agitated or who has struck out at them. These patients are depressed and it should be remembered that this depression is natural and, when the patient adjusts to his changed condition, should improve within a few months. However, in one study two-thirds of patients who were depressed at the initial evaluation remained so seven to eight months later (Lipsey et al, 1984). The best therapy is improvement and any change for the better, no matter how minimal, must be high-lighted by profuse praise and encouragement. There can also be a loss of self-esteem with a refusal to accept a changed body image, sometimes to the extent that the patient will deny that there is anything wrong with him. This state of mind is a serious impediment to progress and the use of portable video equipment may help the patient to adjust his self-concept.

The domiciliary physiotherapist must be able to advise on dressing, and in so doing must remember that attempts at dressing with a paralysed side will involve twisting movements which can in turn cause muscle strain with subsequent pain. Co-operation with the occupational therapist over such matters as how best to put on socks, stockings, trousers, as well as what dressing aids are available, is to be recommended most strongly.

Toilet problems are common: one useful hint is to place a small table by the lavatory pedestal to hold sheets of loose toilet paper; one-handed attempts to pull a toilet roll will invariably result in quantities of paper all over the floor. Although washing is often difficult, self-help must be encouraged. A bath seat is essential, and support rails and uprights can be supplied on loan from the social services department. Patients can be taught to dry themselves by using several small hand towels rather than a large bath towel which would be difficult to handle.

The economic, social and emotional effects experienced by the family as a result of stroke may be expressed in feelings of helplessness and frustration, often projected on to the physiotherapist in the form of criticism or by excessive demands for additional treatment. To counter this the family should be involved in all stages of the rehabilitation and should be encouraged to express their fears and anxieties. The family should also be prepared for the eventual termination of physiotherapy treatment and this process should commence from the first visit. The house-bound stroke patient is not able to mix with other stroke patients as is possible in hospital; such mixing in the ward encourages social skills and will facilitate interaction among the patients. In the case of the stroke patient at home, the physiotherapist will have to ensure that this element of rehabilitation is not overlooked and she may have to advise the family how best to achieve it. The tendency for the family to be protective and over-indulgent to the patient needs to be guarded against.

Although recovery is ultimately dependent upon the underlying pathology, it is evident that the sooner treatment begins, the better the outcome. The age of the patient is not significant although it has been claimed that the younger patient will have a stronger motivation to get better. Elderly patients are as likely to respond as well to treatment as younger ones.

Severe spasticity, if present, may be helped by drugs or by various surgical procedures, while muscle weakness is sometimes treated by electrical stimulators, such as the peroneal stimulator used in cases of foot drop. The painful shoulder, common to many stroke patients, is a constant problem for the domiciliary physiotherapist. She can treat it with positioning, ice, heat, interferential therapy or ultrasound. Connective tissue massage is useful in domiciliary treatment, while support from slings or the use of figure-of-eight bandages may provide some relief. Maitland mobilisations can be effective. In some units biofeedback has been used with varying degrees of success (Williams, 1982).

DISCHARGE

There are certain guidelines governing the discharge from treatment of the stroke patient, and these include:
1. Pressure of new referrals
2. The wishes of the patient and his family
3. Level of progress
4. Availability of follow-up services
5. Lack of further improvement.

For physiotherapists, the lack of progress is likely to be the point at which discharge from treatment is considered. It should be remembered that the idea of 'discharge' is stressful for the patient and his family may respond by demanding further treatment, convinced that improvement will occur. Emotional language is often employed: 'left to rot', 'thrown out' commonly being used to express the fear felt at such a time. Because the domiciliary physiotherapist is often required to face this situation alone, she can experience acute discomfort and personal feelings of guilt. In order to avoid such problems, it is essential that the family is prepared for eventual discharge from the very first visit. This will require continual reinforcement on each subsequent visit and a possible routine is suggested:
1. Explain the nature of the illness and the possible plan of treatment.
2. Reassurance regarding the provision of other supporting services.
3. Praise and encouragement for the relatives.

4. Provide some indication regarding the probable number of weeks' duration of treatment. (The mean number of weeks of treatment in 160 cases within the South Birmingham Health District was 12.)
5. This routine should be repeated on each visit so that the family is conditioned to expect the eventual termination of treatment. There may be cases where treatment will continue indefinitely on a restricted basis as described earlier.

The provision of adaptations within the home, the arrangement of visits to stroke clubs, day hospitals, luncheon clubs and so on may all have to be organised by the domiciliary physiotherapist. Voluntary groups such as the Chest, Heart and Stroke Association (CHSA) volunteer stroke scheme provide valuable support in certain areas and the geriatric health visitor can help at this stage particularly with regard to holiday relief admissions to hospital. It may be necessary to provide certain patients with a wheelchair and to instruct them in its use prior to discharge, with possible adaptation of the home environment, such as the provision of wooden ramps or the removal of some internal doors.

In the case of the patient who will require long-term institutional care in either a young chronic sick unit or in a Cheshire Home, the contact with the domiciliary physiotherapist will assist the patient to endure the stress associated with such a transfer and will help him to adapt more readily to his new surroundings.

The domiciliary treatment of a stroke patient is undoubtedly cost effective although requiring considerable effort, ingenuity and dedication on the part of the physiotherapist concerned. Writing in the *Lancet*, Jarrett (1981) suggests that the patient's home is probably the most appropriate place for the rehabilitation of stroke.

REFERENCES

Brocklehurst, J. C., Andrews, K., Morris, P., Richards, B. R. and Laycock, P. L. (1978). Why admit stroke patients to hospital? *Age and Ageing*, 7, 2, 100.

Frazer, F. W. (1980). Domiciliary physiotherapy – cost and benefit. *Physiotherapy*, 66, 1, 2-7.

Garraway, W. M. (1976). The size of the problem of stroke in Scotland. In *Stroke*, pp. 72-82, (jt. eds. Gillingham, F. J., Maudsley, C. and Williams, A. E.). Churchill Livingstone, Edinburgh.

Garraway, W. M., Akhtar, A. J., Prescott, R. J. and Hockey, L. (1980). Management of acute stroke in the elderly: preliminary results of a controlled trial. *British Medical Journal*, **280**, 1040-3.

Howell, T. H. (1984). How my teaching about the management of stroke would change after my own. *British Medical Journal*, **289**, 35-7.

Isaacs, B. and Evers, H. (eds.) (1984). *Innovations in Care of the Elderly*, p. 71. Croom Helm, London.

Jarrett, S. R. (1981). Stroke patient: home or hospital? *Lancet*, **1**, 46.

Langton-Hewer, R. (1979). How does arm movement recover? *The Practitioner* (December).

Lipsey, J. R., Robinson, R. G., Pearlson, G. D., Krishna, R. and Price, T. R. (1984). Nortriptyline treatment of post-stroke depression. *Lancet*, **1**, 297-300.

Mulley, G. and Arie, T. (1978). Treating stroke: Home or hospital? *British Medical Journal*, **2**, 1321-2.

Tallis, R. (1984). Neurological rehabilitation: the next thirty years. *Physiotherapy*, **70**, 5, 196-9.

Thomas, D. J. (1984). Treatment of acute stroke. *British Medical Journal*, **288**, 2-3.

Wade, D. T. and Langton-Hewer, R. (1983). Why admit stroke patients to hospital? *Lancet*, **1**, 9807-9.

Waters, H. J. and Perkins, J. M. (1982). Study of stroke patients in a single general practice. *British Medical Journal*, **284**, 791-4.

Wild, D., Nayak, U. S. L. and Isaacs, B. (1981). Prognosis of falls in old people at home. *Journal of Epidemiology and Community Health*, **34**, 200-4.

Williams, J. M. (1982). Use of electromyographic feedback for pain reduction in the spastic hemiplegic shoulder. *Physiotherapy* (Canada), **34**, 6, 327-33.

BIBLIOGRAPHY

Caillet, R. (1979). *Hemiplegia of the Shoulder*. F. A. Davis Co, Philadelphia.

Carr, J. H. and Shepherd, R. B. (1983). *A Motor Relearning Programme for Stroke*. William Heinemann Medical Books Limited, London.

Downie, P. A. and Kennedy, P. (1980). *Lifting, Handling and Helping Patients*. Faber and Faber, London.

Frazer, F. W. (ed.) (1982). *Rehabilitation Within the Community*. Faber and Faber, London.

Handling the Handicapped, 2nd edition. Woodhead-Faulkner Limited, Cambridge, in association with the Chartered Society of Physiotherapy. (Regularly up-dated.)

Lubbock, G. (ed.) (1983). *Stroke Care: An Interdisciplinary Approach.* Faber and Faber, London.

Wade, D. T., Langton-Hewer, R., Skilbeck, C. E. et al (1985). Controlled trial of a home-care service for acute stroke patients. *Lancet*, 1, 323–6.

See also Bibliography on pages 217 and 295.

Chapter 13

Spinal Cord Lesions – Clinical

by T. McSWEENEY MCh(NUI), MCh(Orth), FRCS, FACS

The spinal cord may be involved in many diffuse or localised lesions which give rise to a variety of clinical conditions characterised by varying degrees of motor or sensory paralysis. These include developmental, inflammatory, neoplastic, degenerative and demyelinating lesions. Injury to the spinal cord forms a particular sub-group which will be used as the descriptive model in this chapter. Some of these conditions primarily affect the spinal column or the meninges and are therefore extrinsic to the cord. In these patients the resulting impairment in conduction results from direct pressure on the cord or to impairment in its blood supply.

It will be appreciated that the range of disorders so produced is wider than can be conveyed in a short account, but that certain principles of management are applicable to all paralysed patients while the details of treatment may vary depending on the primary condition. The common non-traumatic diseases are briefly mentioned followed by an expanded consideration of traumatic tetraplegia and paraplegia.

DEVELOPMENTAL

Spina bifida is the commonest congenital anomaly and is often associated with other neurological defects. In spina bifida occulta there may be little in the way of physical signs apart from the radiographic evidence that a neural arch has failed to fuse. Differential growth in adolescence may give rise to incontinence with paresis of the lower limbs and sensory impairment. More severe cases (spina bifida cystica) present a formidable social and medical problem. In these babies there is herniation of the meninges or of neural tissue (meningomyelocele) through the skin of the cervical (rare) thoracic or lumbar regions. The spinal cord and nerve roots are often intrinsically abnormal leading to paraplegia, lower limb deformities and paralytic dislocation of the hips (see Chapter 25).

INFLAMMATORY

The advent of antibiotic therapy has greatly reduced the morbidity of bacterial infections of the meninges and the Salk vaccine has been eminently successful in reducing the incidence of anterior poliomyelitis. Nevertheless, the post-viral infections still present a wide spectrum of puzzling neurological syndromes, many of which result in varying degrees of incapacity. Acute disseminated encephalomyelitis is an omnibus term which includes the Guillain-Barré syndrome and other post-viral infections. Recovery may be anticipated in many of these conditions but in others, areas of residual demyelination lead to permanent paralysis.

Infections of the spinal column and of the epidural space are often followed by an advancing paraplegia. Staphylococcal infections usually respond to antibiotic therapy but an acute epidural abscess requires urgent surgical decompression. Tuberculosis is still a scourge in certain countries where Pott's paraplegia remains a common cause of paralysis. Antitubercular drugs and appropriate surgical intervention have greatly improved the prognosis. Regretfully, some patients will remain paralysed because of infarction of the blood supply to the spinal cord; similar remarks apply to other bacterial infections.

Acute anterior poliomyelitis is virtually extinct where a sustained vaccination programme has been carefully followed. Unfortunately, this happy state of affairs is far from universal, and paralytic poliomyelitis is still a widespread and crippling disease. The Sabin attentuated live vaccine is conveniently administered on a lump of sugar and booster doses may be needed at intervals of a few years, especially in endemic areas. The virus may be found throughout the central nervous system but has a particular affinity for the anterior horn cells. Depending on the severity of the illness, many columns of cells will die leading to paralysis of the corresponding muscle fibres; other cells are less damaged so that some recovery can be expected. Recovery may be delayed for many months and the pattern and distribution of the paralysis is often varied. Perhaps one of the commonest sites of infection is in the anterior horn cells of the lumbar enlargement leading to complete or almost complete paralysis of the lower limbs. In young children, contractures and secondary deformities may follow, notably limb-length discrepancies and scoliosis. Respiratory weakness or bulbar paralysis add another dimension to management which is best undertaken by an experienced respiratory team.

NEOPLASIA

The commonest malignant tumour compressing the spinal cord is a secondary deposit from a primary lesion in breast, prostate or bronchus. Local symptoms and girdle pain are common and the paralysis is often of rapid onset. The primary lesion may not be amenable to cure, but surgical decompression of the spinal lesion may be beneficial in lessening the paralysis and sphincter incompetence. The prognosis is largely determined by the sensitivity of the tumour to radiotherapy, chemotherapy or hormonal manipulation.

In contrast, benign tumours can often be completely excised, and the paralysis is reversible even after months of cord compression. Full recovery is often seen after removal of a spinal meningioma and similar remarks apply to the isolated neurofibroma.

DEGENERATIVE AND DEMYELINATING DISEASES

Sub-acute combined degeneration of the spinal cord is one of the few demyelinating diseases which is eminently controlled by treatment. It is due to a deficiency of vitamin B_{12} which also results in Addisonian or pernicious anaemia. The brain and the peripheral nerves are often involved so that the clinical picture may include a mild dementia as well as a peripheral neuropathy. The bone marrow shows a megaloblastic reaction, achlorhydria is present and the diagnosis is confirmed by the low level of serum vitamin B_{12}. The response to vitamin B_{12} therapy is usually satisfactory; in untreated patients the paraplegia quickly becomes irreversible.

MOTOR NEURONE DISEASE (see Chapter 20)

In this disease, the degeneration affects the motor neurones in the cerebral cortex and of certain cranial nerves and in particular the motor neurones in the grey matter of the spinal cord. Three clinical patterns are identified, namely, amyotrophic lateral sclerosis, progressive muscular atrophy and chronic bulbar palsy. As the disease progresses, the various forms merge in a relentless manner and death is often due to suffocation.

Wasting of the small muscles of the hands is a common presentation and this is followed by weakness in the upper limbs and a spastic paresis of the legs. Fasciculation is a constant feature, and this is seen as a rapid (worm-like) contraction of small groups of muscle fibres. While the diagnosis is seldom in doubt, it is important that other conditions such as diabetic and carcinomatous amyotrophy are excluded.

MULTIPLE SCLEROSIS (see Chapter 15)

The myelopathy associated with cervical spondylosis may present a similar picture and to add to the confusion both conditions may co-exist. The localised motor and sensory disturbance of root distribution associated with cervical spondylosis may help to differentiate between the two conditions, and particularly so when there is unequivocal evidence of cranial nerve involvement as in multiple sclerosis.

Other neurological disorders in which the spinal cord is not directly involved, and which may lead to widespread paralysis should be mentioned. These include the muscular dystrophies (see Chapter 27) and the generalised peripheral neuropathies. The primary muscular dystrophies are genetically determined and unfortunately are not helped by specific drug therapy. Some of the metabolic and endocrine myopathies may respond to appropriate treatment. The same is true for certain toxic, metabolic and endocrine neuropathies when treatment can be instituted early.

TRAUMATIC LESIONS OF THE SPINAL CORD

The manifestations of injury to the spinal cord are discussed in Chapter 14 and the peripheral results of complete and incomplete lesions are described. It is important to recognise the effects of cell body destruction (upper motor neurone lesion) in contrast to the signs resulting from interruption of white fibres (lower motor neurone lesion); while recognising that in practice both elements are usually involved.

The significance of these injuries has been recognised from earliest times and manuscripts copied in the seventeenth century B.C. from earlier Egyptian papyri show an awareness of the necessity of rest and support for the injured spinal column. It was Galen, a Roman physician (A.D. 130), who showed that a full cord division abolished all function below the level of transection and that hemi-section resulted in loss of motor function on the same side. He also noted that a mid-line longitudinal section in animals did not produce paralysis. In the nineteenth century the most widely discussed topic was the propriety of surgical exploration. Henry Cline is credited with the first well-documented laminectomy in 1814 but there is good evidence that the operation had been performed by Paul of Aegina (A.D. 625). The difficulties in assessing the place for laminectomy is exemplified in the verbal battles between Sir Astley Cooper who favoured the procedure and Sir Charles Bell who saw no merit in surgical intervention. Not the least of the difficulties stems from the accuracy of the initial assessment about the completeness and extent of the cord lesion and the knowledge that spontaneous improvement can be expected when the damage is incomplete from the start. Laminectomy has few supporters, but at the present time more radical surgical approaches are under trial, and the debate continues.

The modern principles of management and the development of specialised centres were pioneered by Guttmann at Stoke Mandeville Hospital, Bottrill in Toronto and Munro at Boston City Hospital.

Epidemiology

It is difficult to assess the incidence of traumatic tetraplegia or paraplegia in a community. Many factors are involved particularly the prevalence of heavy industry and road traffic conditions. Figures of between 12 and 50 cases per million population per year have been quoted and it is generally agreed that most of the victims of road traffic accidents are between 20 and 24 years. Domestic accidents account for a large proportion of the injuries in elderly patients, while leisure activities are responsible for many of the serious spinal injuries at the other end of life. Diving into shallow water, falls from horses, trampoline and other gymnastic accidents are all too common. Equally tragic are the injuries sustained in hard contact sports, especially in young rugby players.

The necessity of a warming-up period is generally recognised, but gymnastic clubs do not appear to be fully aware of the dangers of faulty equipment and the need for effective shock absorbent safety mats. All contact sports involve some risk but increased aggression quite out of keeping with the spirit of the sport, mismatched age and physical size and breaking of rules are important factors in the alarming rise in the incidence of these injuries over recent years. Physiotherapists can use their considerable influence in the community in lessening these tragedies. Many of the serious spinal injuries caused by road traffic accidents are related to the use of head rests and safety harnesses. On another legislative plane, the enforcement of a speed limit, safety in car design, and the abuse of alcohol are important measures.

Most of the injuries to the spinal column do not affect its inherent stability so that the spinal cord and nerve roots are adequately protected. Forces of greater magnitude and especially those with a torsional element lead to ligamentous disruption and bony injury or displacement. It is in these injuries that the spinal cord may be over-stretched, torn or damaged by direct bony impingement. These extrinsic forces are modified by intrinsic factors, such as the varying strength of bone and ligaments at different ages and whether the related muscles are 'on guard' in anticipation of the injury. Comparatively trivial injuries may have devastating results when the spinal column is weakened as in congenital anomalies, and where the bone has been weakened by neoplastic infiltration or severe osteoporosis. Open wounds and missile injuries are a special group which reflect the violence of society.

Transportation

Special care is required in moving the patient from the scene of the accident to hospital and during the clinical and radiological examinations. Four people are required to lift the patient 'in one piece' and in the supine position on to a firm stretcher. Ideally, a fifth person should be available to supervise the transfer and to apply gentle continuous traction to the head when a cervical injury is suspected. The hazard of vomiting should be recognised in the unconscious or intoxicated patient; the lateral or semi-lateral position is then acceptable, provided an improvised roll or sorbo-rubber pack is used to stabilise the position. Neurological deterioration because of faulty handling and during transportation has been reported. In difficult geographical situations helicopter or fixed-wing aircraft are essential and ambulance crews are usually supplied with special immobilisers and respiratory equipment.

Pathology of the cord injury

The central grey matter is more susceptible to injury than the longitudinal fibres. An area of spreading haemorrhagic necrosis is quickly established in the area surrounding the central canal and depending on the severity of the injuring force this may spread longitudinally over many segments. The process appears to be self-perpetuating for a time. In severe injuries the necrosis and associated oedema spreads into the white fibres. The foregoing is a simplified account of the events in impact injuries and is supported by experimental studies in animals. In the more usual injuries, torsion rather than impact is the injuring force and this results in stretching or severance of the white fibres. Postmortem studies in man suggest that both processes occur. It is interesting to speculate that in the less severe injuries there may be a period immediately following the injury when the white fibres may be salvageable. This would alter the whole course of spinal cord injury. The early infarction is gradually replaced by neuroglial fibrosis which forms an almost impenetrable barrier to regenerating fibres. The fact that axonal regeneration does occur is now generally accepted, but the scar tissue prevents the re-establishment of appropriate continuity. Measures to control the neuroglial scarring would open the possibility of some functional recovery (Fig. 13/1).

Diagnosis

A complaint of pain in the neck, in the interscapular region, in the chest, or in the lower part of the back following an accident should arouse suspicion of a spinal injury. The history of electric shock-like sensations in the limbs, a transient impairment in sensation, or paresis, is very suggestive of cord injury. Unconscious patients, those who have fallen from a height and the victims of road traffic accidents are always suspect. The history should in-

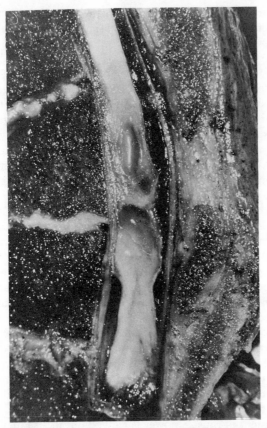

FIG. 13/1 Autopsy specimen, mid-thoracic spine. Shows scarring and cyst formation in spinal cord 25 years after injury. There was some sensory recovery in the intervening years

clude the circumstances of the accident and an analysis of the forces involved. Did the paralysis or sensory loss occur at the time or was there a delay period? The site of bruise marks, lacerations and tender areas may indicate the mechanism of injury. Associated injuries must be assessed; these may take precedence over the spinal injury. Mistakes arise because the possibility of cord damage is not considered.

The examination begins with an assessment of the state of consciousness, and the distribution of any muscle weakness or sensory impairment. This preliminary examination usually separates the serious cases from the patients in whom there is no neurological deficit. A knowledge of the basic anatomy and physiology of the nervous system is essential.

NEUROLOGICAL EXAMINATION

This is done in a quiet area and in a systematic manner. It aims to define the level of the cord injury whether it is complete or incomplete and the nature and extent of the root involvement. The conscious patient may vividly describe the sensory loss and refer to pain (paraesthesiae) in a specific dermatome due to root irritation. The sensory examination proceeds from the innervated to the denervated areas and includes appreciation of light touch, pin prick (sharp/blunt) and joint position sense. Sensory impairment in the upper limbs is tested over the shoulders (C5); on the outer aspect of the forearms, thumb index and middle fingers (C6); in the ring and little fingers (C7); and along the ulnar border of the hand and forearm (C8). Intact sensation along the inner aspect of the arm and axilla indicate that T1 and T2 are intact. It is important to note that the posterior primary rami of C4 supply the skin below the clavicles and become continuous or juxtaposed to the T2 dermatome below this area. The umbilical area (T10), the inguinal area (L1) and the soles of the feet (S1) are important reference points.

Special attention is directed to the sacral area and to the perineum (S3–S5). Preservation of sensation to light touch and pin prick in this area is reassuring evidence that the cord injury is incomplete.

Assessment of muscle power is carried out in a sequential manner. At the initial examination it is sufficient to test the movement of major joints rather than individual muscle action. Thus in the lower limbs where joint movement is not well defined and single muscles are usually innervated from more than one spinal segment the following pattern emerges:

Hip flexion: L1, L2, L3	*Extension:* L4, L5, S1
Knee flexion: L5, S1, S2	*Flexion:* L2, L3, L4
Ankle flexion: L5, S1	*Dorsiflexion:* L4, L5

At a later stage conventional muscle charts based on the MRC scale are essential (see p. 127).

Incomplete lesions exhibit some preservation of sensation or voluntary muscle power below the sites of maximum cord damage. Evidence that the injury is incomplete implies that there may be some if not substantial recovery.

The effects on the autonomic nervous system are more marked in cervical and upper thoracic injuries where lack of sweating, hypotension and a slow pulse are important features. Sphincter control is impaired, paralytic ileus may appear and control of body temperature is often a major problem.

Paradoxical respiration is a striking feature in upper cervical injuries.

RADIOGRAPHY

High quality radiographs of the spinal column are essential. A special problem arises at the cervico-thoracic junction where injuries at this level are all too frequently 'missed'. Having established the site of the vertebral injury other radiological techniques may be arranged in consultation with the radiologist (Fig. 13/2).

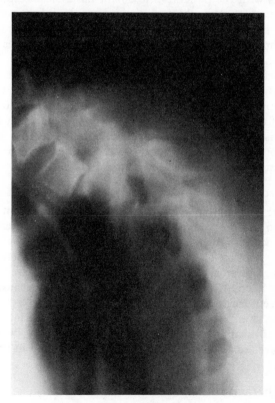

FIG. 13/2 Dislocation at cervico-thoracic junction displayed on Swimmer's view (arm abducted above the head)

Treatment

The paralysis and sensory loss should not be regarded as isolated phenomena; there are respiratory, cardiovascular and metabolic problems quite apart from the profound psychological effect on the patient and on his relatives.

The physiotherapist is part of a team in which the customary lines of professional demarcation are lightly drawn. Communication and co-ordination between therapists and nursing staff are vital as emphasised in Chapter 14. Every opportunity is taken to encourage the patient towards independence and self-reliance; and introducing other patients who have successfully reached a later stage of rehabilitation is of great benefit.

Experience and empathy are essential when discussing the prognosis with the patient. The doctor has a clear responsibility in this regard and an obligation to inform the other members of the team in consultation. It will be appreciated that these patients face unfamiliar and unusual hazards in their daily lives and the professionals have an important teaching responsibility. This requires tact, familiarity with the patient and the level of the lesion, as well as the right amount of firmness in keeping with a humanitarian approach. At times it is easy to forget the catastrophic nature of the disability and to overlook the bereavement reaction. Once this has lessened there often follows a period of latent aggression, lack of co-operation or active rebellion; more serious is the apathy which afflicts a few unfortunate patients.

RESPIRATORY PROBLEMS

These are discussed in Chapter 14. Chest therapy commences on admission and the therapist has a dual role in this context. Apart from direct responsibility for the patient, there is the teaching function whereby all ward staff and relatives are instructed in essential respiratory techniques including assisted coughing and the like. Suction apparatus should be to hand because of the ever-present hazard of atelectasis.

Tracheostomy is seldom required, but a short period of endotracheal intubation (with assisted ventilation) may be required when there are associated chest or head injuries and in bronchitic patients.

GASTRO-INTESTINAL PROBLEMS

Paralytic ileus can be anticipated in many patients, in which instance early passage of a nasogastric tube is required. Only small amounts of fluid are needed in the first 48 hours and solid food is withheld until bowel sounds are present.

CARDIOVASCULAR FEATURES

The low blood pressure and the slowing of the pulse rate in cervical and high thoracic injuries has been mentioned. The unstable cardiovascular system is over-stressed by a large transfusion so that pulmonary oedema is easily produced. When large transfusions are required, as in multiple injuries, monitoring of the central venous pressure is essential.

INCONTINENCE

Intermittent catheterisation carried out with full aseptic precautions has proved a reliable method provided that the patient is admitted promptly to a specialised unit. In young female patients there is increasing support for a modified suprapubic cystotomy. Using these methods in the early weeks it is probable that the long-term vesical and renal problems will be greatly reduced. In many instances a catheter-free life can be anticipated; avoidance of infection and bladder training lead to an automatic pattern of micturition in a substantial number of patients. Evidence of bladder outlet obstruction or a high residual urine will require a transurethral resection or other urological procedures.

CARE OF THE SKIN AND JOINTS

This is considered in Chapter 14 with the essential emphasis on self-discipline and the educational role of the physiotherapist.

Management of the vertebral injury

It is not proposed to give a detailed account of the various bony and ligamentous injuries. In general, a conservative approach is advocated, realising that in the majority of patients the maximum damage to the spinal cord or nerve roots has already occurred (at the time of the accident). It should not be equated with 'doing nothing' and it recognises the need for urgent surgical intervention in certain cases.

There is an urgency to reduce those displacements which significantly encroach on the diameter of the spinal cord. This is especially true in cervical dislocations where prompt reduction is often followed by substantial neurological improvement (Fig. 13/3).

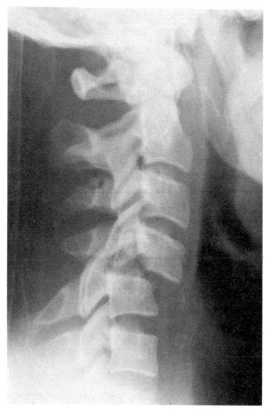

FIG. 13/3 Bilateral facet dislocation C4 on C5. *Note* forward displacement of more than half the diameter of the vertebral body. Considered a 'complete' lesion on admission; substantial recovery followed early manipulative reduction

Open reduction and internal fixation is sometimes indicated in incomplete cord lesions especially at the thoraco-lumbar junction, and when there is a delayed onset of the paralysis. Other indications include inherently unstable injuries, injuries with gross displacement and in multiple injuries as an aid to nursing management.

Conservative management implies postural reduction under radiographic control and in the application of skull traction for certain cervical injuries. Attention to detail and familiarity with the technique are paramount. Bony stability is secured in the majority of cases, and at the present time the results have not been bettered by more elaborate surgical methods.

The treatment of regional injuries is summarised:

Cervical: Skull calipers are applied under local anaesthesia and long-axis traction is instituted. Minor compression fractures and hyperextension injuries in elderly patients do not require skull traction.

In certain circumstances dislocations and subluxations are re-positioned by gentle manipulation under endotracheal anaesthesia and a muscle relaxant. A small number may not stabilise and require bony fusion (Fig. 13/4).

Thoracic: Most of these injuries are stable even when displaced because of the splinting effect of the thoracic cage. Many are accompanied by chest injuries which require intercostal drainage. In exceptional cases re-alignment using Harrington rods is advised.

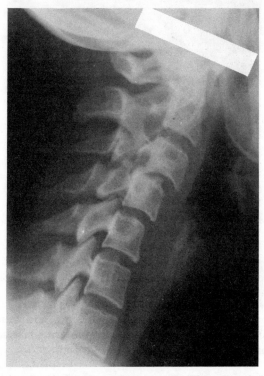

FIG. 13/4 Unilateral dislocation C3 on C4. Less than half the vertebral body displaced forward. Minimal neurological impairment. Unstable at 3 months so that bony fusion was required

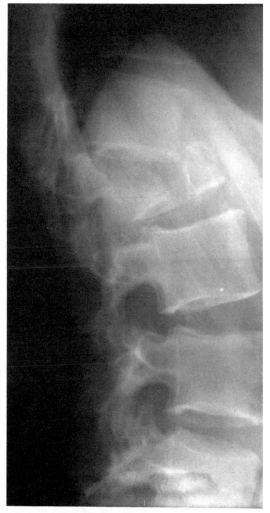

FIG. 13/5 Fracture dislocation at thoraco-lumbar junction

Thoraco-lumbar injuries: Postural reduction usually results in a satisfactory alignment. If this is not achieved, and when there is gross displacement or 'locking' of the posterior facets, open reduction and fixation is required (Figs. 13/5 and 13/6).

Injuries below L2: These injuries are associated with a cauda equina lesion and many require open reduction and internal fixation.

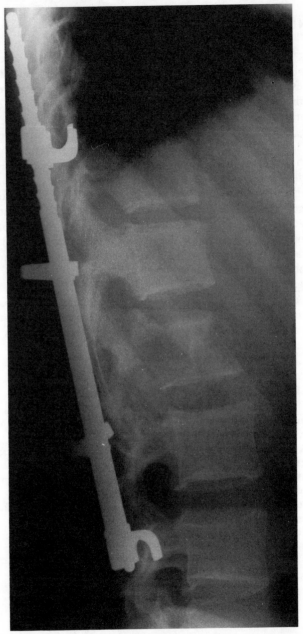

FIG. 13/6 Reduction with Harrington rods of the dislocation in Figure 13/5

CONCLUSION

Many aspects of rehabilitation and resettlement are covered in the following chapter. The physiotherapist has a great influence and responsibility here; co-operation and self-reliance rather than a submissive response must be encouraged. Many patients exhibit indomitable courage right from the start, while in others allowances must be made for unrealistic attitudes, tantrums and periods of child-like narcissism. Re-motivating the patient from within is better than attempting to solve all the problems by outside agencies.

Marital relations and sexual matters are discussed before the patient's return home. Any form of sexual practice that gives satisfaction to the partners and is within the bounds of their religious beliefs and social practice is correct for them. Cultural and racial customs must be recognised and respected, and the patient's spiritual adviser may be a great comfort.

There are many other aspects which will involve vocational members of the team, notably employment and educational programmes. The final aim is to enable the victim devastated by paralysis to live in the community with dignity and as much independence as the disability will allow.

BIBLIOGRAPHY

Bannister, R. (ed.) (1984). *Brain's Clinical Neurology*, 6th edition. Oxford University Press, Oxford.

Harris, N. (1983). *Postgraduate Textbook of Clinical Orthopaedics*, chapter 31. John Wright and Sons, Bristol.

Jeffreys, E. (1980). *Disorders of the Cervical Spine*. Butterworths, London.

McSweeney, T. (1984). Injuries of the cervical spine. *Annals of the Royal College of Surgeons of England*, **66**, 1–6.

Roaf, R. (1980). *Spinal Deformities*, 2nd edition. Pitman, London.

Chapter 14

Spinal Cord Lesions – Management

by B. GOFF MCSP, ONC, DipTP *and* A. EVANS MCSP, ONC

GENERAL POINTS

The causes of cord lesions have been discussed in the previous chapter. Management by physiotherapy will depend on the level, extent and severity of damage to nerve tissue and whether the onset is sudden or gradual. Points to consider include the following:

1. Sudden onset with transient spinal shock.
2. Increase in signs as haemorrhage or oedema can occur after initial injury.
3. A changing clinical picture as spinal shock wears off and oedema subsides.
4. Disparity of bone and cord levels which is minimal in the cervical region but increases at lower levels until, at the lower border of L2, a lesion will not involve the spinal cord but will injure nerve roots (Table 14/1).
5. Cord damage may only be partial leaving some cell bodies and tracts intact. For example, central cord damage may leave the

TABLE 14/1 Examples of anatomical relationships of the spinal cord and bony spinous processes in adults

Cord segments	Vertebral bodies	Spinous processes
C8	Lower C6 Upper C7	C6
T6	Lower T3 Upper T4	T3
T12 L1	T9	T8
L5	T11	T10
Sacral segments	T12 and L1	T12 L1

peripheral tracts unharmed but cause central damage extending up and down from the main level of injury, so-called 'coning' (Hardy and Rossier, 1975). If there is damage to only the right or left half of the cord a Brown-Sequard syndrome will result.

6. There may be damage to nerve roots not only to those emerging from intervertebral foramina at the level of bone damage but also to nerve roots which pass within the neural canal at the site of injury and emerge at lower levels (Fig. 14/1).

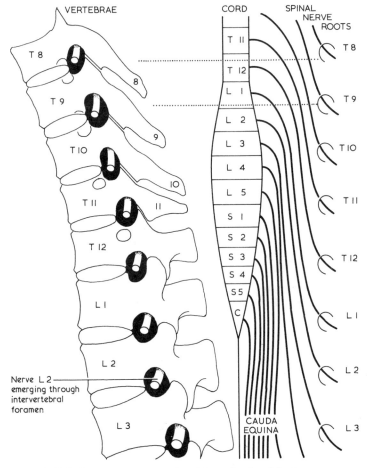

FIG. 14/1 Relative nerve root, cord and bone levels of the lower segments of the spinal cord

7. The changing pathological and resultant clinical signs in progressive conditions, which include multiple sclerosis, syringomyelia, neoplasms, motor neurone disease and Friedreich's Ataxia.

Signs resulting from cell body destruction

At the level of the lesion grey matter is damaged, often permanently.

1. Lower motor cells in the anterior grey column supply skeletal muscle, so destruction results in weakness or flaccid paralysis of muscles in the affected myotomes. Most obvious is the weakness or complete flaccid paralysis of hand muscles if the C7, 8 and T1 cord segments are damaged.
2. Damage to cells in the posterior grey column, or in posterior root ganglions, result in interruptions of afferent pathways with loss of sensation and also of reflex arcs in the spinal cord.
3. Cells in the lateral grey column of the cord segments T1 to L2 are visceral motor cells of the sympathetic system: damage to these interrupts pathways for control of blood pressure and body temperature, and local or general vasodilation may occur.
4. Cells in the lateral grey column of lower lumbar and sacral cord segments are involved in parasympathetic outflow to pelvic viscera. Damage to them may cause flaccidity or spasticity of the urinary bladder, and reflex control of the internal sphincters may be impaired.

Signs resulting from interruption of white fibre tracts

It is thought that when white fibres are destroyed within the central nervous system they do not regenerate, so permanent interruption of nerve conduction occurs.

The ascending tracts convey impulses to the sensorium and also to many other centres in the brain. Interruption of these not only results in loss of all modes of sensation below the level of destruction but also produces a profound effect on centres controlling automatic postural reactions.

The descending tracts convey impulses from the pyramidal, extrapyramidal and cerebellar upper motor systems mainly via the corticospinal, reticulospinal, rubrospinal and vestibulospinal tracts. Interruption of these tracts produces release symptoms because the undamaged motor cells below the level of the lesion are now free to respond, with no modification, to all incoming afferent stimuli. Spinal reflex action is apparent once spinal shock has worn off.

Stimuli which will produce flexor withdrawal, or crossed extensor, reflexes include not only potentially harmful ones such as a pin prick but also constipation with impacted faeces, kidney stones, ingrowing toenails, a sudden change in temperature, a pressure sore, bladder infection, sudden noise, or even the movement of bedclothes. All muscles respond to stretch, so after a flexor withdrawal has occurred and gravity tends to pull the limb down again, a second flexor spasm sometimes occurs elicited by the resulting stretch as the flexors relax. In some cases flexor spasticity is very difficult to prevent and every care must be taken to try to avoid reinforcement and exaggeration of this by such factors as listed above.

Signs resulting from cell and fibre irritation

Some cells and fibres may not be completely destroyed but inflammatory reaction and, later, scar tissue sometimes cause irritation which, especially in the case of sensory cells and fibres, is very troublesome. Girdle pains and phantom limbs are examples.

Signs resulting from involvement of nerve roots

In a minority of cases it appears that many nerve roots are damaged even below the bone damage, possibly from traction on the whole spinal cord at the time of the injury. This may explain the absence of spinal reflex activity which persists permanently in a minority of cases.

Visceral signs

In complete lesions, and in some partial ones, control of the external sphincters of the bowel and the bladder is lost leading to double incontinence. There is also loss of sexual function.

Function loss

Control of active movement is impossible in complete lesions. In partial lesions spasticity is usually present so even if some control of limb movement is spared this is of a mass primitive type. Control of postural stability is absent, or so masked by flexor or extensor mass patterns of movements that normal use of the limbs for stance, locomotion or manipulative skills is impossible.

Postural and equilibrium reactions are lost, and absence of protective pain makes joint and skin damage a serious possibility.

Respiratory function and removal of secretions from the respiratory tract are impaired in all high level lesions.

SECONDARY COMPLICATIONS

Chest

In high level lesions where the intercostal muscles are paralysed, vital capacity and ventilation are reduced, and paralysis of the abdominal muscles makes coughing ineffective or impossible. Secretions collect in the lungs and cannot be removed by the patient's own efforts. In cervical lesions, during the first few days post-injury, there is a thickening of the mucous lining of the nose and the throat resulting in increased secretions and, therefore, difficulty in breathing. This can be relieved with Otrivine nasal drops.

Visceral

Bladder infection, retention or a high residual urine are likely complications.

Circulatory

Vasomotor paralysis, loss of movement and use of the affected parts all impair circulation. Deep vein thrombosis occurs in the trunk or leg vessels of some patients.

Oedema and trophic changes are frequently seen in the hands of tetraplegic patients. Because of interruption of nerve pathways from the vasomotor centre in the medulla oblongata the regulation of peripheral resistance, and therefore of blood pressure, is not adequate. Sudden changes of position from the horizontal to the vertical result in pooling of blood in the abdomen and the legs with the consequence that syncope and vertigo are frequent complications: this is most severe and persistent in high level lesions. Ischaemic necrosis of the cord may occur at mid-dorsal level where there is some restriction of arterial blood supply; this can cause further signs such as a flaccid urinary bladder and other reduced spinal reflexes.

Loss of joint range and soft tissue range

Unless treatment is carried out regularly joint range becomes limited and soft tissue contractures soon prevent good functional positioning.

Deformity

This may be defined as a malalignment of body segments which impairs or prevents function. It is related to loss of range of both joint and soft tissues. Impaired circulation, deposition of calcium salts in soft tissue around joints, the persistent pull of spastic muscles or the unopposed pull of spared muscles whose antagonists are flaccid, all contribute to the risk of deformity. Certain muscle groups are stronger than their antagonists or are more likely to be involved in spastic reflex actions, and the force of gravity mitigates against some joint positions.

Joint and skin damage

Unrelieved pressure quickly impairs the circulation on weight-bearing surfaces. The loss of protective pain is devastating in its effect and because he is unaware of it the patient does not move to relieve pressure. Sunburn, extremes of temperature, scratches and strain on ligaments can all readily cause skin or joint damage. Prominent nails in shoes and failure to dry the skin carefully after washing are other examples of how easily skin damage can occur. Poor circulation reduces the resistance to infection so abrasions or small pressure sores easily become infected. Careless handling of paralysed and insensitive parts can also contribute to joint and soft tissue damage or even fractures.

Calcification of soft tissue

In some cases calcium salts are laid down in soft tissue around joints (Fig. 14/2). The reasons for this are not fully understood but some disturbance of local circulation or trauma are possible causes (Goldman, 1980).

Spasticity

The uncontrolled activity of lower motor neurones in undamaged segments of the spinal cord below the level of the lesion produces

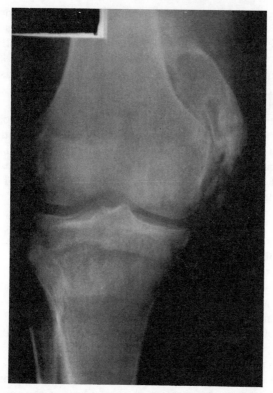

FIG. 14/2 Radiograph of a knee joint showing calcified soft tissues

a number of problems. The result may be severe spasticity which predisposes to pressure sores, contractures, deformity and greatly reduced function. Even in partial lesions, with some control of movement of the trunk and limbs, spasticity prevents normal postural reactions and normal use of the part.

Psychological factors

This is discussed finally not because it is the least important but because all other signs, symptoms and complications revolve around the degree of acceptance by the patient of his disability. The sudden complete loss of function, dependence on others and uncertainty about the future inevitably have a profound effect on the mental and emotional state of the patient. Even in patients whose lesion is at a low cord level, or where the onset is gradual, psychological problems may arise.

In the case of some tetraplegic patients the dependence, which lasts for many weeks and may be permanent, includes not only total care of bladder and bowel function, turning and all personal hygiene, but also feeding with fluids and solid food.

Concern about dependants, relatives and friends, future occupation and, indeed, all domestic and social affairs can cause great distress to all but the very young.

The emotional state fluctuates: after an initial depression a period of reactionary optimism usually occurs followed later by the most difficult period of more penetrating realisation of the predicament. The psychological complications are frequently aggravated by a well-meaning but unhelpful attitude of relatives and friends.

PROGRESSIVE CORD LESIONS

As more nerve tissue becomes involved in pathological changes dysfunction gradually increases. A variety of symptoms and signs occur as more cell bodies and tracts are damaged.

Loss of sensation is partial and may only include cutaneous or kinaesthetic sensation because interrupted impulses resulting in such loss normally travel in different tracts in the cord.

The motor signs are very variable but the most common sign is that caused by interruption of some fibres of the corticospinal tracts. This produces a spastic state of muscles similar to that in the leg of a patient with spastic hemiplegia.

The plantar response is extensor, ankle clonus occurs on slight stretch of the calf and gradually control of learned patterns of movement with selective control of individual joints is lost. Instead of the limbs taking part automatically in postural reactions to changing stimuli, only limited patterns of total movements are available.

Normal functions such as rising from sitting and normal gait are difficult or impossible. At first the extensor thrust pattern predominates, there being a combination of extension, adduction and medial rotation at the hip joint, extension at the knee joint, plantar flexion at the ankle joint and inversion at the subtalar joint. Later, as the control from the brain is further reduced by more extensive cord involvement, the predominant pattern is of total flexor withdrawal of the leg or legs. It should be noted that these two patterns are produced by superficial muscles passing over two joints and the postural reactions of deeper muscles passing over only one joint are not elicited.

The reasons for this failure of normal postural reaction are complex. The spastic total patterns prevent normal stimuli occurring in the deep pressure-bearing area of the heel or in the structures composing joints, thus abnormal afferent input elicits mass movement of withdrawal or thrust instead of postural stability for weight-bearing. There may also be interruption of some tracts of the spinal cord from the extrapyramidal and cerebellar centres, thus further reducing modification of spinal reflexes. If existing nerve pathways for postural reflexes are not used, synaptic resistance increases and the normal responses become less and less easy to elicit. Expressed differently this means that if spasticity is not relieved or reduced it becomes more severe. The flexor withdrawal reflex, being the most primitive protective reflex, is the most persistent and vicious reflex, once it is released from modification.

Circulatory disturbance occurs, which aggravates the sensory and motor disability. Secondary complications also produce further loss of function unless prevented by adequate treatment. Examples of this are contractures of the soft tissues, particularly the strong flexors of the hip and knee joints, the adductors of the hip joint and the calf muscles.

TEAMWORK

This is essential to co-ordinate the activities of medical, nursing and paramedical personnel. Each must have some knowledge of the role of other team members. Treatment involves nurses and therapists working together and the timing of turns, chest care or, in later stages, activities by the patient, need co-ordinating. The medical social worker, local authorities, follow-up co-ordinator, who is usually a nurse or occupational therapist, and the disablement resettlement officer (DRO), will all be involved in the long-term welfare of the patient. The DRO can contact employers and attempt to re-establish in suitable employment all patients who were wage earners previous to their illness or injury.

Relatives and the patient

The relatives, and the patient, are as much part of the team as the professionals, and must be considered at all times. Eventually it is they and the patient himself who will share the responsibility for the success or otherwise of attempts to restore him to an independent life in the community. In the case of the most severely disabled patients the relatives may be able to undertake nursing care at home after suitable instruction and with the necessary equipment. The services of district nurses and health visitors may be required, and, where there is one, the follow-up co-ordinator will maintain the link between home and hospital.

PRINCIPLES OF TREATMENT COMMON TO SPINAL CORD LESIONS OF SUDDEN ONSET

Early stage

1. To prevent movement of unstable spine causing further cord damage.
2. To maintain a clear airway.
3. To prevent damage to skin and joints.
4. To care for bladder and bowel function.
5. To give support and try to help acceptance of the situation by the patient and the relatives.

Stage when weight-bearing through the spine is permitted

1. The emphasis is on activity to gain as much independence as possible.
2. Adjustment to sitting and standing positions must be acquired; balance and posture training are given.
3. Responsibility for care of the patient's own skin, joints, bladder and bowel health must be encouraged.
4. Transfers, without damage to skin or joints must be learned.
5. Locomotion in a self-propelled or powered wheelchair is acquired; in some cases ambulation in orthoses and using crutches may be learned (see pp. 359–63).
6. Resettlement at home and, if possible, in a suitable occupation should be aimed for.
7. Follow-up and after-care will be needed when patients are discharged. Regular reviews are necessary and a system of domiciliary visiting by a specially trained nurse or therapist has been found helpful in many spinal units.

Procedures

SURGERY

This may be performed to reduce the risk of further cord damage and to stabilise the spine. A general anaesthetic may add to respiratory problems and additional care will be required to avoid complications developing. Tendon transplants may be done in selected cases involving the cervical cord, for example, the posterior deltoid tendon to triceps, or if the wrist extensor muscles are strong, one of these may be transplanted to give some finger flexion.

POSITIONING

The principal aim of careful positioning is to hold the spine in such a position that further cord damage is prevented. This principle should be observed by the personnel who convey the patient from the scene of the accident to a hospital. It should continue to govern the subsequent procedures until the spine is considered sufficiently stable to allow trunk movement and weight to be taken through it in a vertical position. This is usually not until 8 to 12 weeks after injury. Such positions must be maintained during all radiographic examinations, throughout all nursing and therapeutic procedures such as washing, attendance to bowel and bladder functions, clearing secretions from the chest and necessary change in position or passive movements of the limbs.

Secondary aims of careful positioning are to prevent circulatory complications, prevent deformity and damage to skin, joints, or soft tissues. Prevention of compression of veins especially in the calf and prevention of pressure on bony prominences help to achieve these aims.

Details of positions and methods to maintain them vary according to several factors. The level of the lesion is one factor; skull traction and support for the neck by sandbags, a cervical collar or a special head rest is used for patients with cervical cord lesions. In the case of patients with a dorsal or lumbar vertebral level of lesion, support for the neck is not essential but the lower parts of the spine must be prevented from moving and the lumbar lordosis maintained. This is usually achieved by the placing of pillows (Fig. 14/3). It is vital for all team members to be meticulous about positioning and in each case they must know which method is used and why it has been selected.

Another consideration in choosing a method of positioning is

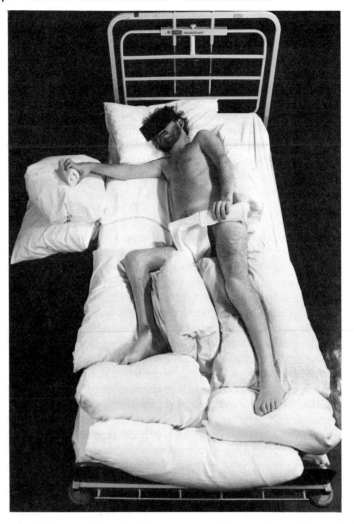

FIG. 14/3 The position of pillows on a bed for a patient with a spinal injury

the number of people available to turn the patient at regular intervals. A method which has proved to be effective is the use of firm pillows and small mattress sections carefully placed under the head, the trunk and the legs and to separate the legs and support the feet. A minimum of three trained persons is needed to execute each turn to a different position while maintaining the immobility of the spine. Details of this method may be found in nursing textbooks (see p. 380).

Special beds have been designed to achieve maintenance of appropriate positions and to allow automatic and/or continual turning. The Rota-Rest bed is an example; its mechanism, electrically operated, turns the bed slowly through 130°, thus pressure on any point is never prolonged. A beneficial effect is also achieved for the lungs and, possibly, the kidneys. When the motor is switched off the bed remains stationary in any desired position so that nursing or physiotherapy procedures can be carried out. An advantage of this type of bed is that a team is not needed for turning – therefore it is useful where there is less staff available and also in the home, on discharge, for the tetraplegic patient who cannot turn himself.

TURNING

Turning the patient in rotation from right side lying to supine, to left side lying and back to supine position is necessary during the early stage of bed rest. At first the turns are at 2-hourly intervals throughout each 24 hours, but gradually this may be reduced to 3- or 4-hourly turns providing there are no signs of threatened skin breakdown on pressure-bearing points such as the sacrum or the femoral trochanters. During the turn the position of the spine must be maintained and special instruction and training must be given to all personnel on the ward who at any time help to form the turning team. The senior nurse present will direct the team and ensure that the turn is correctly done; she also gives commands so that the timing of the turn is co-ordinated. During the turn linen may be changed, the undersheet straightened and meticulous care taken to ensure that no crumbs or other abrasive material are left in the bed. The skin must be inspected to detect any signs of threatening pressure sores. Care must be taken not to disturb the catheter, if present, or other intubation such as a naso-oesophageal tube or tracheostomy tube. Details of treatment for respiratory complications will be discussed later but it should be noted that physiotherapy techniques to help clear secretions and to assist coughing are frequently needed before, and after, turning.

The nursing and physiotherapy staff should work in close co-operation at all times but in the early stages of care of the cervical cord cases this is particularly necessary, not only to avoid too many disturbances for the patient, and to make the contribution of each team member more effective, but also because they often act as a substitute for each other. Physiotherapists frequently act as members of the turning or lifting team; and all personnel working on a spinal unit should be taught how to make the patient cough to help clear secretions.

Another important feature of the turn is that the limbs are repositioned at each turn. This not only ensures relief of pressure on bony points but helps maintenance of circulation and joint and soft tissue mobility. It is a disadvantage of the use of the automatically turning bed that the limb joints are not moved as it turns. For this reason physiotherapy care for patients on these beds needs to be more frequent. Special types of bed in spinal injuries units include water beds, low air-loss beds and automatic-turning beds.

CHEST CARE

Respiratory complications can occur in patients with spinal cord lesions for many reasons, for example, pre-existing chronic respiratory disorder, lowered resistance to infection, paralysis of muscles of inspiration or those needed for effective coughing. An added factor is paradoxical respiration caused by paralysis of intercostal muscles. Details of physiotherapy will be found on page 349, but any case of spinal cord injury, or dysfunction from other causes, may require treatment to prevent internal secretions causing obstruction, and to improve the ventilation of the lungs. All cases should have regular respiratory function tests and the results recorded so that comparisons can be made. Vital capacity (VC) measurements with a spirometer and peak flow measurements using a Wright's peak flow meter or a Vitalograph machine are routine procedures in spinal injuries units. A fall in VC can be caused by the development of a haemothorax, a pneumothorax, a paralytic ileus, or by a rise of cord level damage which may occur in cervical lesions resulting in weakness of the diaphragm.

CARE OF THE URINARY BLADDER AND THE BOWELS

Although this care is essentially a nursing and medical concern the physiotherapist needs to be aware of the management required to avoid retention of urine or bladder infections; and how to avoid damage to urinals by careless handling during positioning and other activities, and during the application of splintage.

Tact is needed to help patients accept the complication of double incontinence, and to become responsible ultimately for the care of their bladder and bowel function; they need to be helped to realise how vital such care is to their general well-being.

TRANSFERS

Certain fundamental points relating to transfers apply equally whether the patient can achieve them himself or has to depend on others to lift him (p. 355).

All members of the team concerned in any way with patient care should know how to lift patients alone or with help, and how he should lift himself, if possible, without damage to skin or joints. The physiotherapist can help instruct other personnel such as orderlies and nursing aides in this important procedure.

ASSESSMENT AND RECORDS

The capabilities of the patient, his control of movement, the extent of motor and sensory loss and, later, his ability to compensate for motor loss must be assessed at regular intervals. Joint range and the presence of any deformity likely to impair function should also be considered. The examination of the patient and tests for functional ability including the respiratory function tests are likely to be carried out by several members of the team; doctors, physiotherapists and occupational therapists all share this responsibility. Charts of function achievement specially prepared for paraplegic and tetraplegic patients are helpful.

Nurses take and record body temperature, pulse and respiratory rate, arterial blood pressure, fluid intake and output.

All records must be dated and filed and be freely available to other team members. Regular consultation between all team members is helpful and will be more effective if records are available.

Complete Cord Lesions

Physiotherapy management for low level lesions (paraplegia) will be discussed. Additional requirements for high level lesions (tetraplegic) and partial lesions will follow where the management is different.

PARAPLEGIA: EARLY STAGE WHILE ON BED REST

1. *Passive movements* to the legs are carried out at least twice daily in the first three to six weeks and possibly reduced to once a

day later if good circulation and range are being maintained. Because it is not possible from the neutral position, to carry out hip extension on the under leg when the patient is in side lying it may be necessary to visit the patient several times so that each leg can be treated when it is uppermost.

Sensitive handling is needed because damage can occur to soft tissue around joints especially during the stage of spinal shock. It is also necessary later to guard against eliciting spinal reflexes. The physiotherapist must learn to feel when the limit of joint and soft tissue range is approached. Movements should be in normal patterns; they should be performed slowly and, eventually, in their full range at least twice at each handling. During the first few weeks pain at the site of the lesion may limit slightly the range obtained on passive movement.

Maintenance of the length of some structures which pass over more than one joint is especially important to prevent deformity which would later hamper good function such as long sitting, standing, or crutch walking.

Overstretching of soft tissue is harmful, but functional length must be maintained in the following structures: muscles, tendons, ligaments, and fascia. For long sitting, length is needed in the hamstrings. For standing there needs to be full hip and knee extension, and the length of calf muscles and fascia must be sufficient to allow at least 90° at the ankle with the knee straight and the foot flat on the floor. The toes should not be allowed to curl or claw so that shoes can be put on easily and not cause pressure sores.

To improve circulation passive leg movements are repeated for at least three minutes to each leg and for this purpose need not be in the full range. The legs are moved one at a time and care is taken not to allow sufficient hip flexion to cause movement of the lumbar spine. After treatment the pillows supporting the legs and feet are replaced correctly.

If there is any sign of oedema careful measurement of the girth of the calf should be made, recorded and repeated subsequently for comparison. Blood will be taken for the prothrombin time to be estimated, and leg movements stopped until the doctor says they may be restarted.

The number of treatments required each day depends upon such factors as the method of nursing and turning the patient, his age and the probability of circulatory complications. When the automatic turning bed is used, limb movements by physiotherapists are needed more frequently than for patients who are turned manually as in the latter case leg positions are changed at each turn.

When spinal shock wears off, muscle tone returns to the leg muscles and careful nursing and handling during physiotherapy are needed to prevent reinforcement of spasticity. The physiotherapist's hands should be smooth and warm and care taken not to elicit either a flexor withdrawal or an extensor thrust (Fig. 14/4). Pressure through the heel and the long axis of the limb together with slow smooth movements tend to elicit a postural response of all deep muscles acting on the knee and ankle. These then work in combination to stabilise the joint as they do in normal weight-bearing and total spastic movements are inhibited.

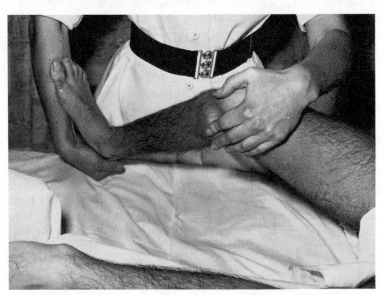

FIG. 14/4 Position of the hands when handling a leg with spasticity

2. Only those patients with pre-existing chronic chest disorders, or who sustained trauma to the chest at the time of injury, are likely to need intensive physiotherapy to maintain or improve respiratory function.
3. Strengthening exercises for the upper limbs may be permitted.

Additional requirements in tetraplegia

PASSIVE MOVEMENTS

Passive movements are essential for all the joints of the upper limb over which the patient has no voluntary control. Unless great care is taken range of movement is rapidly lost in the hands. If the biceps muscle is active but the triceps muscle paralysed then flexor contracture of the elbow will present a problem. Some form of splintage to maintain elbow extension is advocated and can be achieved by using (a) Orthoplast, (b) pneumatic splints, (c) plaster of Paris, or (d) a Robert Jones pressure bandage.

In lesions with the C6 cord segment intact but damage to C7, some radial wrist extension is often spared allowing a 'tenodesis action' of passive finger flexion as the wrist is actively extended. This can be of use to the patient providing the long finger flexors are *not* overstretched but they need to be sufficiently long to give satisfactory results if tendon transplants are contemplated. Functional length of the finger and wrist flexors and of biceps muscle should be such that it allows the hand to be placed flat on a surface with the elbow extended to act as a prop. If the arms are to be placed behind a patient in long sitting then the length of the biceps muscle must allow extension at the glenohumeral joint; elbow extension and forearm pronation. Full shoulder-girdle and shoulder joint range must be maintained. In some spinal injuries units the patient's arms are placed in full elevation for a period each day, full protrusion is also maintained by placing the arms across the chest but care is taken not to restrict breathing. In very high cervical lesions spasticity of the muscles of the hand, forearm and elbow may occur.

CIRCULATION

In tetraplegics circulation to the hand is frequently very poor, and trophic changes, oedema and Sudeck's atrophy may result.

One method of trying to control oedema in the hand is by the use of inflatable plastic splints. These are placed around the hands and forearms, care being taken to see that the whole hand is encircled; the splints are inflated until a comfortable gentle squeeze is experienced on the fingers of the physiotherapist when she places them within the grip of the splint. These splints are left on for up to 20 minutes once or twice a day. Ideally, a pump should be connected to the valve of the splint so that an intermittent pumping action is obtained. Care is needed to ensure that the pressure is not too high, for the patient cannot guard against this as the hands have no sensation. In some units the hands are bandaged in the 'boxing glove splint' devised by Professor J.I.P. James and developed by Dr Cheshire and Glenys Rowe (Bromley, 1980; Cheshire and Rowe, 1970). Even later when the hands are left free by day, the bandaging is continued at night.

CARE OF THE RESPIRATORY TRACT

The combined resources of medical, nursing and physiotherapy personnel are needed if serious respiratory complications develop. The physiotherapist uses vibrations and rib-springing to clear secretions from the periphery of the lungs and when secretions have collected in the upper respiratory tract she is able to assist coughing by careful placing of her hands, or hands and one fore-arm, and by giving firm pressure on the upper abdomen and lower parts of the chest in time with the patient's effort to give a forced expiration. This procedure needs experienced care both to be effective and to avoid damaging the chest cage or the contents of the abdominal cavity. Figures 14/5 and 14/6 show the position of the hands for assisted coughing.

Auscultation and chest radiographs are used to locate areas especially involved in the collection of secretions or atelectasis and the physiotherapist will learn by experience to palpate the chest to locate abnormalities of air entry. Respiratory function tests are carried out daily if necessary. Co-operation with the nursing staff is essential as secretions are cleared before and after each turn. Suction through an endotracheal tube may be neces-sary and in some cases a tracheostomy is performed.

DIAPHRAGMATIC PACING

In some high cervical lesions above C3, C4, the spinal cord has been injured above the cell bodies of the phrenic nerve leading to loss of power to the diaphragm. In these cases it may be possible to stimulate the phrenic nerve by implanting electrodes and thus producing a diaphragmatic contraction, with the aim that the patient will ultimately become free from mechanical ventilation. Most people with this level of lesion are usually totally ventilator dependent.

The placing of electrodes is specialised and is only performed on selected patients following a thorough pre-operative assess-ment, screening and percutaneous stimulation of the phrenic nerves. A strong contraction of the diaphragm must be obtained for a successful result. There are various reasons for a poor result

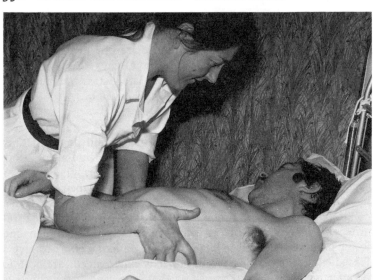

FIG. 14/5 Position of the hands and forearm for assisted coughing

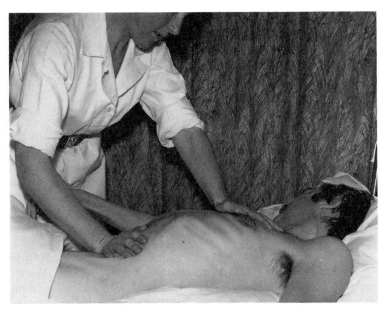

FIG. 14/6 Position of the hands for assisted coughing

including anterior horn cell or nerve root damage of C3, 4, 5, in which case the patient is not suitable for this procedure. If phrenic nerve electrodes are able to be implanted each hemidiaphragm is paced either one at a time or simultaneously. The duration of pacing commences for a few minutes each hour and is gradually increased. Between pacings the patient is reconnected to the ventilator until the full 24 hours is able to be covered (Glenn, 1980).

STRENGTHENING EXERCISES

These are given using manual resistance to all spared muscles in the arm, taking care not to cause undue movement of the cervical spine.

PARAPLEGIA: STAGE WHEN WEIGHT-BEARING THROUGH THE SPINE IS PERMITTED

Treatment is rapidly progressed to increasing activity by the patient. The nursing staff are usually responsible for sitting the patient up in bed, e.g. using a crank to raise the top of the bed to support the spine. Physiotherapy is given with the patient sitting up in bed to commence balance training and lifts to relieve pressure.

When the patient is allowed to sit out in a wheelchair the aims of treatment are as follows:

Readjustment of postural sense and equilibrium reactions

The patient must learn to retain a good posture and to maintain balance in many positions without the support of a back rest or his arms (Fig. 14/7). The physiotherapist must appreciate that until the patient sits up for the first time with no support or contact with a supporting surface for his head, trunk or arms he cannot fully realise the consequence of the sensory loss in the lower part of his body.

Posture correction and balance is trained with the patient sitting on a pillow on a low plinth. The feet should be supported on the floor or a low platform so that the thighs are fully supported and the hips, knees and ankles are at a right angle. The physiotherapist should take great care that the patient does not fall or damage his buttocks or legs. Until he is strong and has learned to

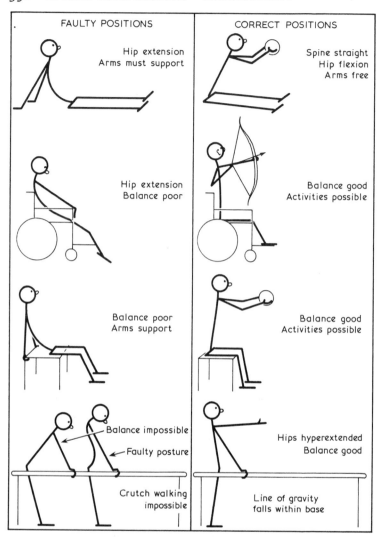

FIG. 14/7 Faulty and correct postures

transfer himself safely the patient is lifted to the plinth by two people. Use of a mirror may be helpful at first and any suitable method of balance training is used. Arm movements are given when balance is good and activities including ball games are added as soon as possible.

Balance is also practised in the wheelchair. Use of the chair,

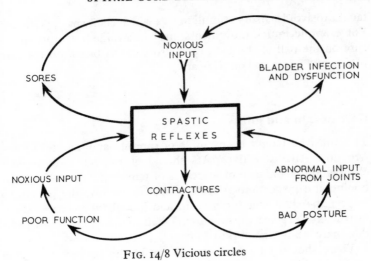

FIG. 14/8 Vicious circles

negotiation of slopes, curbs and picking up objects from the floor are all taught.

Spasticity

The severity of spasticity varies with the efficiency of early treatment, with the position of the patient and in response to incoming stimuli from the skin, deep structures of the legs and from the urinary bladder. If involuntary spasms occur the risk of pressure sores is increased. Sores, bladder infection, and contractures in soft tissue all increase stimuli likely to elicit spasms and aggravate spasticity. A vicious cycle may result increasing the risk of complications and to poor posture and function (Fig. 14/8). Psychological stress also increases spasticity and is much more troublesome in some patients than in others. Although many factors influence the severity of spasticity an attempt should be made to evaluate this: Goff (1976) describes a method of grading the severity of spasticity. It must be remembered that there is a great risk of dominance by the flexor withdrawal reflex in complete cord lesions unless adequate treatment is given.

Kuhn (1950) stated 'alterations in dominance of postural and protective reflexes may occur but extensor spasms are the natural outcome of complete transection of the cord in man if complications can be avoided'. Periods of standing in a standing frame help to reduce spasticity (p. 366). Physiotherapy techniques to reduce spasticity are described in Chapters 7 and 8. Patients are taught to avoid sensory stimuli to legs which elicit spastic reflexes. For example, quick movements must be avoided, as must pressure on the ball of the foot. (See also sections below on the care of skin and joints and on self-care.)

Care of skin and joints

This must be taught by example of careful handling and by instruction. All insensitive parts should be protected by vigilant observation, avoidance of extremes of temperature, careful positioning and inspection. A hand mirror is used by the patient to inspect the skin over the sacrum and ischial tuberosities. He is instructed to report to the nursing staff immediately he suspects that there is any sign of skin damage.

There should be a firm base to the bed to prevent a sagging mattress which causes creases in the sheet. During long periods of sitting in a wheelchair the skin over the ischial tuberosities must be protected by using a wooden-based, sheepskin covered, firm sorbo-cushion or cushions with a convex base which compensate for the sag in the wheelchair seat. Other types are available. Regular lifts performed by the patient himself, relieve pressure and allow return of circulation to the skin. The lifts must be maintained for 15 to 30 seconds and are needed every 15 minutes when the patient sits up. Some patients eventually need to lift at less frequent intervals but the relief of pressure soon becomes an automatic action.

The patient learns to turn himself in bed and a habit of doing so becomes established. Regular reminders by the night staff may be needed until turning is automatic. The patient is taught to use the prone lying position to eliminate sacral pressure.

The length of time that the patient is allowed up is gradually increased. He must be taught to observe the position of his legs and to lift them carefully when moving.

Self-care

The patient must be able to wash, dress, attend to his own urinal, maintain joint range in the legs by doing his own passive movements and apply his orthoses. These activities are taught by several members of the team but balance in the long-sitting position must be achieved to facilitate good function.

Transfers (Figs. 14/9 to 14/12)

These are taught from and to the wheelchair and the bed, plinth, bath, lavatory seat, and motorised vehicle. Also taught is safe transfer from and to a mat for treatment sessions. Various methods are tried out and the best for the individual is finally selected.

In teaching safe transfers the principles include correct positioning of the chair, ensuring that the brakes are fully on and lifting the legs with the hands on to the plinth, bed or floor from the footplates of the chair. During these manoeuvres care must be taken not to knock the legs or drag them along a hard surface. When the legs are positioned correctly the trunk is lifted so that the buttocks are clear of the support and will not be dragged or knocked as the transfer is completed.

In transferring from a wheelchair to a plinth the approach can be from the side or one end. In the former case the chair is placed slightly obliquely alongside the plinth, the arm of the chair on the near side is removed and if necessary a pillow placed over the top of the large wheel of the chair; the brakes are applied securely.

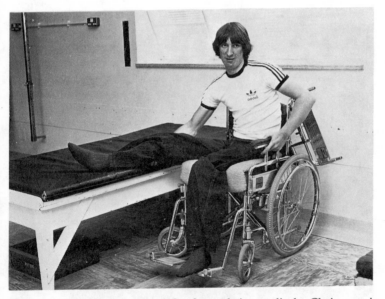

FIG. 14/9 Preparation to transfer from chair to plinth. Chair arm is removed; the chair is alongside the plinth; the near leg is lifted to the plinth

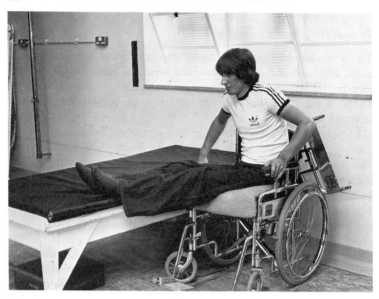

FIG. 14/10 The far leg has been lifted to the plinth; the arms are ready to lift

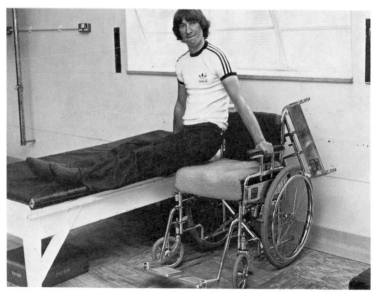

FIG. 14/11 A high lift is necessary to clear the chair wheel as the trunk is lifted to the plinth

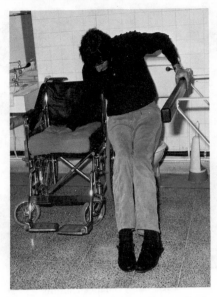

FIG. 14/12 Transfer from a wheelchair to the lavatory

Next the legs are lifted and placed on the plinth, the far leg is sometimes crossed over the other. Then the near-side hand is placed on the plinth sufficiently centrally to allow room for the buttocks to be placed on the plinth also, the other hand is placed on the far side-arm of the chair. A good high lift of the trunk follows and it is swung over on to the plinth and the long-sitting position is thus obtained.

Whatever method of transfer is used there is a risk of the chair moving if the tyres are worn or the floor slippery. The patient soon learns to be cautious and to position the chair correctly to avoid slipping between the chair and the plinth and to avoid too much sideways thrust with the off side arm which may cause the chair to slip sideways (Fig. 14/9).

Exercise and activity (Figs. 14/13 and 14/14)

This is arranged for all spared muscles. Mat work, transfers, use of weight and pulley circuits including the use of a Westminster pulley circuit and also proprioceptive neuromuscular facilitation (PNF) techniques of manually resisted trunk and limb patterns of movement are all useful. Rookwood Hospital, Cardiff and

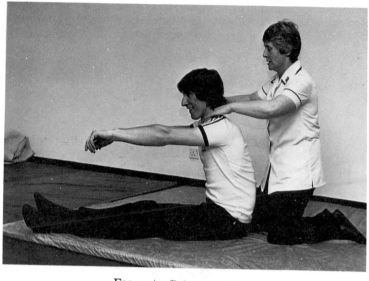

FIG. 14/13 Balance training

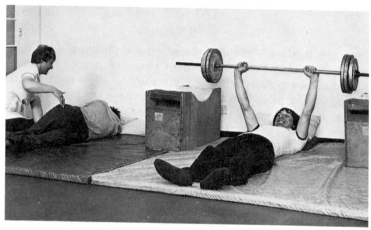

FIG. 14/14 Rolling and weight lifting

Oswestry, use a Gympac System for resisted exercises (see p. 381).

Stance and gait

These are trained as soon as sitting balance is good. Standing balance in leg orthoses is taught in parallel bars. Various styles of orthoses are used and a universal orthosis is available to assess the potential for walking.

The posture is very important as the weight must be over the feet to keep upright without the control of muscular power in gluteal muscles and hamstrings. The patient must learn to pay attention to sensation in the upper trunk and compensate for loss of equilibrium reactions in the legs and lower trunk. The hips must be slightly hyperextended and the dorsal spine straight. Many patients can maintain good balance for short periods without the support of both arms. This skill is essential for a good 'swing-to' or 'swing-through' gait.

To get to standing from the wheelchair the patient first extends the knees passively and locks the knee hinges in extension. Some patients need to place the leg on a support to achieve this, others manage by a 'high kick' type of lift or by extending the leg out in front of the chair with the foot on the floor. When both knees are locked in extension, and the chair correctly placed with the brakes on, the buttocks are lifted forward to the front of the chair seat, the hands grip the parallel bars or wall bars and a lift up and forward takes the body into the standing position. Care is needed to see that the feet do not slip forwards.

In the early stages of training, weak patients, or those with short arms, may need assistance and the physiotherapist stands in front of the patient, between the bars, placing her feet in front of the patient's shoes and if necessary gripping the top of trousers or slacks to assist the action of standing.

Gait is trained at first in parallel bars then progress to using a rigid walking frame, 'the plough' (Fig. 14/15) then to one crutch and one bar as the patient gains confidence and proficiency. Finally, two crutches are used and steps, slopes, curbs, rough surfaces and stairs are negotiated if possible. The four-point gait is the most elegant and takes least room in a crowded place. However the swing-to or swing-through gait is quicker and most young patients with strong arms can achieve this method of crutch walking. Elbow crutches with swivel tops are used so that the patient can stand and rest his forearm on the upturned arm support and have his hand free to open doors. 'Canadian' type ring top crutches with the ring above the elbow have been found useful. The hand can be used to open doors, and the crutch remains on the arm (Fig. 14/16). Some patients use rigid walking frames instead of crutches.

When the patient is proficient in crutch walking he learns to get up from the chair to standing, turn and walk away. This

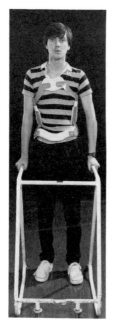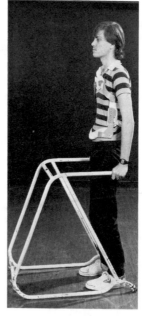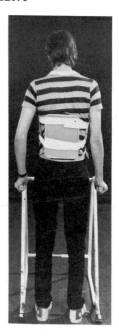

FIG. 14/15 Anterior, lateral and posterior views of a patient who has an L1 lesion wearing a Jowett brace and using the 'plough' walking aid

activity needs careful planning, strong arms and upper trunk and good equilibrium reactions to gain balance once upright. The exact method is usually worked out by each patient to suit his or her particular abilities. The physiotherapist uses her experience to help each patient learn this activity. Wheelchairs with arms that can be raised assist the patient to get to standing. A demonstration by a more experienced patient, such as one back in hospital for review, can be most helpful.

One method of standing from the wheelchair with no other support than the chair will be described. The turn can be to either side to suit the individual's abilities but will be described as for turning to the left. The chair is placed with the back against a wall or firm support and the brakes secured, the foot plates raised and turned to the sides. The orthoses are locked in extension and the right leg lifted across the left. The shoulders and trunk are twisted to the left so that the left hand is placed behind the patient's trunk on the right chair arm and the right across in

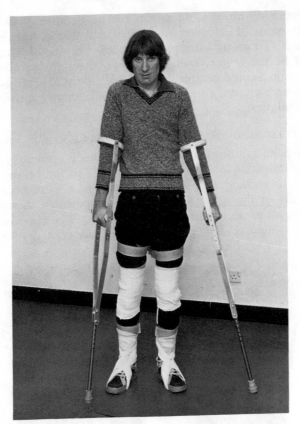

FIG. 14/16 Standing with the aid of Canadian crutches and back splints

front of the trunk on to the left arm of the chair. A good high lift follows with a twist of the pelvis to bring the patient to standing facing the chair. He then achieves balance in standing so that he can release one arm to reach and place his crutches ready to back away from the chair and walk.

Other methods may be possible, each patient should be encouraged to find the most suitable method for his ability. The crutches must be placed near or leaning against the chair so that they are within reach when stance is achieved. Patients should be encouraged to discuss their achievements and difficulties during treatment sessions, and group activities are of great psychological value.

Overcoming physical difficulties can be a source of great fun and the sense of achievement is similar to that of learning any new skill. To create a happy atmosphere but one of hard work should be the objective of every physiotherapist working in a spinal unit. Several centres in the USA and the UK are carrying out research projects using electrical stimulation to improve walking techniques.

THE 'ORLAU' HIP GUIDANCE ORTHOSIS (PARAWALKER)

A four-point gait using orthoses and crutches is commonly taught to patients with a low level of paraplegia (T10 and below), but a competent walking style can be difficult to achieve because of instability at the hips. This may cause adduction, flexion and rotation, all of which are difficult to control. The Hip Guidance Orthosis (hgo) (Figs. 14/17 and 14/18) has been developed in

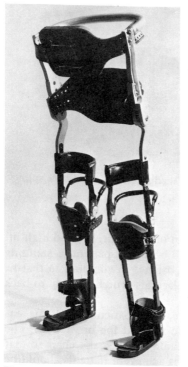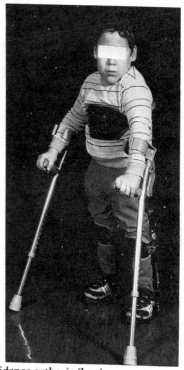

FIG. 14/17 (*left*) The ORLAU hip-guidance orthosis (hgo)

FIG. 14/18 (*right*) A patient with a high paraplegia using the hgo and crutches response to this problem and provides a means of achieving a safe low energy four-point (step by step) gait for both low and high levels of paraplegia. The latissimus dorsi muscles must be functioning (C6, 7, 8 nerve supply) together with the arm and hand muscles required for crutch walking.

The essential features of the orthosis are:

1. A rigid body brace which helps to maintain the relative abduction of the legs during the swing phase of the gait cycle.
2. A hip joint with a limited flexion/extension range and friction free operation.
3. Stabilisation of the knees and ankles.
4. A shoe plate incorporating rocker sole.
5. Simple fastening arrangements to ease putting on and taking off the orthosis.

The hgo is of use in both congenital and traumatic paraplegia. A four-point gait is useful in confined spaces, such as the home or school, with the advantage of providing a cosmetic style of walking. Some users choose to use a swing-through gait in addition where greater speed is required and this facility is still open to them with this orthosis. Patients quickly achieve independence in walking, sitting and standing and car transfers.

(The 'Orlau' hgo takes its name from the unit which designed it, namely, The Orthotic Research and Locomotor Assessment Unit (ORLAU), The Robert Jones and Agnes Hunt Orthopaedic Hospital, Oswestry, Shropshire.)

Sport and recreation

Swimming, team ball games in wheelchairs, archery and field events can all be included. These achieve objectives such as strong exercise, balance training, stimulation of increased exercise tolerance and an opportunity for social activities in the evenings and at weekends in competition with other patients.

Transport

This should be encouraged in either a car supplied by the Department of Health and Social Security to a disabled driver or in a specially adapted car of his own. Transfers to and from these and lifting a transit chair into and out of the car must be taught and arrangements made for driving instruction.

Assessment of patient's ability and preparations for resettlement

Function charts are useful to record this. Regular reassessments are helpful, not only to note progress but also to stimulate the patient's interest and to help to wean him from dependence on physiotherapy or nursing staff. Detailed sensory charts may be completed by the medical staff or by a physiotherapist. Tests of voluntary power are only appropriate for those muscles completely or partially denervated by loss of lower motor neurones at the level of the lesion. Power in spastic muscles cannot be graded on a voluntary power scale but the severity of spasticity should be evaluated and recorded (see p. 353).

During the time of increasing activity the social worker and the occupational therapist will discuss possible occupational training which may be needed, and, with the relatives, the need for any necessary alterations to the home. Physiotherapists should also show the relatives how to help the patient care for his skin and how to maintain full joint and soft tissue range.

As can be seen by the variety and extent of the new skills the patient must learn, there should be very little time for inactivity. A full day's programme 5 or 6 days a week is helpful in maintaining a work habit and is of immense psychological value. All patients should be responsible for their own timekeeping as this helps to restore self-respect and leads to independence.

Before a patient is finally discharged he is usually allowed home for weekends. This allows for gradual adjustment to a new lifestyle, and on his return any problems encountered can be discussed. Time spent at home is eventually increased to periods of a week or longer before final discharge.

Follow-up

Follow-up after discharge by frequent reviews is needed to provide continuing support when the patient returns to the community.

At each review the following must be checked: the range of joints and soft tissue, the health of the bladder and of the skin, also the state of splints, crutches and the wheelchair. Any problems which have occurred can be discussed and all help given to maintain full independence.

ADDITIONAL POINTS FOR HIGH PARAPLEGICS AND TETRAPLEGICS WHEN WEIGHT-BEARING THROUGH THE SPINE IS ALLOWED

A sorbo collar or other support is needed for tetraplegics.

Postural hypotension is almost inevitable: an abdominal binder assists control of this problem and gives a measure of stability to the lower trunk. Support stockings are used also to aid venous return.

A tilting table is useful, especially one with a mechanical device to tilt it. The patient is lifted on to the table which is covered with a suitable soft mattress or foam rubber pad, a pillow is placed under the head, one over the hips and one at chest level. Straps secure the patient to the table at the chest, hips and the knees and it is then raised at the head-end until it is almost vertical. Two attendants must be present to help keep the patient firmly and correctly positioned and to ensure that the table can be swiftly lowered to the horizontal position should the patient suffer from syncope. The upright position is only maintained for a very short period at first. The time is gradually increased as the patient's tolerance of the vertical position improves.

Postural training

Adjustment of posture and balance must be taught. Extreme patience and encouragement are needed on the part of the physiotherapist and she must be vigilant in her care to ensure that the patient does not fall or become frightened of doing so. These patients must be helped to be more aware of subtle changes of position of the head than is usual and to compensate quickly if their balance and stability are threatened. Slight head movements and arm movements may correct the alignment of body segments sufficiently to maintain a sitting position or the arms may be used in a saving reaction.

A good position of the legs with the feet on the floor under the knees, a right angle at ankle, knee and hip and the legs in slight abduction gives a measure of stability to the trunk even though the patient has no control of movement and has no sensation below neck level.

Balance is practised in long sitting and in the wheelchair once the patient has gained sufficient confidence and adjustment of vasomotor function to allow this.

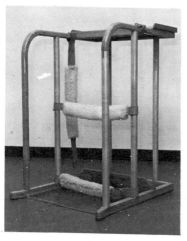
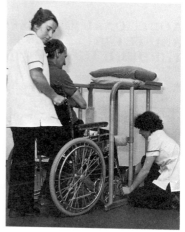

FIG. 14/19 (*left*) Standing frame. Lowest strap is placed behind the feet; centre strap in front of the knees; highest strap is fixed behind and below the buttocks

FIG. 14/20 (*right*) The wheelchair is placed ready for the lift to standing, the feet being placed in front of the lowest strap

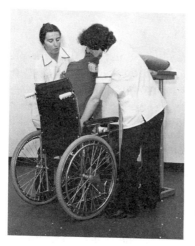
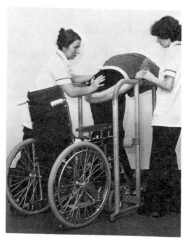

FIG. 14/21 (*left*) The patient is lifted to lean standing

FIG. 14/22 (*right*) The top strap being fixed

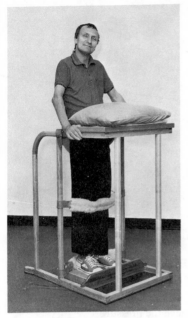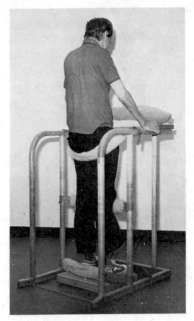

FIG. 14/23 (*left*) The patient can stand alone supported in the frame. Balance training, ball games, etc. can be carried out

FIG. 14/24 (*right*) Posterior view of the patient in the standing frame

A standing frame may be used; the construction of which, together with the use of sheepskin covered straps, enables a patient to stand without using leg supports (Figs. 14/19 to 14/24). Balance training is given, the kidneys benefit, spasticity in the legs is reduced and the patient derives psychological benefit from the periods of standing.

Care of the skin

In the case of high thoracic and cervical lesions skin care is vital even if the patient cannot actually do it for himself. The responsibility is his for seeing that he is lifted at frequent intervals. He must request the nursing staff or other therapists who are with him to lift him so that the circulation can return adequately to areas taking his weight. One method of lifting a seated paralysed patient to relieve the weight on the ischial tuberosities is as follows:

The patient folds his arms, the lifter stands behind with her

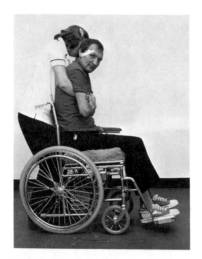 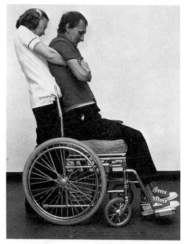

FIG. 14/25 (*left*) Preparation to lift a patient in order to relieve pressure. *Note* the physiotherapist's grip under the axillae and over the folded arms of the patient

FIG. 14/26 (*right*) The actual lift to relieve the pressure

arms under the patient's shoulders and hands gripped over the patient's forearms (Figs. 14/25 and 14/26). It is then possible to give a sufficiently high lift to allow the return of circulation to the buttock region. The lift must last for at least 15 seconds. It is repeated as frequently as necessary to keep the skin in a healthy condition. Later the patient is taught to relieve pressure himself by lifting upwards or by rolling on to one buttock and then on to the other (Figs. 14/27, 14/28 and 14/29).

Training in the care of the hands is included. Gloves or special palm mittens are worn while wheeling the chair. Cigarette holders must be used if the patient smokes. Hot plates and mugs must not be placed in the hand or rested on the legs. Gloves must be worn in cold weather and for activities such as gardening and propelling a chair.

The patient is responsible for requesting that the skin is inspected daily and that the urinal is not causing friction.

Self-care

The precise level of the lesion influences the degree of self-care possible. There is a great difference in functional ability of a

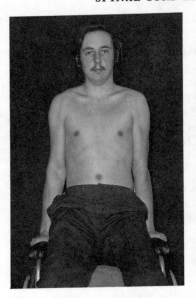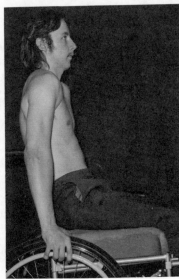

FIG. 14/27 (*left*) Patient lifting himself to relieve pressure by pushing up from the arms of the chair

FIG. 14/28 (*right*) Patient lifting himself to relieve pressure by pushing up from the wheels of the chair

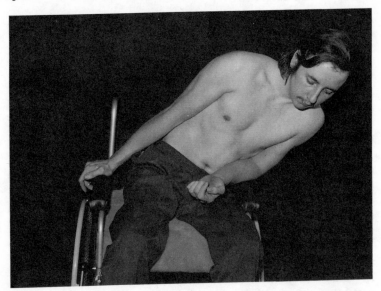

FIG. 14/29 A low cervical tetraplegic rolling sideways to relieve pressure

patient with voluntary control of elbow extension and one who has none.

A patient with control of an active triceps can support himself firmly on one or both arms, lift safely to relieve pressure on his seat and wheel his chair strongly even with no active control of the hand. If the triceps muscle is active some use is usually possible in the wrist extensors as these share the segmental supply from C7. With gadgets strapped to the hand, feeding, shaving, smoking, attention to personal hygiene and hair grooming are possible.

Morale is aided by helping each patient to take a pride in his or her own appearance. A wig should be provided for a patient who has had to have the scalp shaved during the period on skull traction. Girls are helped to make up and men to shave with special adapted electric razors.

Transfers

Some low cervical lesions can achieve transfers unaided, others learn to transfer using a sliding board or with an attendant who is taught standing transfers.

Exercise and activities

A regime of strengthening exercises for all spared muscles in the upper limb is needed for all cervical lesions according to the level. Paralysed hands are bandaged to handles for weight and pulley circuit exercises.

Activities are commenced as soon as the patient has adjusted to sitting up. Mat work is very valuable. The patient must be lifted on to the mat carefully and mat activities such as rolling, balance training in long sitting and modified cross sitting are taught (see Figs. 14/13 and 14/14).

Some patients, particularly those with active elbow extension and radial wrist extension achieve a remarkable degree of control of activities. Some can hook their thumbs into their trouser pockets and sit up using the shoulder adductors and extensors and in the same way raise the trunk. Others get to forearm support and then to arm support.

The patient without active elbow extension, is much more disabled; as he must rely on the force of gravity to extend his elbows he cannot keep them stable in any position except possibly a vertical position with the hand on a firm surface directly below the shoulder. The shoulder adductors are weak also, so the arm cannot be firmly pressed over the hand.

Standing

Standing is recommended for all patients with high thoracic or cervical lesions (see Figs. 14/19 to 14/24). Standing with leg support in some form of splint such as plaster of Paris shells or a specially designed standing frame is to be encouraged. The patient gains a psychological uplift from a period of standing which may not be understood by those of us who have never had to lie flat or sit immobile throughout days, weeks and years. Physiological benefits of standing include better drainage of the kidneys, some beneficial stimuli to keep the leg bones strong, a position which maintains length of hip flexors, knee flexors and calf and a means of reducing spasticity. In many cases standing improves the activity of postural muscles of the neck and upper trunk. The patient can have some apparatus supplied so that they can stand for a period daily at home when they are discharged from the spinal unit.

Sport and recreation

With adapted apparatus archery, table tennis and swimming are arranged for tetraplegics. Art therapy is valuable; gadgets can be used to hold pencils or brushes or special dental devices used to allow the patient to paint using his mouth. Apparatus, such as POSSUM/POSM (patient-operated selection mechanism), which is controlled using the mouth by pneumatic control can be supplied to enable a patient to switch on and off lights, electric fires, radio or television sets, control a telephone, page turner or electric typewriter.

Other apparatus designed for a tetraplegic patient include a ball-bearing feeding device, an opponens splint and flexor hinge splints.

Transport

Motorised transport can be controlled by a tetraplegic patient who has active use of the elbows and wrists but the patient has to be lifted into and out of the car. This is facilitated by the use of a sliding board.

Resettlement and follow-up

For patients with cervical lesions resettlement presents many difficulties and the relatives must be thoroughly trained to care for the patient at home. This is the responsibility of all members of the team and should begin as soon as is practicable.

Follow-up and frequent review is necessary and domiciliary visits from experienced nurses, occupational therapists, or physiotherapists are of great value.

Although patients need a personal attendant the prognosis is more favourable for tetraplegics who return to the community than for those forced by circumstances to remain in institutional care. The future is grim for those young patients who must depend entirely on others to be fed and for all personal care and who have no family able and willing to do so.

Even those patients who can achieve some degree of self-care need adapted buildings, accommodation and some supervision, if they are to live away from home or institution. The road to independence does not depend solely on physical disability but ultimately on the will of the individual to achieve his potential.

FEMALE PATIENTS WITH CORD LESIONS

Treatment for female patients is as described above but some added problems arise. One example is the relative shortness of arms and heavier pelvis and legs of a woman compared to that of a man. These factors make transfers difficult for all but the most slender and youthful females.

Another problem is that relating to double incontinence – no really satisfactory urinal is available. Bladder training is therefore of vital importance to the female patient. Nurses are responsible for attempting to establish a regular automatic reflex emptying of the bladder. Fluid intake is carefully regulated both in the quantity and the times when it is taken. The patient must understand the aim of the training and if possible learn to express the bladder manually to ensure good emptying. Menstruation brings special problems and may upset the automatic bladder function. Young patients often achieve a remarkable success in bladder training. The physiotherapist should understand the aim of training. Intermittent self-catheterisation is now taught to some patients.

In spite of these physical difficulties women show great determination and courage and many paraplegics achieve complete independence.

CHILDREN WITH COMPLETE CORD LESIONS

Children with cord lesions present a challenge but no greater problems than adults, if care is taken to prevent deformity.

Because growth is retarded when normal use of a part is prevented, the lower limbs of a child with paraplegia are relatively short. This factor is an advantage as transfers and gait are facilitated if the arms are long and the lower part of the body lighter than normal.

Many children show great adaptability to physical defects and are very rewarding to train in new skills. They become almost recklessly proficient in the use of wheelchairs, take to swimming eagerly, learn swing-through gait and develop speed and expertise in this rapidly. Many children can get up from the floor unaided, gain balance in standing, place the crutches for use and walk off. Orthoses are needed for these activities but do not need to be hinged at the knee for very young children.

Regular, frequent review is needed, however, to ensure that good function is preserving both the joint range and the length of soft tissue.

As the child grows, new splints are needed and the older child needs hinged orthoses to enable him to sit correctly on a stool or chair. A check of the spine is needed as scoliosis can develop.

Bladder training is as essential as it is for adults, and regular checks are made by the urologist to see that kidney function is good. Parents should be instructed in the care of the skin, the bladder, the use of splints; they should be shown how to give passive movements to preserve joint and soft tissue range.

If possible, normal schooling should be arranged but the school authorities must be instructed in precautions against skin damage from extremes of temperature or from abrasion.

Incomplete lesions

TRAUMATIC PARAPLEGIA

In the early stages medical, nursing and physiotherapy management are as for complete lesions which at first the incomplete lesions may appear to be. However, spared muscle activity and the early onset of spasticity may make maintenance of stability of the trunk problematic. Both in early stages and when the patient is allowed to sit up a careful assessment is needed to identify precise signs and potential of each individual and to recognise problems which may be caused by spasticity, muscle imbalance and partial or complete sensory loss. The patient is asked to attempt movements of the legs and observation of these will indicate if selective movements are possible or if only spastic synergies occur. Spontaneous, or readily elicited, ankle clonus and brisk phasic stretch reflexes indicate spasticity. Sensory testing of cutaneous and kinaesthetic sense is performed and records kept for comparison.

Physiotherapy will be dictated by the degree of sparing and severity of spasticity but broadly follows the regimes as described for complete lesions. In cases where spasticity is a problem the extensor thrust pattern usually predominates unless the patient is inactive, gets severe bladder complications or pressure sores in which circumstances a flexor withdrawal reflex becomes dominant. If the hip flexors and abdominal muscles are weakened or denervated completely the flexor withdrawal is not as strong as it is if these muscles are innervated and therefore play a part in the withdrawal reflex. Sometimes upper motor tracts from the basal ganglia, reticular formation and the vestibular nuclei are still partially intact and so release of tonic reflexes influences the spinal reflexes. An example of this can be observed if the patient has a much stronger extensor thrust in the supine position than in side lying or prone lying which indicates some release of the tonic labyrinthine reflexes.

As previously described (p. 353) a vicious cycle can develop if spasticity is allowed to increase the risk of sores and contractures.

Because the cord lesion is partial the neurological signs may change rapidly as inflammation subsides. The physiotherapist must be observant as she performs passive movements to the legs. Any change in muscle tone, sign of voluntary control of movement or of return of sensation should be recorded and reported to the consultant. Prognosis depends on the extent and rate of recovery of neurological function in the first weeks after onset.

If there is sensory sparing the patient should be encouraged to think of the movements of the legs as the physiotherapist performs them passively. Similarly, if some voluntary control of movement returns at this stage he should be encouraged to try to assist leg movements as the physiotherapist performs them. The physiotherapist should attempt an explanation of spasticity to the patient, as the difficulty in controlling a spastic limb with imperfect voluntary movement is more frustrating to some patients than is the acceptance of a completely paralysed one. Quick movements must be avoided and the placing of skin contacts selected with care (see Fig. 14/4, p. 347). Methods to reduce spasticity and to elicit postural reactions are described in Chapter 8.

The time needed for healing of the spinal injury is as for a complete lesion.

Stage when weight-bearing through the spine is permitted

As with complete lesions the patient has to acquire sitting balance, learn to care for insensitive skin and joints and how to avoid eliciting spasticity.

A position which has been found useful for patients with spasticity is a modified cross sitting. The hips are flexed, laterally rotated and abducted, the knees flexed and the soles of the feet are in contact. This must be accompanied by a posture of erect spine, not a rounded spine and only in a sitting position so that it is not a flexor-withdrawal pattern of legs and trunk.

Another important consideration is that strong muscle work in the unaffected parts may cause overflow to the lower segments of the cord. This may elicit spasms or reinforce spasticity so the programme of muscle strengthening for the arms may have to be modified.

Points to consider when the patient is more active include the following:

1. The flexor withdrawal and the extensor thrust are both mass movements and neither is suitable to support the weight of the body or useful for activities, such as standing from sitting, standing or walking.
2. Every consideration must be given to providing afferent stimuli which produce a stabilising co-contraction of the deep muscles whose activity results in providing a mobile but stable postural background. If this can be achieved the patient will be able to realise his potential for independence.
3. Preparation must be planned for good postures of sitting, prone kneeling, kneeling and standing (see Fig. 14/7, p. 352). The patient must learn to elicit a postural response rather than a spastic total movement. For example, the spasticity of the calf is often a great nuisance, preventing a good stance and

making walking almost impossible. The length of the soleus muscle is the key, and a slow maintained lengthening must be achieved by the physiotherapist and by the patient before standing is attempted. Even if long leg orthoses are needed, and even if an attempt is made to control the extensor thrust by ankle control on the orthosis, a reduction of spasticity prior to standing will be of great benefit. If an orthosis is not needed the patient should sit in a good position with the heels firmly on the floor, and some weight through the tibiae should be provided by pressure on the knees. The pressure should be maintained for 5 minutes or until the calf relaxes.

Insufficient hip flexion to get the weight of the trunk well over the feet is another fault of sitting posture. This is likely if the extensor thrust is strong and is also contributed to by too much decline in the angle of the back of the chair (Fig. 14/7, p. 352). The patient must learn to lean well forward, keeping the spine straight and head posture good. When the correct starting position is achieved the patient is instructed and helped if necessary to stand, pushing the heels down, the hips forward and the shoulders up and back. The physiotherapist should keep the patient stable by pressure on the iliac crests down through the legs.

When a good standing position is achieved the trunk should be moved, keeping an upright posture, so that weight is transferred from side to side, from before backwards and in a turning motion rocking over the feet. At all times the aim is to keep good pressure on the heels and to avoid a sudden stretch of the ball of the foot.

Standing with or without orthoses with the support of parallel bars or a standing frame is helpful to reduce spasticity providing a good normal alignment of feet, legs and trunk can be achieved (see Figs. 14/19 to 14/24). Some patients may not need long orthoses but may find a below-knee splint useful to control the ankle position. In the training stage a Swedish knee cage is useful to teach control of a spastic limb.

Most patients with incomplete low paraplegia can walk well eventually but need the use of crutches, sticks or a rigid walking frame. They learn to negotiate stairs and obstacles but many need a wheelchair for long distances.

Resettlement problems are similar to those of patients with complete lesions and everyone concerned in their care can assist in solving difficulties. Follow-up is essential for these patients, and at review a careful re-assessment must be made especially of the spasticity and any problems it may create. Length of soft tissues must be assessed to ensure that contractures are not developing. Good function, once achieved, is the best way to prevent deterioration.

Additional points in cases of tetraplegia

Because the cervical spine is relatively mobile and also vulnerable, injury is common and frequently produces a partial cord lesion. As discussed previously, partial lesions present with great variation and the precise treatment needed depends on the clinical symptoms.

In all but the most mild cases some residual flaccid paralysis of the hands will make manipulative skills difficult or impossible. This factor with the added problem of imperfect control of the spastic trunk and lower limbs, leads to a very frustrating situation. The use of crutches or sticks may be almost impossible for a patient with weak or insensitive hands. The spasticity of the legs can be reduced by the patient's own handling if he has normal use of his arms, but this is usually impossible for incomplete tetraplegics.

As for all partial lesions, assessment of the individual abilities and difficulties of each patient is essential.

A plan of treatment must be made and co-operation is needed with the occupational therapist and the social worker to try to help each patient to realise his potential for rehabilitation.

CHILDREN WITH PARTIAL CORD LESIONS

Partial cord lesions may be caused by trauma, developmental errors, infection or severe bone disease.

Treatment follows the principles of treatment for the cause and should be appropriate for the individual neurological symptoms.

Assessment should be attempted but in very young infants the examiner needs a knowledge of the normal motor behaviour and experience of handling young children with neurological defects.

Prognosis is made by the medical personnel but is aided by a concise report of examinations and observations by the physiotherapist. The habitual posture or response may be difficult to assess in a short examination session and the physiotherapist who handles the child for a longer time and more often, should be able to give a valuable account of her observations. Methodical examination and simple, clear, well-documented, dated reports are required. Management is basically that which is described in Chapter 23.

PROGRESSIVE CORD LESIONS

Treatment for these lesions depends upon the cause, rate of progression and the precise signs and the dysfunction of each individual. (See Chapters 8 and 16.)

CAUDA EQUINA LESIONS

A lesion of the spine below the second lumbar vertebra may cause damage to the roots of spinal nerves passing from the lower segments of the cord within the neural canal until they emerge at the corresponding intervertebral foramina.

As the nerve roots contain only nerve fibres, these may regenerate and conduction of nerve impulses along them will be restored. However, dense scar tissue sometimes prevents good recovery of function, and if regeneration does occur it takes up to two years for nerve axons to grow to the most distal muscles and skin.

Treatment of the initial injury follows the principles for fractures of the spine, and treatment for neurological symptoms must be appropriate for severe and extensive lower motor neurone lesions.

If the tip of the lowest segment of the spinal cord is involved the lesion is known as a combined conus and cauda equina lesion. In these cases some partial or complete loss of control of the external sphincters may create problems of incontinence which are permanent.

Loss of skin sensation over the buttocks may also occur and be permanent, thus appropriate training is needed in skin care.

REMINDERS FOR PATIENTS WITH SPINAL INJURY, AND FOR THEIR ATTENDANTS

Care in bed

1. See there are no creases in the bottom sheet.
2. Use a firm mattress on a firm support so that the mattress does not sag.

3. Turn regularly as instructed by the nurses.
4. Do not use hot water bottles.
5. Inspect the skin each night and morning. Use a hand mirror to see posterior parts. If any redness occurs, investigate and take necessary measures to prevent breakdown of skin.
6. Inspect skin of legs when orthoses are removed.
7. If sheets are wet these must be changed at once.

Care while dressing

1. Do not use safety pins.
2. Do not wear tight clothing, trousers, stockings or shoes. Avoid holes in socks.
3. Keep finger and toenails short and smooth.
4. Check temperature of bath or washing water with a thermometer to avoid scalds. Water must be below 36.5°C (98°F).
5. Check inside shoes before putting them on to ensure there are no nails or other harmful objects inside. Inspect feet when shoes have been removed.
6. Be careful not to have sharp objects in trouser pockets.

Transfers

1. Always move the legs carefully, lift them and do not drag them along, place down carefully.
2. Always lift high enough to avoid dragging buttocks over hard surfaces.
3. See the brakes are on and the wheelchair secure.
4. Do not sit on hard surfaces, use a cushion or rubber seat in the bath and lavatory.

Care when in the wheelchair

1. Lift every 15 minutes for 15 seconds.
2. High cervical lesions must be lifted every 30 minutes.
3. Do not sit too near a fire or radiator.
4. Tetraplegics should wear gloves when wheeling chair.
5. Take care while smoking not to drop hot ash or cigarette ends; tetraplegics should use a cigarette holder.
6. Avoid exposing the legs to extremes of temperature, e.g. wrap up in a rug if outdoors in cold weather.
7. Do not expose insensitive skin to strong sunlight.
8. Do not rest hot plates or mugs on your legs. Tetraplegics should use insulated mugs.

Care in motorised transport

1. Transfer with care.
2. Use a cushion.
3. Do not use a car heater.
4. Wrap up legs if weather is cold.

REFERENCES

Bromley, I. (1980). *Tetraplegia and Paraplegia*, 2nd edition, p. 15. Churchill Livingstone, Edinburgh.

Cheshire, D.S.E. and Rowe, G. (1970). The prevention of deformity in the severely paralysed hand. *Paraplegia*, **8,** 1, 48–56.

Glenn, W. (1980). The treatment of respiratory paralysis by diaphragmatic pacing. *Annals of Thoracic Surgery*, **30,** 106–9.

Goff, B. (1976). Grading of spasticity and its effect on voluntary movement. *Physiotherapy*, **62,** 11, 358–61.

Goldman, J. (1980). Heterotopic ossification in spinal cord injuries. *Physiotherapy*, **66,** 7, 219–20.

Hardy, A.G. and Rossier, A.B. (1975). *Spinal Cord Injuries, Orthopaedic and Neurological Aspects*. Georg Thieme, Stuttgart.

Kuhn, R.A. (1950). Alteration in dominance of postural and protective reflexes. *Brain*, **73,** 1–51.

BIBLIOGRAPHY

Books

Bedbrook, G.M. (ed.) (1981). *The Care and Management of Spinal Cord Injuries*. Springer, New York.

Bromley, I. (1980). *Tetraplegia and Paraplegia*, 2nd edition. Churchill Livingstone, Edinburgh.

Burke, D.C. and Murray, D.D. (1975). *A Handbook of Spinal Cord Medicine*. Macmillan Publishers, London.

Cloward, R.B. (1980). Acute cervical spine injuries. *Ciba Clinical Symposia*, **32,** 1.

Fallon, B. (1976). *So You're Paralysed*. Spinal Injuries Association, London.

Ford, J.R. and Duckworth, B. (1974). *Physical Management for the Quadriplegic Patient*. F.A. Davis and Co, Philadelphia.

Guttmann, L. (1976). *Spinal Cord Injuries*, 2nd edition. Blackwell Scientific Publications Limited, Oxford.

Hardy, A.G. and Rossier, A.B. (1975). *Spinal Cord Injuries, Orthopaedic and Neurological Aspects*. Georg Thieme, Stuttgart.

Nixon, V. (1985). *Spinal Cord Injury – Rehabilitation Institute of Chicago Procedure Manual*. William Heinemann Medical Books Limited, London.

Roaf, R. and Hodkinson, L. (1977). *The Paralysed Patient*. Blackwell Scientific Publications Limited, Oxford.

Rogers, M. A. (1986). *Living with Paraplegia*. Faber and Faber, London.

Rossier, A. (1973). *Rehabilitation of Spinal Cord Patients*. Documenta Geigy Acta Clinica, Basle.

Spinal Injuries Association (1980). *People with Spinal Injuries: 1. Nursing Management in the General Hospital*. Spinal Injuries Association, London.

Vinken, P. J. and Bruyn, G. W. (jt. eds.) (1976). *Injuries of the Spine and Spinal Cord*, Parts I & II. North Holland, Amsterdam.

Walsh, J. J. (1964). *Understanding Paraplegia*. Tavistock Publications, London.

Papers

Abrahams, D., Shrosbree, R.D. and Key, A.G. (1979). A functional splint for the C5 tetraplegic arm. *Paraplegia*, **17**, 198–203.

Lamb, D.W. and Chan, K.M. (1983). Surgical reconstruction of the upper limb in traumatic tetraplegia. *Journal of Bone and Joint Surgery*, **65B**, 3, 291–8.

Journal

Paraplegia – the official journal of the International Medical Society of Paraplegia. Obtainable from Churchill Livingstone, Edinburgh. Published bi-monthly.

EQUIPMENT

Gympac System Limited
Unit 5, Ty Verlon Industrial Estate
Cardiff Road, Barry, South Glamorgan CF6 3BE

Rancho caliper – available through the hospital appliance officer
Described in:
Duffus, A. and Wood, D.J. (1983). Standing and walking for the T6 paraplegia. *Physiotherapy*, **69**, 2, 45–6.

Standing frame – available from:
Theo Davies, Argoed, Glyn Ceriog
Llangollen, Clwyd LL20 7HN

Swedish knee cage – available through the hospital appliance officer

Universal Brace – available through the hospital appliance officer

ACKNOWLEDGEMENT

Both authors thank their colleagues at the Robert Jones and Agnes Hunt Orthopaedic Hospital, Oswestry for their help in the revision of this chapter. They are particularly grateful to Mrs P. Butler MSc, MCSP for writing the section on the ORLAU hip-guidance orthosis. They thank all the patients who have allowed their photographs to be used in the chapter without the masking of their features. They thank the photographic department for their help, the secretaries for typing and the Shropshire Health Authority for permission to publish the photographs.

Chapter 15

Multiple Sclerosis – Clinical

by J. M. SUTHERLAND MD (Glas), FRCP (Edin), FRACP

Multiple sclerosis (MS), also known as disseminated sclerosis, is primarily a disorder of myelin sheaths, nerve axons being affected in a secondary manner. Myelin, derived from oligodendroglia, envelops nerve axons in a winding process and has two functions: it controls the passage of ions on which transmission of nerve impulses depend; second, it has an insulating action. Thus, myelin sheaths are responsible for the normal propagation and conduction of nerve impulses. The process of myelination is completed in childhood and thereafter there is a slow metabolic turnover, replacement keeping pace with degradation.

Multiple sclerosis is characterised by the occurrence of patchy areas of demyelination (plaques) occurring in a widespread manner throughout the central nervous system (hence 'multiple' or 'disseminated'). This active demyelination is usually followed by gliosis – 'scarring' (hence 'sclerosis').

PATHOLOGY (pathophysiology)

The characteristic pathological features of MS is the occurrence of plaques of demyelination, active and sclerotic, in the white matter of the brain, cerebellum, cranial nerves and spinal cord, the optic nerves and around the third and fourth ventricles. The relationship of many plaques to small veins and to periventricular areas suggests that the agent responsible for demyelination may invade the nervous system from the blood and from the cerebrospinal fluid.

In an area of active demyelination, myelin sheaths fragment and disintegrate. There is considerable oedema and cellular proliferation in the region and related axis cylinders show some evidence of degenerative change. The loss of myelin and the oedema are responsible for the delayed conduction of nerve impulses and this is aggravated by even slight elevations in body temperature. This is reflected in the symptomatology of the disorder when a slight rise in body temperature due to exertion may produce a temporary exacerbation of a symptom, while hyperthermia produced by a heat cage may result in temporary aggravation of symptoms and thus have a diagnostic significance.

In old plaques there is no inflammatory reaction. The plaques are grey and shrunken; myelin has disappeared; axis cylinders are reduced in number; there is a lack of cellularity and a marked gliosis. It is possible that in some instances active demyelination may be followed by re-myelination rather than gliosis so that nerve conduction in the region is restored to normal or at least is not accompanied by obvious symptomatic effects. Thus, after an attack of optic neuritis subsides the patient may experience no residual defects although, usually, visually evoked cerebral responses will show some abnormality in the affected eye.

Periventricular plaques may not give rise to any symptoms. Such plaques can sometimes be detected by CT brain scans but it would appear that nuclear magnetic imaging is much more sensitive in demonstrating these 'silent' lesions. In a patient presenting with a monosymptomatic onset of, for example, weakness in one leg, the ability to demonstrate multiple lesions in the central nervous system is of great diagnostic value.

A concept of the pathogenesis of MS is summarised in Figure 15/1 (Lumsden, 1973; Adams, 1977).

AETIOLOGY

Sex incidence

In most series, female patients predominate slightly over the males and this is particularly marked in low incidence areas. On the other hand, when the age of onset is over 40 years male patients outnumber female.

Age incidence

Multiple sclerosis is a disease of early adult life. The age of onset is between 20 and 40 years in some 70 per cent of patients. Approximately 20 per cent develop the disease after 40 years of age but an onset over 50 years, while not unknown, is unusual. Only some 10 per cent of cases occur in the second decade of life.

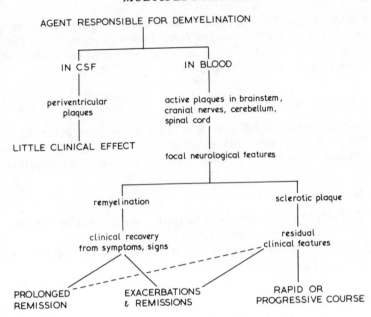

FIG. 15/1 Pathogenesis of multiple sclerosis

Prevalence and geographic distribution

One of the most remarkable features of MS is the increased incidence and prevalence in temperate as opposed to tropical and subtropical climates. This is true for both the Northern and Southern hemispheres. For example, high-risk areas with a prevalence in excess of 30–50 per 100 000 of the population can be defined in Northern Europe, Canada, Northern United States of America and New Zealand, while low-risk areas with prevalence rates less than 15–20 per 100 000 occur in the Mediterranean littoral, the deep South of the United States of America, South Africa and Northern Australia.

In the United Kingdom, in general, the prevalence rate is 50–80 per 100 000. However, in north-east mainland Scotland there is a high prevalence rate of 127 per 100 000 rising to 184 per 100 000 in the Shetland Isles while in the Orkney islands the prevalence rate of 309 per 100 000 is the highest reported in the World.

Epidemiological studies have furnished evidence suggesting that if an individual migrates from a high-risk area such as the Orkney Islands to a low-risk area such as Northern Australia, the migrant retains the high risk of his country of origin unless migration occurs in childhood, probably before 15 years of age. This suggests that the critical time for exposure to some environmental factor or factors occurs in the first 15 years of life.

Ethnic factors

Independent of latitude, MS appears to be more prevalent in Northern European stock than in other ethnic groups such as Indians, Fijians, New Zealand Maoris and Australian Aborigines.

Heredity

Although MS is usually sporadic the disease occurs some 20 times more often in first-degree relatives of MS patients than in the general population at risk. There is, however, no Mendelian pattern in the genetic predisposition.

Other factors

It is difficult to determine the precise significance of factors such as trauma, emotional upset, intercurrent infections and pregnancy. While statistical proof is lacking, most neurologists have encountered instances which have persuaded them that in some patients one or other of these factors may trigger-off the onset of the disease or an exacerbation. While it is recognised that pregnancy is potentially harmful, it is probable that physical fatigue and emotional tensions associated with the puerperium, rather than the pregnant state, are responsible.

The aetiology – a hypothesis

Available evidence suggests that two factors are important in the aetiology of MS – an environmental factor and a genetically determined predisposition.

ENVIRONMENTAL FACTOR

Although conclusive evidence is lacking it seems probable that infection with a virus or viruses, widespread in nature, is responsible. Exposure to this agent in early life leads to the formation of protective antibodies and immunity. In adult life, the result of re-infection or infection will depend on genetic vulnerability, ethnic factors or possibly exposure to an overwhelming infection.

GENETIC PREDISPOSITION

A genetic susceptibility to MS appears to exist and is linked with the human leucocyte antigen (HLA) system, the major histocompatibility complex of man. This system consists of closely linked genes some of which control the expression of antigen. In Europe, North America and Australia HLA-A3 and HLA-B7 and related antigens DW2 and DR2 occur in a significant proportion of MS patients and their relatives. On the other hand, the frequency of HLA-DW2- and DR2-positive individuals is much less in a control population and in ethnic groups in which MS is uncommon.

A disturbance of immune responses in MS is also suggested by the abnormality of cerebrospinal fluid immunoglobulins found in the majority of patients. The gamma globulin is increased; the proportion of the total protein which consists of IgG is increased; following electrophoresis, diffuse protein bands (the oligoclonal pattern) occur in the gamma globulin region.

Given such an alteration in immune responses of the body, the subsequent progress of the disease (a prolonged remission after one or two exacerbations; a course characterised by exacerbations and remissions over many years; an acute course is probably an expression of the degree and nature of autoimmune reactions. This concept of the aetiology is summarised in Figure 15/2

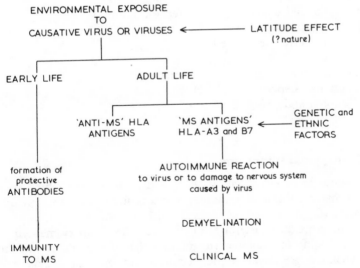

FIG. 15/2 Aetiology of multiple sclerosis – a hypothesis

(Acheson, 1972 and 1977; Leibowitz and Alter, 1973; Fraser, 1977; Batchelor, 1977; McLeod, 1982; Thompson et al, 1983).

CLINICAL FEATURES

The onset

The initial symptom of MS may appear suddenly or insidiously and is generally referable to a single lesion in the white matter of the nervous system. The common initial symptoms are motor disability in one or more limbs, impaired vision in one eye, double vision, or paraesthesiae. After a number of weeks the initial symptom clears or improves, often, however, to return in the future on one or more occasions or to be supplanted by evidence of a lesion elsewhere.

The symptoms commonly encountered in the course of MS and the structures involved are indicated in Table 15/1.

TABLE 15/1 Symptoms of multiple sclerosis

SYMPTOMS	NEUROLOGICAL STRUCTURE INVOLVED
Blurred vision	Optic nerve(s)
Double vision	III or VI cranial nerves
Weakness of leg(s)	Pyramidal tract(s)
Paraesthesiae: ataxia	Posterior column(s)
Inco-ordination, ataxia, intention tremor, slurred speech	Cerebellum
Incontinence of urine	Spinal cord
Emotional changes (euphoria: depression)	Hypothalamus

Paroxysmal symptoms

Distinct from exacerbations of the disease process which may improve or clear over a number of weeks and distinct from symptoms which worsen or appear with elevations of the body temperature due to exercise or exposure to heat, paroxysmal symptoms lasting for moments to minutes may occur. These include trigeminal neuralgia, tonic seizures and episodic ataxia and dysarthria. Lhermitte's sign, an electric shock-like feeling, tingling or vibration experienced down the back or in the limbs produced on flexion of the neck, could be included under this heading. Although not diagnostic of MS (it may occur in cervical spondylosis, tumour and arachnoiditis), the occurrence of Lhermitte's sign in an appropriate clinical setting strongly suggests MS.

Physical signs

In an established case of MS the results of neurological examination reflect the scattered nature of the lesions. Thus, there may be evidence of atrophy of one optic nerve, impaired ocular movements or nystagmus, intention tremor in one hand, evidence of bilateral pyramidal tract dysfunction and impaired vibration sense and joint position sense in one leg. A change in emotional expression is common and although euphoria out of keeping with the patient's disabled condition may be striking, depression is more frequent.

At an early state in MS symptoms may outstrip physical signs of disease giving rise to an erroneous diagnosis of hysteria. Conversely, in some patients, physical signs such as unequal knee jerks and an extensor plantar response may occur in the absence of related symptoms. However, the therapist should be on the look out for weakness in a leg after exercise followed by recovery after rest as probably indicating MS.

THE COURSE AND PROGNOSIS

The course of MS is very variable but the following comments may serve as a guide to a therapist treating a patient with MS in the absence of any specific therapy being available.

1. Some 80–90 per cent of cases run a course characterised by exacerbations and remissions.
2. In this group of patients the average duration of life is some 30 years from the onset.
3. About 33 per cent of patients in this group will show little evidence of progression of the disease for a period at least in excess of 10 years, in some instances 30–50 years.
4. The group of patients with a good prognosis tend to have an early age of onset (30 years or below) and a low relapse rate particularly after the second year.
5. The average patient in the exacerbation-remission group tends

to have a relapse once every two years. In this group 50 per cent will be disabled but still ambulatory in six years, non-ambulatory in 18 years, and deceased in 30 years.
6. Some 10–20 per cent of cases progress from the onset. These patients tend to have a later age of onset (35–45 years) with short remissions between the first few relapses and thereafter a progressive course resulting in death within months to a year or two.
7. A change from a relapsing to a progressive course may occur at any time but is more common after early relapses than later ones.
8. In long-standing cases it is not uncommon after the age of 50 years for death to be due to causes quite unrelated to MS. (McAlpine, 1961; McAlpine, 1973; Confavreux et al, 1980.)

The Kurtzke Disability Scale (Table 15/2) is widely employed to indicate a patient's status, progress, and response to therapy. Employing this scale, Stages 3–4 can be expected in 5–6 years; at 10-years duration Stages 5–6; after 18–20 years duration, Stages 7–8 will be reached and Stages 9–10 in 30 years. It must be emphasised that these views are based on a large number of patients. They give a general outline but are of only limited value in individual patients.

TABLE 15/2 Kurtzke Disability Scale (Rose, Kuzma, Kurtzke et al, 1968)

0 Normal neurologic examination
1 No disability, minimal signs (e.g. Babinski's sign; decreased vibration sense)
2 Minimal disability (e.g. slight weakness; mild gait, sensory or visual disturbance)
3 Moderate disability though fully ambulatory (e.g. monoparesis, moderate ataxia)
4 Relatively severe disability though fully ambulatory, able to be self-sufficient and up and about for some 12 hours per day
5 Disability severe enough to preclude working a full day
6 Assistance required for walking (e.g. canes, crutches, braces)
7 Restricted to a wheelchair – able to self-wheel and enter and leave chair alone
8 Restricted to bed but with effective use of arms
9 Totally helpless bed patient
10 Death due to MS

LABORATORY DIAGNOSIS

There is as yet no specific laboratory test for MS. In established cases a history of the occurrence of symptoms scattered in time, and neurological findings indicative of lesion scattered in space throughout the central nervous system, strongly suggests the diagnosis. In such circumstances the 'great imitators,' neurosyphilis and neurological systemic lupus erythematosus, merit consideration and can be excluded by laboratory tests. Similarly, laboratory evidence may furnish evidence which will support the diagnosis of MS in an early case with, perhaps, a monosymptomatic onset (Table 15/3).

TABLE 15/3   Laboratory studies in multiple sclerosis

TEST	SIGNIFICANT FINDINGS
Lumbar puncture – CSF	
Cells	Lymphocytes normal – 50/mm^3
Protein	Normal – 100mg/dl
Gamma globulin	Increased
IgG/albumin ratio	In excess of 27%
Electrophoresis	Oligoclonal bands
VDRL	Negative
Electrophysiology	
Evoked potentials – visual	Abnormal in 70–80% of cases
– somato-sensory	Abnormal in 60–70% of cases
– auditory	Abnormal in 50% of cases
CT brain scan	May show old plaques as low density areas, and recent demyelination as high density areas – positive yield low
Nuclear magnetic resonance (NMR)	Very effective in demonstrating subclinical lesions in CNS
Artificial heating (heat cage or hot bath)	May render overt a latent symptom, visual, motor or sensory. Use with caution.

DIFFERENTIAL DIAGNOSIS

Multiple sclerosis together with modified neurosyphilis and neurological systemic lupus erythematosus, is one of the great imitators of nervous system diseases. As indicated in Table 15/4, MS can enter into the differential diagnosis of many other conditions depending on the level of the nervous system involved.

TABLE 15/4 Differential diagnosis

MS: SITE OF DEMYELINATION	PRESENTING FEATURES	CONDITIONS ENTERING INTO DIFFERENTIAL DIAGNOSIS
Spinal cord	Paraplegia ± sensory ataxia	Spinal cord compression by tumour, spondylosis Friedreich's ataxia Motor neurone disease B_{12} neuropathy Syringomyelia Myelo-radiculitis
Optic nerve	Impaired vision	Other causes of optic neuritis Optic nerve glioma
III, VI cranial nerves	Diplopia	Aneurysm of circle of Willis Intracranial tumour Myasthenia gravis
Cerebellum	Ataxic gait ± Intention tremor Slurred speech	Tumour, abscess involving cerebellum Alcohol Friedreich's ataxia
Combination of above		Neurosyphilis Encephalomyelitis Carcinomatous neuropathy Systemic lupus erythematosus

TREATMENT

In the sense of affecting a cure or preventing future exacerbations, there is at present no specific treatment for MS. This is not to be taken that nothing can be done for patients with MS. In this section current therapies, treatments being evaluated, and symptomatic measures will be discussed.

In Table 15/5 a number of treatments in current use, or being evaluated, and their rationale are summarised. With reference to the section 'Aetiology – A Hypothesis' (p. 386), it will be apparent

TABLE 15/5 Some therapies in multiple sclerosis (*after* Waksman, 1983)

RATIONALE	THERAPY
Antiviral agents (destruction of hypothetical virus)	amantadine: acyclovir: interferon
Immunosuppressive therapy (auto-immunity suppressed)	corticotrophin (ACTH): cortico-steroids: azathioprine cyclophosphamide antilymphocyte serum: plasma-pheresis
Immunopotentiating therapy (remedy defect in immune mech-anism)	Transfer Factor: interferon
Other	low fat diet with linoleic acid sup-plements vitamin B_{12} hyperbaric oxygen

that in theory the disease process could be interrupted at various levels. The putative virus could be destroyed. Anti-viral drugs, thus far, however, have not proved successful and there is no specific vaccine available as the nature of the virus or viruses has not been established.

If an auto-immune reaction is responsible for demyelination, immunosuppressive drugs should be useful. Certainly ACTH and corticosteroids appear to shorten exacerbations but they have no influence on the progress or course of the disease. Azathioprine has been reported to be of some limited value.

An inability of the body to mount an effective immunological response has led to the use of Transfer Factor and interferon. Transfer Factor is a dialysable leucocyte extract which has the capability of transferring cell-mediated immunity from an immune donor to a non-immune recipient. Interferon is also derived from leucocytes and has both anti-viral and immunological properties. These substances are at present being evaluated as is the value or otherwise of hyperbaric oxygen.

CURRENT THERAPY

Although dietary measures have been shown to be at the best of only marginal benefit, a low animal and dairy fat diet supplemented by unsaturated vegetable oils and the fat soluble vitamins seems to result in some reduction in the number and severity of exacerbations. Linoleic acid, in the form of sunflower seed oil, 30ml twice daily, and vitamins A, D and E are employed to supplement the dietary restriction of low saturated animal fats.

Vitamin B_{12} is necessary for normal myelination, and, although statistically of no proven value, vitamin B_{12} (cyanocobalamin, 1mg) can be given intramuscularly, once or twice weekly, with advantage as an acute exacerbation subsides.

For an acute exacerbation, prednisone 100mg once daily on alternate days, orally, or tetracosactrin (Synacthen Depot) 1mg intramuscularly daily-weekly are of value in lessening the damage, and shortening the duration of acute exacerbations of MS. These drugs are of no value given chronically over long periods. They do not influence the course of the disease and because of potential side-effects continuous therapy is not recommended.

SYMPTOMATIC TREATMENT

Measures employed to alleviate some of the symptoms of MS are indicated in Table 15/6. It should be noted that the dosages given are 'average' for adult patients and because of side-effects dosage has to be individualised for each patient. This is particularly true of baclofen and dantrolene and it should be recalled also that these drugs may increase locomotor disability by reducing the 'splinting' effect of extensor muscle spasm in a weakened leg.

GENERAL MEASURES

What to tell: In the early stages when the diagnosis is only 'possible' there seems little point in alarming the patient unless specific questions are raised. In an established case it is usually better to discuss the diagnosis openly with emphasis on the favourable course in many instances.

In some instances suggesting, or helping the patient contact, the local MS Society may be of value.

Maintenance of optimal general health, adequate exercise and adequate rest (even to the extent of one day per week in bed) is beneficial.

Advice regarding marriage: There is of course no contra-indication to marriage but it is advisable for both partners to have a frank discussion with a doctor about the disease and possible consequences.

TABLE 15/6   Symptomatic treatment in multiple sclerosis

SYMPTOM	TREATMENT	DOSE
Spasticity and muscle spasms	baclofen (Lioresal)	15–30mg bd
	dantrolene (Dantrium)	100mg bd
	diazepam (Valium)	5mg bd-tds
	phenol in glycerine	1ml 2% solution intrathecal
Precipitancy of micturition	belladonna alkaloids (Atrobel: Donnatab)	1–2 tabs bd or tds
	propantheline (Probanthine)	15mg bd-tds
	baclofen (Lioresal)[1]	5mg qid
	Percutaneous electrical stimulation, lower dorsal-sacral region	
Incontinence of urine	Urinal	
	Permanent catheterisation	
	Percutaneous stimulation, lower dorsal-sacral region	
	Subtrigonal phenol injection[2]	
Paroxysmal symptoms	carbamazepine (Tegretol)	200mg bd or tds
	clonazepam (Rivitrol)	2mg bd
Depression	amitriptyline (Tryptanol)	25–75mg nocte
	imipramine (Tofranil)	25mg bd

[1] Taylor, 1979
[2] Ewing, Bultitude and Shuttleworth, 1983

Pregnancy, or more likely the puerperium, carries with it an increased risk of an exacerbation of the disease, but provided the patient is not disabled and has been in remission for two years, a pregnancy is not strongly contra-indicated. Oral contraceptives have no adverse effect on exacerbations.

Might my baby develop MS? Although some 11 per cent of MS sufferers have a near relative similarly affected, and the number of first-degree relatives is some 20 times the expected number, there is no Mendelian pattern and genetic counselling is impossible. The incidence of MS in relatives of patients, in descending order of frequency is siblings, parents, children, other relatives (McAlpine, 1973). The genetic factor is probably a defect in immunological response linked to the HLA system. The risk of a child of a patient with MS ultimately developing the disease is quite small and would not contra-indicate a patient having a family.

REFERENCES

Acheson, E. D. (1972). Epidemiology. In *Multiple Sclerosis: A Reappraisal*, pp. 3–80, 2nd edition. (eds. McAlpine, D., Lumsden, C. E. and Acheson, E. D.). Churchill Livingstone, Edinburgh.

Acheson, E. D. (1977). Epidemiology of multiple sclerosis. *British Medical Bulletin*, **33**, 9–14.

Adams, C. W. M. (1977). Pathology of multiple sclerosis: progression of the lesion. *British Medical Bulletin*, **33**, 15–20.

Batchelor, J. R. (1977). Histocompatibility antigens and their relevance to multiple sclerosis. *British Medical Bulletin*, **33**, 72–7.

Confavreux, C., Aimard, G. and Devic, M. (1980). Course and prognosis of multiple sclerosis assessed by the computerised data processing of 349 patients. *Brain*, **103**, 281–300.

Ewing, R., Bultitude, M. I. and Shuttleworth, K. E. D. (1983). Subtrigonal phenol injection therapy for incontinence in female patients with multiple sclerosis. *Lancet*, **1**, 1304–6.

Fraser, K. B. (1977). Multiple sclerosis: a virus disease? *British Medical Bulletin*, **33**, 34–9.

Leibowitz, U. and Alter, M. (1973). *Multiple Sclerosis: Clues to its Cause*. North Holland Publishing Company, Amsterdam, London. American Elsevier Publishing Company, New York.

Lumsden, C. E. (1973). The clinical pathology of multiple sclerosis. In *Multiple Sclerosis: A Reappraisal*, pp. 311–621, 2nd edition. (eds. McAlpine, D., Lumsden, C. E. and Acheson, E. D.). Churchill Livingstone, Edinburgh.

McAlpine, D. (1961). The benign form of multiple sclerosis. A study based on 241 cases seen within three years of onset and followed up until the tenth year or more of the disease. *Brain*, **84**, 186–203.

McAlpine, D. (1973). Clinical studies. In *Multiple Sclerosis: A Reappraisal*, pp. 83–307, 2nd edition. (eds. McAlpine, D., Lumsden, C. E. and Acheson, D. E.). Churchill Livingstone, Edinburgh.

McLeod, J. G. (1982). Multiple sclerosis – a review. *Australia and New Zealand Journal of Medicine*, **12**, 302–8.

Rose, A. S., Kuzma, J. W., Kurtzke, J. F. et al (1968). Co-operative study in the evaluation of therapy in multiple sclerosis. ACTH vs placebo in acute exacerbations: preliminary report. *Neurology*, **18** Supp., 1–20.

Taylor, M. (1979). The idiopathic unstable bladder and its management. In *Proceedings of a Symposium*, Southern General Hospital, Glasgow, 30 November 1979. Published in collaboration with the Scottish Medical Journal, Longman.

Thompson, E. J., Kaufmann, P. and Rudge, P. (1983). Sequential changes in oligoclonal patterns during the course of multiple sclerosis. *Journal of Neurology, Neurosurgery, Psychiatry*, **46**, 547–50.

Waksman, B. H. (1983). Rationales of current therapies for multiple sclerosis. *Archives of Neurology*, **40**, 671–2.

BIBLIOGRAPHY

Barnes, M. P., Bates, D., Cartlidge, N. E. F. et al (1985). Hyperbaric oxygen and multiple sclerosis: short-term results of a placebo-controlled, double-blind trial. *Lancet*, **1**, 297-300.

Buonanno, F. S., Kistler J. P., Lehrich, J. R. et al (1983). H nuclear magnetic resonance imaging in multiple sclerosis. In *Neurologic Clinics: Symposium on Multiple Sclerosis*, pp. 757-64, vol. 1. (ed. Antel, J. P.). W. B. Saunders Co, Philadelphia.

Capildeo, R. and Maxwell, A. (eds.) (1982). *Progress in Rehabilitation: Multiple Sclerosis*. Macmillan Press, London.

Dworkin, R. H., Bates, D., Millar, J. H. D. and Paty, D. W. (1984). Linoleic acid and multiple sclerosis: a re-analysis of three double blind trials. *Neurology*, **34**, 1441-5.

Fischer, B. H., Marks, M. and Reich, T. (1983). Hyperbaric oxygen treatment of multiple sclerosis. A randomized, placebo controlled, double blind study. *New England Journal of Medicine*, **308**, 181-6.

Liversedge, L. A. (1977). Treatment and management of multiple sclerosis. *British Medical Bulletin*, **33**, 78-83.

McFarlin, D. E. (1983). Treatment of multiple sclerosis (editorial). *New England Journal of Medicine*, **308**, 215-17.

Matthews, W. B. (1980). *Multiple Sclerosis: The Facts*. Oxford University Press, Oxford.

Matthews, W. B., Acheson, E. D., Batchelor, J. R. and Weller, R. O. (eds.) (1984). *McAlpine's Multiple Sclerosis*, 3rd edition. Churchill Livingstone, Edinburgh.

Moulin, D., Paty, D. W. and Ebers, G. C. (1983). The predictive value of cerebrospinal fluid electrophoresis in 'possible' multiple sclerosis. *BRAIN*, **106**, 809-16.

Poser, C. M., Paty, D. W., Scheinberg, L. et al (1983). New diagnostic criteria for multiple sclerosis: guidelines for research protocols. *Annals of Neurology*, **13**, 227-31.

Powell, H. C. and Lampert, P. W. (1983). Pathology of multiple sclerosis. In *Neurologic Clinics: Symposium on Multiple Sclerosis*, pp. 631-44, vol. 1. (ed. Antel, J. P.). W. B. Saunders Co, Philadelphia.

Sutherland, J. M. (1982). Multiple sclerosis: 50 years on. *Clinical and Experimental Neurology*, **19**, 1-12.

Chapter 16

Multiple Sclerosis – Management

by J. M. TODD BSc, MCSP

The previous chapter has described the clinical aspects of multiple sclerosis and this chapter will concentrate on the role of the physiotherapist in the care of multiple sclerosis (MS) patients. It is accepted that there are many MS sufferers who will never need physiotherapy because their disease process is either too mild or so slow that their activities are not restricted; nevertheless, advice for those with minimal signs is included.

Close interdisciplinary teamwork is necessary to ensure the most effective management of the disability as well as sufficient support to allow the patient and his family to make the emotional and physical adjustments required to cope with a progressive handicap.

Hospital based therapists often encounter more people who are deteriorating or who already have established problems and consequently there is a tendency to think only of the progressive nature of the disease; a pessimistic attitude may, therefore, be adopted towards the efficacy of treatment and overall management when a more positive approach would be of greater benefit to the patient. It has been observed that MS patients respond well to an active programme and positive atmosphere provided by a rehabilitation unit or spinal injuries unit where staff and patients face the problems of handicap with an optimistic and enthusiastic attitude (Carr and Shepherd, 1980; Davies, 1975; Ritchie Russell and Palfrey, 1969). If the symptoms presented by MS are treated as they would be if they were the result of trauma or other disease, a more active and positive management will result with the focus on strengths rather than problems.

Where the disease leads to disability the patient is, from the earliest, encouraged to take the responsibility for his own well-being, particularly with regard to skin care generally, bowel and bladder function, prevention of pressure sores, contractures and the avoidance of infection.

The motor dysfunction seen in these patients arises from the disorganised neurological mechanisms of posture, balance and movement, and treatment is aimed primarily at these central mechanisms. However, management of the disabled MS sufferer needs to be continuous and not confined to 'treatment' sessions. If certain postural mechanisms are stimulated during treatment and not reinforced between sessions, they will need to be retaught every time. If treatment aimed at prevention of deformity is counteracted by bad positions and abnormal movement for the rest of the day then the effect will be wasted. It is therefore most important to consider the handling and equipment used throughout the 24 hours and not just during the treatment period.

The therapist must allow time to explain the rationale of treatment to the patient, his relatives and to any staff who may be involved, as well as teaching specific handling or positioning necessary to stimulate required responses. All those caring for MS sufferers are shown which postures and movements to encourage, and which to avoid, i.e. which positions will make certain movements easier so that independence can be retained. Wherever possible, it is more effective if these activities can be incorporated into the daily routine so that a way of life is established which allows for continuous therapy.

Appropriate treatment will lessen the effect of any symptoms and, therefore, the earlier it is started the more opportunity is given for re-educating whatever potential abilities exist for decreasing deficit and avoiding secondary preventable complications. The therapist should encourage good relations with the neurologists and general practitioners who refer patients, to ensure they understand the role that the therapist can play in advising about ways of reducing to a minimum the effects of new symptoms or overcoming any functional difficulties, and the advantages of early contact with the therapist in the prevention of secondary handicap.

Periods of immobility for whatever reason should be stringently avoided. Special care is necessary at the following time: influenza, colds or infection; surgery; pregnancy; fracture or sprain of a joint and following the provision of a walking aid or wheelchair. At such times early activity and the need to be out of bed is normally stressed but MS sufferers tend to be kept immobile for longer. The need to stand, walk and balance in sitting on the side of the bed each day is vitally important. A refresher course of intensive physiotherapy after such an event will be required to ensure the former level of function is regained.

ASSESSMENT

According to the site of the lesions the clinical picture can present a broad spectrum of dysfunction. Damage can occur anywhere in the brain or spinal cord resulting in malfunction of any of the neurological mechanisms. As MS is usually a progressive disease with gradually increasing neurological deficit (Patzold and Pocklington, 1982), the signs and symptoms are not static and may also vary from day to day.

It is a complex condition, not just a motor problem. As motor function cannot be isolated from other functions (Affolter and Stricker, 1980), it is important for the therapist to recognise that she is dealing with a multiple handicap. There will be handicaps arising from the original lesion and often secondary handicaps arising directly from these or resulting from inadequate management of basic defects. To illustrate this, paucity of movement leads to limited sensation and perception of everyday things. This reduced activity may also lead to apparent defects of perception such as agnosia or apraxia. If there is decreased movement in the legs and the patient is allowed to transfer like a paraplegic his ability to use the legs becomes further reduced. Lack of experience can also affect speech and lead to more rapid deterioration of language.

In addition to the complexity is the long-term and fluctuating nature of the course of the disease. Accurate recording of the symptoms is vital both to understand the problems so that their management can be planned, and for the evaluation of treatment to guide future management. For assessment, general information about the patient's medical history and social circumstances is noted, and this usually provides an opportunity to find out how much the patient knows about the disease and also his own views about any problems. The information needed to make a thorough assessment of the neurological impairment can be divided into various sections.

Joint range

A full assessment of the passive range of motion in each joint is recorded, noting reasons for any limitation.

Soft tissue shortening

A special note is taken of any 'tightness' or any shortening, remembering that two-joint muscles are more vulnerable.

Sensory disturbance

Disturbances such as paraesthesia or numbness and tingling are frequently early clinical signs. Sensory deficit may be due to the actual disease process or due to lack of experience or awareness. Abnormal afferent information will give rise to abnormal responses. Without correction, repetition of abnormal movement will eventually be learned and accepted as the normal.

Vision

Unfortunately, impaired vision and nystagmus are added complications in a multiple handicap where eyes may have to substitute for proprioceptive loss.

Tone

Alteration of tone may be of supraspinal or spinal origin and may present as hypotonia or hypertonia which is usually in the form of spasticity but rigidity is often found. The therapist notes the distribution of the abnormal tone and the factors which influence its increase or decrease, such as a specific posture or a particular movement.

Voluntary movement

Once tone is normalised the active movement itself may vary in strength and co-ordination and it may not automatically occur during balance and maintenance of posture. The quality of the movement is recorded, for example whether selective movement is available. Frequently, full use is not made of all available isolated movement for functional activities and disuse will often result in reduced ability, e.g. persistence in locking the knee in hyperextension when walking may contribute to loss of ability to take weight on a mobile knee. Using the better arm exclusively, because it is quicker, for feeding or dressing may lead to a more rapid deterioration of the other arm. If actual weakness is present, a muscle chart to show grading of strength may be helpful (see p. 127).

Involuntary movement

Involuntary movement may be present and can be general or isolated to one joint or limb. A distinction is made between ataxia, athetosis, chorea and tremor; a note is made of any abnormal reflex activity such as the influence or use of the ATNR.

Posture and balance mechanisms

Postural reactions cannot be separated from voluntary movement (Bobath, 1978), but they deserve special consideration because training voluntary activity does not necessarily re-educate or stimulate the necessary postural reactions (see Chapter 3) which also do not seem to correlate with tone.

Prevailing abnormal postures

Abnormal postures may be as a direct result of abnormal tone, or may be because of excessive use of the influence of reflex patterns or attitudes, particularly the influence of the labyrinthine reflex, the symmetrical and asymmetrical tonic neck reflex either to aid movement or to achieve postural stability. It is important to ensure that any habitual postures do not become fixed contractures as a result of adaptive shortening of soft tissues.

Perception

As perceptual processes are involved with motor performance and considered to be prerequisites for learning (Affolter, 1981), it is useful if the therapist is aware of any impairment.

Memory

A memory deficit may necessitate adaptation to the programme of physical management.

Behavioural and intellectual disturbance

This may be apparent, again as a direct result of pathology or due to inadequate emotional and social experience for which movement is necessary. Most people coping with a physical disability will experience increased anxiety, irritability or changes of mood from time to time.

Function

A full assessment of functional ability is carried out normally with the occupational therapist, and a home or work assessment may also involve the social worker.

PRINCIPLES OF PHYSIOTHERAPY

The information gathered from the different areas is used to compile a list of problems, and an appropriate plan for their management is drawn up. In recent years the role of the physiotherapist in the general management of long-term disability has undergone a change in emphasis. In addition to applying specific treatment techniques the therapist is more involved in the overall physical management and in advising about the prevention of secondary handicap.

The successful treatment of the neurological defects found in MS requires a combination of the skills developed in other specialised areas particularly from the treatment of stroke, head injury, spinal injury and cerebral palsy. The physiotherapist may be involved from the earliest signs to the terminal stages of the disease and she therefore needs to be acquainted with all the appropriate techniques required to treat any of the many possible signs and symptoms (Bobath, 1978; Goff, 1972; Knott and Voss, 1969). At each stage specific techniques will be required to treat the neurological deficit and to allow any potential a chance to reveal itself. Every attempt must be made to facilitate normal movement or co-ordination which may have been lost during an exacerbation or period of immobility. Prompt intervention will reduce to a minimum the deficit and avoid the effects of forgetting due to lack of experience.

General principles of assessment and treatment are described in the early chapters of this book and readers are advised to refer to specialised sections for help with specific problems. Here, general advice for the planning of treatment will be given and, for convenience, special advice and points for emphasis will be indicated as though the course of the disease could be divided into four stages, although in practice one will merge with another.

AIMS OF PHYSIOTHERAPY

1. To re-educate and maintain all available voluntary control.
2. To re-educate and maintain normal postural mechanisms.
3. To maintain full range of motion of all joints and soft tissues and to teach the patient and/or his relatives suitable stretching procedures to prevent contractures.
4. To incorporate treatment techniques into the way of life by relating them to suitable daily activities thus providing a means of maintaining any improvement.
5. To offer advice about sensible use of energy.
6. To prevent the use of abnormal movement which is inefficient and tiring in itself and may inhibit function.
7. To inhibit any abnormal tone.
8. To stimulate all sensory and perceptual experience and maintain the experience of normal movement throughout the course of the disease not only to exploit potential but to enable the patient to feel safer and move more freely when the assistance of relatives or helpers is required in the later stages.

General preventive measures

No two patients are alike in either their circumstances or their symptoms, thus no two treatments can be the same. However, whatever approach is adopted, there are certain problems seen in most patients with disability which are possible to anticipate and prevent.

PLANTAR FLEXED FEET

Shortening of the tendo calcaneus can be prevented by avoiding the use of a total pattern of extension for weight-bearing; by attention to the posture of the feet when sitting; and by daily standing if walking is no longer functional.

A PREDOMINANT PATTERN OF EXTENSION AND ADDUCTION IN THE LOWER EXTREMITIES

A pattern of total extension can be inhibited by training correct weight-bearing through a mobile knee; by attention to adequate flexion at the hip joint when sitting; and by the use of tailor-sitting to stretch the adductors.

KNEE FLEXION CONTRACTURE

Contracture at the knee can be prevented if the hamstrings are stretched by touching the toes in long sitting while keeping both knees extended.

HIP FLEXION CONTRACTURES

Shortening of the hip flexors can be prevented by ensuring good hip extension when walking or standing. Daily prone lying should be encouraged.

FLEXED THORACIC SPINE

Poor trunk posture can be avoided by active dorsal extension in sitting and when prone; stretching by supine lying over a pillow, or in sitting with hand support behind.

FLEXION AND INTERNAL ROTATION AT THE SHOULDERS

Limitation at the shoulders can be counteracted by training balance reactions and by self-assisted full range shoulder elevation.

FIXED HEAD POSITIONS

Use of fixed head positions may be avoided by training adequate balance and postural reactions and preventing the use of abnormal movement patterns.

SPECIAL EMPHASIS NEEDED AT DIFFERENT STAGES

Early advice

Initially the patient may complain of poor balance on the stairs, difficulty with fine finger movements or heaviness of one leg, and eye symptoms or some sensory disturbance may be present.

1. If the patient is referred to a physiotherapist at this stage, however minor the deficit appears to be, a thorough assessment of movement in all positions will enable suitable advice to be given about any potential lack of symmetry in posture, movement or balance which is observed.
2. If appropriate, emphasis can be given to certain activities in daily life which would stimulate postural and balance responses, e.g. going up and down stairs one foot after the other

and standing from sitting without using the hands for balance; lifting one leg across the other when putting on shoes and socks; emphasis of dorsal extension during dressing or when reaching for objects. If suitable activities can be introduced as part of the daily routine it saves devoting time to a special programme of exercises with which people have difficulty continuing (Carr and Shepherd, 1980). If more specific emphasis is required additional work using a balance board or large therapy ball can be practised at home (see Chapter 11).

3. The benefit of resting in a position of side lying rather than supine can be explained, also that the patient must learn to lie in a prone position either over a pillow, foam wedge or suitable cushion, perhaps while reading or watching television, or even while sleeping.

4. The usual occupation and pastimes should be continued: during the assessment, work and leisure activities may be discussed with a view to conservation of energy; this is similar to the consideration which is given to joint preservation with arthritis sufferers. For the MS sufferer the danger of doing too much seems less than the danger of doing too little but slight adjustments made in the organisation of the daily routine may avoid undue fatigue and conserve energy for more enjoyable pursuits.

5. The patient should be advised to keep fit and healthy and encouraged to pursue some form of active exercise. Participation in sport such as tennis, badminton, swimming or riding provides valuable recreation as well as keeping the patient active. Any abnormal patterns of movement observed during these activities should be corrected because if continued they will reinforce the abnormal at the expense of the normal.

6. After initial and intensive re-education and instruction during the early stage, patients find it helpful to attend follow-up sessions every three or six months to evaluate the programme and to discuss any other problems. Many departments now provide a long-term reviewing system so that outpatient physiotherapy should not be necessary nor encouraged if adequate adaptation has been made to daily activities.

Slightly more marked signs but walking unaided

If the signs and symptoms increase, reassessment is necessary and adjustments made to their management. It is helpful to involve relatives and, if necessary, visit both home and work to make further suggestions about sensible use of energy and ways of overcoming particular problems. The physiotherapist should be ready to ask the help of other members of the team, e.g. social worker, nurse, occupational and speech therapist and dietitian. The same principles of physical management are continued but special attention may be needed in the following:

1. Nutritional counselling may be given both because of the link between nutrition and multiple sclerosis and in the interests of general health (Crawford and Harding, 1982). In addition, advice may be sought for weight control as an increase of only 1kg (2.2lb) can affect mobility in a person with even minimal increased tone in the legs. Paradoxically, when ataxia is a feature, energy output is increased and this, in combination with tiredness and laboured feeding, could result in a gradual reduction in weight.

2. As the signs become more marked, concern about the future increases and social and psychological problems may arise. Frequently, some of the fear and depression can be relieved if the patient and family are given a fuller understanding of the symptoms, or practical guidance to overcome the physical or financial problems connected with employment, mobility or domestic arrangements. Occasionally, skilled counselling may be helpful to overcome specific marital, family or sexual difficulties (Burnfield and Burnfield, 1982). If some of the psychological stress can be alleviated, energy can be channelled more constructively towards enjoyment of life in spite of the handicap.

3. If the function of the bladder or bowel is affected the patient should understand that correct management of them could influence the amount of tone throughout the body. Urodynamic assessment may demonstrate that the bladder is hypertonic or hypotonic and increased irritability or retention or any infection will increase tone generally which, in its turn, could affect mobility. Bowel function can be managed as for a spinal cord lesion to avoid constipation, as this will cause increased tone and may also affect bladder function.

4. Particular attention will be required to overcome undesirable ways of moving or performing functional activities, and to teach the specific stretching activities already mentioned to prevent any adaptive shortening.

5. Whatever type of abnormal tone is present there will usually be reduced rotation in the trunk in an attempt to maintain stability; therefore, activities to encourage facilitation of this

must be incorporated into treatment sessions and into home or work activities. For example, always turning on to the side before sitting on the edge of the bed to get up will facilitate rotation and head and trunk righting reactions. A suitable self-activity could be in side sitting to inhibit extensor thrust, rolling both knees together from one side to the other – and if the arms are clasped above the head this will emphasise much needed dorsal extension. When ataxia is present the activity may be adapted during treatment so that approximation can be given through the arms in a 'lifting' pattern.

6. Use of walking aids: Great care must be taken when an aid for walking becomes necessary. Suitable activities which will counteract the inevitable detrimental effects will need to be encouraged. These effects may not be immediately apparent. Where possible, aids should be given during a refresher course so that proper instruction and evaluation may be carried out and arrangements made for a further follow-up. Typical points to watch would be:

   (a) alteration in posture due to leaning on the stick or crutches;
   (b) marked reduction in balance reactions of head and trunk through using the hands for balance resulting in increased difficulty with other functional activities in lying and sitting;
   (c) possible alteration in distribution of tone throughout the body requiring extra care to maintain all the isolated movement available.

In a wheelchair for part of the time

The chair should not be used full time until absolutely necessary and every effort must be made to keep ambulant if at all possible. However, it may be advisable to use a wheelchair for long distances in order to save time and to avoid unnecessary fatigue. This is a very dangerous period in management and many complications are directly related to insufficient guidance at this time. The inevitable reduction in amount of activity and increased use of the sitting posture usually lead to an alteration in patterns of spasticity and movement which will need specific treatment if potential problems are to be avoided.

1. The prescription of the wheelchair requires full consultation between the user, his relatives and all members of the team. There are many guides to assist the necessary decisions, but a few points will be mentioned, as simple basic mistakes are

frequently made with rather serious consequences. If the chair is not correctly measured it can cause or increase abnormal postures, especially if it is too wide. The height of the foot plates is particularly important; they should be able to be adjusted to achieve a right angle at the hips and knees. Some elevating leg rests which do not allow this should be avoided. Heel straps which are fixed to the foot plate are frequently ordered; unless altered they hold the forefoot in an unsupported position and this leads to increased flexion of toes. The slightest tightness of toe or plantar flexors increases spasticity and could prevent walking or, later, the vital use of standing for transfers and maintenance. A strap behind the legs is more practical. Some reclining back rests will not raise sufficiently to allow a right angle at the hips – a fact which may alter management of tone and posture in the trunk and legs (Pope, 1985).

2. Wheelchair management should be very carefully taught. It is as important for the MS sufferer to receive the same detailed preparation and instruction in the use of the wheelchair which would be given to a person with traumatic paraplegia. This means meticulous attention to symmetry of posture with even weight distribution on both buttocks. The patient should be warned not to maintain asymmetrical positions for long periods, for example, always leaning on the same arm could lead to a scoliosis and affect the tone in the trunk and legs. The degree of flexion at the hip will influence both the position of the head and trunk and the pattern of spasticity in the leg. Too much extension at the hip can increase extensor thrust in the leg. Hip retraction on one side can produce a pattern of flexion, adduction and medial rotation with corresponding decrease in functional ability. The automatic use of the wheelchair arms should be avoided, unless necessary for safety; this will stimulate a more active sitting posture which will help to retain balance mechanisms. Sitting in a suitable ordinary chair makes a change from the wheelchair.

3. The period when there is increased use of the sitting position requires close supervision not only to ensure adequate management of the tendency of hypertonus to change from extension to flexion but also to prevent contractures. The patient must walk each day and if extra support is required in the way of gaiters, splints, bracing, a suitable walking aid or parallel bars, these should be readily available. Any interruption in the routine may mean not only losing the skill for ever but a risk of introducing a vicious circle of complications (p. 353).

4. Extra care with stretching of muscle groups which tend to shorten is vital. A pause to give an extra stretch each time a transfer is executed will help to maintain the length of the calf muscles and the hip flexors. The prone position and tailor-sitting will maintain range at the hip but specific stretching of hamstrings in long sitting is required. It is usually necessary to check full shoulder elevation, especially if ataxia is present, because this movement is performed so rarely in daily life (see pp. 269–70).

5. There may be considerable changes during this period. Probably even part-time work will no longer be practical and alternative pursuits must be found to continue an interesting and stimulating life and to continue a responsible role within the family and social circle. Guidance may also be needed on various aspects to retain personal independence; this may include advice about suitable clothing and footwear as well as other aids which will enable the person to remain independent for as long as possible.

FULL TIME USE OF A WHEELCHAIR

1. Once walking is no longer feasible even for maintenance, additional provision must be made for standing. The physiological benefits of standing include reduction of spasticity, maintenance of length of hip and the knee flexors and calf muscles, more efficient drainage of the kidneys and possible benefits to counteract osteoporosis. Support for the knees in standing could include gaiters, plaster of Paris or polythene back slabs, or long-leg bracing. If needed, suitable apparatus, such as a standing frame, must be supplied to assist standing at home (see Chapter 14).

   In residential care or hospital a tilt table may be used with the patient prone or supine but care is required to obtain equal weight-bearing through both legs. It is of more benefit if standing can be an active and not just a passive experience. Correction of symmetry and posture, and activities to encourage balance can be practised while in the upright position.

2. Additional help may be needed to improve independence at home. Modifications to the bed or bathroom may retain independent turning and transfers or make it easier for helpers to assist. If the standing transfer has been maintained it is usually

possible for relatives to manage a pivot transfer even when the disease is advanced (see pp. 263–4).

3. If necessary the patient may have to ask relatives to assist with positioning, stretching and pressure relief. If he is no longer able to correct the sitting posture himself extra care is needed to check that there is equal weight distribution and good alignment of the trunk and limbs. This is particularly important on some air-filled cushions which make balance more critical. Vigilant attention to such details will frequently overcome problems of balance and posture of the head and trunk which affect feeding and speech, or asymmetry in the lower limbs which could be the start of a vicious circle of complications.

MANAGEMENT OF SPASTICITY

Spasticity and its management has been discussed in Chapter 7 but it needs to be reiterated that managing spasticity in multiple sclerosis is of the utmost importance. The following points need to be continually remembered:

1. Diligent attention to educating the need for avoidance of positions and activities which increase tone or reinforce abnormal movement patterns.

2. Daily walking or standing for weight-bearing which has an inhibiting effect on hypertonus.

3. Constipation, bladder infections, pressures sores must be avoided.

4. Regular stretching of all potentially tight structures, especially at danger times such as illness or the transition to a wheelchair. Contractures must be prevented at all costs; action must be taken as soon as there is any difficulty in obtaining full range of passive movement. An increase in the amount of treatment or an additional activity or use of another adjunct may be indicated.

5. Prolonged application of ice either locally or for total immersion can be used effectively for temporary reduction of hypertonus (Lee and Warren, 1978).

6. The inhibitory effect of drugs such as baclofen and diazepam is sometimes helpful but close monitoring is required as they may reduce arousal and active ability.

7. Use of splinting needs careful consideration as, without extra treatment, it may actually increase the problem. Removable splints are usually ineffective because the corrected position is

not maintained and they are difficult to re-apply. However, at danger times splinting in the form of an all-round plaster of Paris cylinder for the leg or a below knee weight-bearing plaster can sometimes be considered to inhibit spasticity. If contractures do occur application of serial plasters can be used to correct the shortening.

8. Intrathecal injections of phenol may be useful but require knowledge of the neurological mechanisms involved as well as an understanding of the implication of any imbalance in a movement disorder. If ataxia is also present the possible reduction in stability should be considered.

9. Surgery may be required either to divide or to lengthen tendons, e.g. the hamstrings or tendo calcaneus, or in the form of a partial or total neurectomy, e.g. obturator. However, unless the original cause of the problem is eliminated or a different management is introduced the difficulty is likely to recur.

MANAGEMENT OF ATAXIA

Ataxia and its management has been discussed in Chapter 7 but, as with spasticity, ataxia requires understanding and continual treatment. The following points need to be remembered:

1. Attention to ensuring adequate experience of movement can easily be overlooked because the voluntary control present makes the lack of use less obvious to the therapist.

2. Many patients voluntarily restrict movement of the head and trunk to gain more stability and extra emphasis needs to be given to the stimulation of balance and righting reactions during treatment and throughout the day.

3. Instability and difficulty in performing activities against gravity often leads to the use of abnormal patterns of movement or reflex attitudes in an attempt to increase tone and achieve stability. This may appear to be an acceptable short-term answer but later it may contribute to reduced functional ability, e.g. pressing the head into extension and rotation against the back of the chair can affect tone in the limbs and reduce the demand for already poor head control. Always folding the arms or pushing one arm into extension and medial rotation may assist sitting balance but will prevent use of the arms for more skilled functions and predispose to contracture. Improving the postural mechanism gives a better background to movement and therefore facilitates functional ability.

4. A person with poor co-ordination tends to push against any available surface to achieve stability; therefore, any straps, aids or props used to assist certain functional activities, if permanently fixed, may actually increase abnormal movement and could eventually prevent the original function they were aiding. To counteract this an alternative position or extra work to stimulate the postural mechanism may be required to balance the management.

5. Some approaches to the relearning of motor control, for example those developed by Frenkel, Peto, Carr and Shepherd (1982), have emphasised the use of cognitive control. Greater understanding of memory and control of action, current theories of learning and neural plasticity enables the therapist to provide and monitor a more appropriate programme of maintenance which will retain maximum functional ability.

ADDITIONAL MANAGEMENT

Respiration

Breathing exercises should be incorporated into the programme at all stages. If the muscles involved in respiration are affected, the patient and relatives can be shown suitable positions for postural drainage and how to assist coughing to clear secretions. In advanced cases, the use of suction to remove secretions may be more effective if coughing is tiring.

Feeding

It is particularly important to be aware of the effect of position and posture on a patient's ability to eat independently. Training balance reactions, head control, eye/hand co-ordination, could help to retain the basic motor skills required to bring the food to the mouth. Techniques to normalise tone, increase sensation and facilitate voluntary control within the mouth help to maintain patterns of chewing and swallowing necessary for efficient eating.

Whenever possible the patient must be encouraged to feed himself and adaptations to cutlery, non-slip mats, and thermal plates can be helpful.

In many instances a liquid diet is given when what is really required is advice about suitable positions and instruction in facilitation of chewing and swallowing. With the right help it should be possible for a normal diet to be enjoyed. Solid food will help to retain the ability to chew, and stimulate lip closure and tongue and cheek movements. Maintaining good oral feeding patterns will also help to maintain speech patterns.

Communication and mobility

A variety of systems to assist with the use of telephone, radio, typewriter and other communication aids can be supplied to allow more independence. Various forms of motorised transport are available for those who cannot manage a hand driven chair.

Bladder and bowel function

Incontinence can cause much embarrassment but problems arising from such distressing complications must not be accepted as an automatic outcome of MS. Adequate management is possible and dignity can be maintained. Much help can be gained by reference to the careful management accorded to bladder and bowel function in spinal injuries units. The initial responsibility for accurate diagnosis causing the incontinence belongs to the doctor but the therapist may be involved in establishing a suitable training regime of appropriate exercises (Mandelstam, 1977). The therapist must be aware of the need to avoid infection of the bladder or retention of urine, as this can damage the kidneys and also have a marked effect on spasticity. The use of drugs, surgery or stimulation may be considered (Hawkes, Beard and Thomas, 1982).

Constipation is a frequent problem with MS; it is aggravated by reduced mobility and has a marked effect on spasticity. It can be helped by allotting a regular time of day for bowel movement, a larger fluid intake and a high residue diet. If this is insufficient, regular aperients and suppositories every two or three days are used to train a convenient and regular routine.

The therapist can help the patient and his family to accept that effective management is possible in most instances and is of vital importance both medically and socially.

Prevention of pressure sores

Pressures sores can be prevented: if attention is given to stressing special positioning to inhibit spasticity and to the importance of relieving pressure in bed and in the wheelchair, the patient need no longer fear that pressure sores are inevitable. (See Chapter 14 for preventive measures.)

REFERENCES

Affolter, F. (1981). Perceptual processes as prerequisites for complex human behaviour. *International Rehabilitation Medicine*, **3(1)**, 3–9.

Affolter, F. and Stricker, E. (eds.) (1980). *Perceptual Processes as Prerequisites for Complex Human Behaviour*. Hans Huber, Bern.

Bobath, B. (1978). *Adult Hemiplegia: Evaluation and Treatment*, 2nd edition. William Heinemann Medical Books Limited, London.

Burnfield, A. and Burnfield, P. (1982). Psychosocial aspects of multiple sclerosis. *Physiotherapy*, **68**, 5, 149–50.

Carr, J. H. and Shepherd, R. B. (1980). *Physiotherapy in Disorders of the Brain*. William Heinemann Medical Books Limited, London.

Carr, J. H. and Shepherd, R. B. (1982). *A Motor Relearning Programme for Stroke*. William Heinemann Medical Books Limited, London.

Crawford, M. A. and Harding, J. (1982). The role of diet in multiple sclerosis. In *Progress in Rehabilitation: Multiple Sclerosis*. (eds. Capildeo, R. and Maxwell, A.). Macmillan Press, London.

Davies, P. M. (1975). A physiotherapist's approach to multiple sclerosis. *Physiotherapy*, **61**, 326–8.

Goff, B. (1972). The application of recent advances in neurophysiology to Miss M. Rood's concept of neuromuscular facilitation. *Physiotherapy*, **58**, 12, 409–15.

Hawkes, C. H., Beard, R. and Thomas, D. G. (1982). Surgical aspects of multiple sclerosis. In *Progress in Rehabilitation: Multiple Sclerosis*. (eds. Capildeo, R. and Maxwell, A.). Macmillan Press, London.

Knott, M. and Voss, D. E. (1969). *Proprioceptive Neuromuscular Facilitation*, 2nd edition. Harper and Row, New York.

Lee, J. M. and Warren, M. P. (1978). *Cold Therapy in Rehabilitation*. Bell and Hyman, London.

Mandelstam, D. (1977). *Incontinence*. Heinemann Health Books Publication, London.

Patzold, U. and Pocklington, P. R. (1982). Course of multiple sclerosis. First results of a prospective study carried out of 102 MS students from 1976–1980. *Acta Neurologia Scandinavica*, **65**, 521–9.

Pope, P. M. (1985). A study of instability in relation to posture in the wheelchair. *Physiotherapy*, **71**, 3, 124–9.

Ritchie Russell, W. and Palfrey, G. (1969). Disseminated sclerosis – rest and exercise therapy – a progress report. *Physiotherapy*, **55**, 8, 306–10.

BIBLIOGRAPHY

Affolter, F. and Stricker, E. (eds.) (1980). *Perceptual Processes as Prerequisites for Complex Human Behaviour*. Hans Huber, Bern.

Bach-Y-Rita, P. (1980). *Recovery of Function: Theoretical Consideration for Brain Injury Rehabilitation.* Hans Huber, Bern.

Barton, A. and Barton, M. (1981). *The Management and Prevention of Pressure Sores.* Faber and Faber, London.

Basmajian, J. V. (1979). *Muscles Alive. Their Functions Revealed by Electromyography,* 4th edition. Williams and Wilkins, Baltimore.

Hewer, R. L. (1980). Multiple sclerosis – management and rehabilitation. *International Rehabilitation Medicine,* **2,** 116-25.

Incontinence 1. (1983). *Physiotherapy,* **69,** 4, 104-13.

Incontinence 2. (1983). *Physiotherapy,* **69,** 5, 144-9.

Wilson, B. A. and Moffat, N. (eds.) (1984). *Clinical Management of Memory Problems.* Croom Helm, London.

Chapter 17

Parkinsonism – Clinical

by R. B. GODWIN-AUSTEN MD, FRCP

Parkinson's disease and the parkinsonian syndrome comprise a group of disorders characterised by tremor and disturbance of voluntary movement, posture and balance. Parkinson's disease was first described by James Parkinson in 1817; its pathology was defined about 100 years later and the treatment has been revolutionised since the 1960s by the introduction of levodopa.

The 'parkinsonian syndrome' is that group of disorders in which the characteristic symptoms and signs of parkinsonism develop but are secondary to another neurological disease (e.g. encephalitis lethargica, Alzheimer's disease). Thus, whereas Parkinson's disease is a primary degenerative condition occurring in the latter half of life and following a progressive course, the parkinsonian syndrome has a natural history dependent on the cause. The word 'parkinsonism' is used to describe the symptoms and signs irrespective of the cause of the disease state. Where the parkinsonian syndrome is complicated by some generalised degenerative process (e.g. cerebral arteriosclerosis) treatment may be less satisfactory than in the uncomplicated case.

CLINICAL FEATURES

The patient with parkinsonism may present with the characteristic tremor. The diagnosis is then easily established although it is important not to label other forms of tremor 'parkinsonian'. More than 50 per cent of patients with Parkinson's disease do not have any tremor and the presenting symptoms are then much more diverse. The patient usually attributes the symptoms of the disease to 'old age' and is correspondingly grateful when treatment relieves them. Common presenting symptoms are slowness of walking and disturbance of balance with occasional falls or difficulty with fine manipulative movements such as dressing or shaving. Pain is a common presenting complaint and patients may attend a physiotherapy department for the treatment of cervical spondylosis, frozen shoulder, backache or osteoarthritis of the hip when their symptoms are in fact due to parkinsonism. The pain is rapidly relieved by appropriate treatment for their parkinsonism.

The general slowing up, associated as it often is by an apathy with depression, may lead friends and family to conclude that the patient is dementing. This is seldom the case. Patients with parkinsonism retain intellect and are the most co-operative patients to treat.

Early symptoms of the disease may include difficulty with specific movements such as writing; difficulty in turning over in bed or rising from a low chair; an excessive greasiness of the skin or an unusual tendency to constipation; and an inability to raise the voice or cough effectively. And all the symptoms tend to be disproportionately worse when the patient is under stress. Furthermore most patients discover that they have become much more subject to the effects of what would formerly have been regarded as trival stresses. The patient therefore tends to avoid social engagements and to reduce the amount of work he does. The family may then conclude that it is all due to 'laziness' or psychological causes.

SIGNS

Posture

The patient with Parkinson's disease usually shows some disorder of posture. When standing there is a slight flexion at all joints leading to the 'simian posture' with the knees and hips slightly flexed, the shoulders rounded and the head held forward with the arms bent across the trunk (Fig. 17/1). More rarely the abnormality of posture will be a tendency to lean backward with a rather erect stance.

When sitting the patient tends to slump in the chair often sliding sideways until supported by the arm of the chair. The head again may fall forward on the chest.

The abnormal posture can be voluntarily corrected but only temporarily and with considerable effort and concentration.

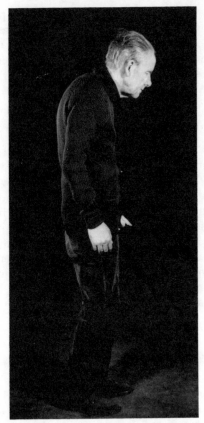

FIG. 17/1 The typical posture of a man with Parkinson's disease

Balance

When standing, these patients characteristically have a tendency to topple forwards. They are unable to make the quick compensatory movements to regain balance and so are easily knocked over. When they start to walk there is difficulty in shifting the centre of gravity from one foot to the other so their paces become short and shuffling – and the patient may lean too far forward in walking so that he has to 'chase' his centre of gravity if he is to avoid falling forward.

There are specific difficulties in turning round or initiating the movements of walking. The patient describes the feeling 'as if the feet are glued to the floor'. If he is pulled, he will fall over and an important part of physiotherapy is to teach the patient and his family how to overcome these problems (see Chapter 18).

Getting out of a chair may be difficult because the patient can no longer automatically judge how to place his centre of gravity over his feet. Thus he falls back into the chair each time he attempts to rise.

Learnt and voluntary movements

All movements are reduced in range and speed (akinesia). In walking the patient tends to take small paces and to walk more slowly. Speech becomes slower and softer. Handwriting tends to get smaller and after writing a few words slows down and becomes increasingly untidy. Cutting up food may become impossible and buttons and shoelaces likewise. Repetitive movements such as stirring and polishing are often particularly affected.

By contrast some complex co-ordinated movements such as driving a car may be relatively little affected. And similarly the preparation of meals and tasks such as cleaning a house or using a typewriter may pose few problems, although slower than normal.

Automatic movements

These are specifically reduced or lost in Parkinson's disease. The patient blinks infrequently and has an expressionless 'mask-like' face giving the spurious appearance of stupidity. There are none of the restless associated movements of the hands seen in the normal. When walking the patient does not swing his arms but instead walks with them hanging slightly flexed at the elbow.

Automatic swallowing of saliva is also impaired so that these patients tend to dribble involuntarily particularly when they sit with the head flexed on the chest.

Coughing as an automatic reflex response to clear the airway may be defective and there is therefore a risk of respiratory infection.

Unfortunately treatment does not restore any of these defects of automatic movement to any significant degree.

Rigidity

Muscle tone is increased in parkinsonism but the resistance to passive movement at a joint is uniform throughout the range of the movement (in contrast to spastic hypertonia). Two types of parkinsonian rigidity are described - 'lead pipe' where the resistance is smooth or plastic; and 'cogwheel' where the resistance is intermittent.

Although rigidity does not account for the poverty of movement which characterises parkinsonism it undoubtedly contributes to it. Similarly it is the rigidity which plays a part in the causation of the muscle pain already described. Relief of the rigid hypertonia is an important part therefore of the treatment.

Rigidity may be very asymmetrical or even unilateral. It may occasionally only affect one group of muscles to any significant degree - such as the neck muscles, forearm or thigh muscles. And it increases with nervous tension or in a cold environment.

Tremor

Like rigidity, tremor is usually asymmetrical or unilateral. It consists of an alternating contraction of opposing muscle groups causing a rhythmical movement at about 4 to 6 cycles per second. Tremor is usually maximal at the periphery and affects the arm more frequently than the leg.

Tremor is more of an embarrassment to the patient than a handicap because it is maximally present at rest but reduces or disappears on voluntary movement. Thus the patient is able to lift a glass to his mouth steadily without spilling the contents but the hand when relaxed on the lap is constantly shaking. Furthermore any anxiety or self-consciousness increases the tremor so that the embarrassment of any social occasion may become intolerable.

AETIOLOGY

The symptoms and signs of parkinsonism stem from a disturbance of function in two regions of the basal ganglia - the substantia nigra and the corpus striatum (caudate nucleus and putamen). These central nuclear masses of grey matter contain practically all the dopamine in the human brain. Dopamine is a chemical substance and one of the neurotransmitter amines (like adrenaline and noradrenaline) which carry the electrical message from one neurone to the next across the synapse. In parkinsonism there is a specific reduction of dopamine concentration at the synapse. This lack of dopamine results from a degeneration of neurones in Parkinson's disease or in the degenerative parkinsonian syndromes (such as Alzheimer's disease) or from focal damage in the parkinsonian syndromes following encephalitis lethargica, head injury or manganese poisoning. There is a chemical block to the action of dopamine in parkinsonism due to phenothiazine drugs.

Parkinson's disease accounts for the great majority of cases of parkinsonism. The cause of the degeneration in the substantia nigra and corpus striatum is unknown but it is a progressive process with a time course from onset to death between 10 and 15 years. Some cases progress more rapidly. Others so slowly that deterioration may be undetectable. And modern treatment has so improved the prognosis that there is now no overall excess mortality from Parkinson's disease when comparison is made with individuals of the same age.

In the worst cases increasing immobility leads eventually to weight loss, pressure sores and respiratory complications which are the usual cause of death.

In parkinsonism secondary to phenothiazine drugs or following encephalitis lethargica (now very rare) involuntary spasms of the eyes (oculo-gyric crises) may occur. Post-encephalitic parkinsonism is often non-progressive and may be associated with widespread brain damage causing behavioural disorder, spastic weakness and visual disturbance.

Features of the parkinsonian syndrome may occur in patients following a single severe head injury or following multiple head injuries (e.g. in boxers). Such cases are generally resistant to drug treatment, and like those cases in whom parkinsonism is part of a generalised degenerative process there is commonly intellectual impairment further reducing therapeutic responsiveness.

TREATMENT

The treatment of the patient with parkinsonism must be multi-disciplinary and, above all, designed to be appropriate to the individual case. Thus the patient with only tremor is going to require very little treatment, whereas disturbance of locomotion or severe slowness of movement of the hands (bradykinaesia) may require treatment involving drugs, physiotherapy and occupational therapy. The more disabled patients usually require the advice and assistance of medical social workers, welfare officers and disablement resettlement officers.

Drug treatment and physiotherapy are the most important forms of treatment in this condition with surgical treatment being only occasionally appropriate.

Drug treatment

The depletion of brain dopamine characteristic of this condition causes a reactive increased production of acetylcholine in the basal ganglia. Treatment is designed therefore to replenish the dopamine by administering the dopamine precursor levodopa – and reduce the acetylcholine with anticholinergic drugs such as benzhexol (Artane) or orphenadrine (Disipal). Levodopa is usually given in combination with a chemical which prevents its metabolism outside the brain and these combined tablets are marketed as Sinemet (levodopa plus carbidopa) and Madopar (levodopa plus benserazide).

Levodopa-containing drugs are the most effective treatment for the severe case and provide relief from most of the symptoms and signs especially the slowness and poverty of voluntary movement which is the main cause of disability. They also relieve the rigidity and substantially reduce the tremor. While on treatment with these drugs many patients lose all the manifestations of the disease and appear 'cured' although as soon as the treatment is stopped symptoms recur. On this treatment improvement may increase over many months.

Side-effects may be troublesome at the start of treatment (nausea and vomiting, postural hypotension, confusional states) or become manifest only after months or years of treatment (choreiform involuntary movements of the face or limbs, and 'on-off' attacks in which for periods of 30 minutes to 2 hours the patient becomes profoundly akinetic and unable to move).

Anticholinergic drugs, while less effective than levodopa, have an additive therapeutic effect with particular benefit to rigidity. They produce dryness of the mouth, slight blurring of near vision and occasionally hesitancy of micturition and confusional states.

The side-effects of both types of drug are dose dependent, disappearing when the dose is reduced.

Amantadine is sometimes used in the mild case. It acts by releasing dopamine in the brain but it is less potent and effective than levodopa.

Bromocriptine is a synthetic compound which mimics levodopa in all its actions and side-effects but has a slightly longer period of action.

The value of destructive surgical procedures on the thalamus in cases of parkinsonism was discovered in 1958 by a happy accident. During an operation on the brain of a patient with Parkinson's disease a small blood vessel had to be tied because of a haemorrhage. The resulting 'stroke' far from increasing the patient's disability led to the abolition of tremor and reduction of rigidity on the other side of the body. Tremor continued to be treated by surgical means until the advent of levodopa which is a more effective and safer method of treatment in most cases.

General care

None of the drug therapy is effective unless the patient takes advantage of his improvement and returns to more normal activity. The slowness of movement and difficulties with walking make the patient disinclined to be active and tend to make him over-ready to accept help and become dependent on others. This leads to a dependent state of mind and chronic invalidism. Furthermore, relatives tend to be over-anxious to help, and must be advised to allow, and indeed encourage, the patient to remain independent however long it takes him, for example, to dress or wash. Regular exercise should be encouraged, and the patient should remain at work if possible and continue to maintain an interest in hobbies, sport and social activities.

It is rarely necessary, even for the most severely afflicted cases, to require hospital care - even on a day basis. Home nursing is normally satisfactory following advice by an occupational therapist on aids and appliances - such as a high chair (and raised lavatory seat), zips and Velcro fastenings to clothes, electric razor and toothbrush.

The occasional patient is bed or wheelchair-bound but here the nursing care required is no different from that of any other patient unable to stand or walk. In such cases particular attention has to be paid to respiratory infection and pressure sores since intercurrent illness greatly exacerbates the parkinsonian disability, and reduces the benefits of drug treatment.

Physiotherapy

See Chapter 18.

BIBLIOGRAPHY

Godwin-Austen, R. B. (1984). *The Parkinson's Disease Handbook.* Sheldon Press, London.

Marsden, T. D. and Parkes, J. D. (1977). Success and problems of long-term therapy in Parkinson's disease. *Lancet*, **1**, 345.

Parkinson's Disease: A Booklet for Patients and Their Families, by R. B. Godwin-Austen and published by the Parkinson's Disease Society.

Parkinsonism – Management

by S. FRANKLYN MCSP

Idiopathic Parkinson's disease is usually a slowly progressive condition spanning many years. During this time the patient may become gradually less independent and more reliant on outside help. The aim of physiotherapy should be to help the patient maintain his independence for as long as possible and to advise relatives and helpers how to handle the affected person as the disease progresses and the disabilities become more established.

The symptoms of Parkinson's disease are wide ranging and combine to substantially restrict the patient's functional independence (see Chapter 17). Posture is affected. In the early stages of the disease the only abnormality may be a protruding head but as the disease progresses, kyphosis of the thoracic spine, flexion and adduction of the hips and shoulders, flexion of the knees and elbows and shortening of the calf muscles become apparent (see Fig. 17/1, p. 419).

As these postural changes slowly occur the patient's balance reactions are affected and he complains of falling and feeling unsteady. This is hardly surprising as the centre of gravity is now over his forefoot, or even in front of his feet, and his base has contracted, that is, his feet are adducted and he may be weight-bearing through his fore foot. Thus, if he moves out of this narrow base he is likely to fall. In addition the righting reflexes are affected.

Gait is affected. The normal heel-toe gait is compromised; the patient walks with a flat foot or a toe-heel gait (Fig. 18/1). This reversal of the normal gait pattern in conjunction with the postural changes cause the symptoms of festination and freezing. When *festinating*, the patient walks with a progressively shortened stride until he runs uncontrollably. When *freezing* occurs the patient is unable to move his feet and complains that they appear

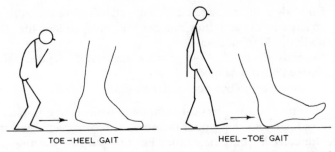

TOE–HEEL GAIT   HEEL–TOE GAIT

FIG. 18/1 Gait mechanism: toe-heel gait in Parkinson's disease; heel-toe gait in normal health

stuck to the ground. This frequently occurs in narrow spaces and doorways. In addition he may have difficulties initiating movement.

Rising from a chair, rolling over in bed, and activities involving fine hand movements, such as writing and sewing, are among some of the activities that may eventually be affected. All these activities may be classed as automatic movements, that is, they are movements not under conscious control.

When a parkinsonian patient performs an affected activity the movement may begin normally, but one or more components of the total movement may be faulty making it difficult or impossible for the movement to be completed satisfactorily. As the disease progresses, rotational movements are lost, flexion of the spine, elbows, hips and knees becomes more noticeable and difficulties and abnormalities of movement patterns become more apparent. In severe cases, performance of the desired activity becomes impossible, unaided.

Disability grading

As there is such a wide range of disability, a grading system is necessary to identify the patient's overall disability. The Yahr Scale (Haehn and Yahr, 1967) categorises the stages of the disease as follows:

  I. Unilateral involvement only, usually with minimal or no functional impairment.
 II. Bilateral or midline involvement without impairment of balance.

III. First signs of impaired righting reflexes. Functionally restricted in his activities but can lead independent life. Disability mild to moderate.

IV. Severely disabled. Able to walk and stand unaided but is markedly handicapped.

V. Confinement to bed or wheelchair unless aided.

In addition to the physical symptoms patients are frequently depressed, anxious, have poor memory for recent events and may have difficulty learning new tasks. For this purpose learning may be divided into three functions: learning the information, retaining it and recalling it for use. Laboratory experiments have shown that parkinsonians can learn a task (Marsden, 1982), thus the defect is thought to be in one or both of the latter functions. This aspect of the disease may well have a profound effect on the patient's response to physiotherapy for if a patient is unable to remember or recall a task he has been taught, he will be unable to use the information when necessary. For example, when a patient freezes he is taught to put his heels to the ground. He is able to do this when told but often has difficulty recalling and initiating the activity when alone.

In the early stages of the disease it is possible to teach the patient to overcome some of his functional difficulties, but as the disease progresses treatment may become less successful as faulty movement patterns, postural and other symptoms become more firmly established.

Physiotherapy is always given in conjunction with drug treatment and occupational and speech therapy should they be necessary.

ASSESSMENT

The assessment should be designed to give the therapist a general impression of the patient's medical condition, his social circumstances and a detailed description of his physical problems.

General information

It is important to take a full medical history to determine whether there are other factors besides Parkinson's disease that affect the patient's general health and mobility, e.g. arthritis, hemiplegia.

A history of the disease itself, its duration and physical signs and symptoms should be noted. These include tremor, akinesia, dyskinesias, rigidity, pain, particularly around the thighs, 'on-off' symptoms, excessive salivation, difficulty swallowing and poor balance (for further details see Chapter 17).

The patient's medication should be noted with particular emphasis on anti-parkinsonian drugs and their dosages. These may be adjusted as the patient's condition alters, often with a resultant change in performance. A full social history is necessary to record whether a patient is working or retired, what his work is, what his hobbies are and how he fills his day. A person who is working or who has active interests will be more motivated towards helping himself than someone who does nothing all day. The type of accommodation and whether the patient lives alone or not are relevant, as are any services the patient receives, such as meals-on-wheels.

The patient's difficulties and the reasons for them must be noted in detail so that suitable treatment and advice may be given to overcome them when possible.

Physiotherapy assessment

A patient's posture, balance and functional performance are recorded. Many patients' functional performance varies during the day so it is important to note the time of the assessment and the time since the last dose of drugs was taken. This is particularly important when patients experience the 'on-off' symptom. In order to reduce the effects of these symptoms on the assessment results, the assessment should be carried out at the same time of day on subsequent occasions. If a patient is 'off' on the first assessment but 'on' on the subsequent assessment the difference in performance will be enormous and may be attributed to treatment rather than the 'on-off' symptom.

POSTURE

As posture is invariably affected this should be assessed using a 1 to 4 scale. Pictorial grading is the easiest method to use (Fig. 18/2). Similar gradings may be used to assess posture in sitting and lying should this be relevant to the individual.

BALANCE

To test balance reactions, the patient is asked to:
1. Sit unsupported for 1 minute.
2. Stand without an aid for 5 seconds.
3. Stand on one leg and then the other without an aid for 5 seconds.

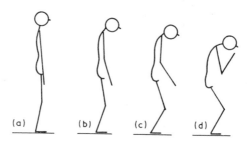

FIG. 18/2 Posture grading. (a) 1. Normal. (b) 2. With head protruding. (c) 3. Head protruding, with marked kyphotic thoracic spine, slight flexion at knees and elbows. (d) 4. Marked flexion of the trunk, elbows, hips and knees

FUNCTIONAL ASSESSMENT

Common difficulties such as turning over in bed, sitting from lying and standing from the sitting position should all be timed and graded. The grading scale used is:
1. Normal.
2. Can complete a task with difficulty but without an aid.
3. Can complete task with the use of an aid, such as pulling on the side of the bed.
4. Unable to complete task.

The same grading and timed assessment may be used to record performance for other functional difficulties as appropriate.

Gait should be assessed by allowing the patient to walk a fixed distance and recording the number of steps and the time taken to cover the distance. The quality of the heel strike should be noted and may be divided into three categories: (1) heel-toe; (2) flat-footed, and (3) toe-heel.

In addition, the patient's ambulatory posture should be noted and whether he experiences difficulty initiating movement. Note should be taken of any walking aid used.

Finger dexterity may be assessed by allowing a maximum of 3 minutes to button up three shirt buttons. The number of buttons and the time taken should be noted.

At the end of the assessment the therapist should be in a position to categorise the patient's disease severity using the Haehn and Yahr Scale and list the aims of treatment.

At the beginning of each subsequent assessment any change in drug regime must be noted.

Additional assessments

These easily administered tests may be useful to help assess a patient's learning disabilities.

1. *The Verbal Learning Test* is used to test immediate memory span, learning and delayed recall for verbal material (Lezak, 1976). It consists of a list of 15 words which are read to the patient who must repeat the list at intervals during the assessment.

2. *The Verbal Comprehension Test* is used to test the patient's comprehension of verbal instructions (Boller and Vignolo, 1966). It consists of giving sets of increasingly complex instructions which the patient must follow.

Once the assessment has been completed the therapist should have a clearer understanding of the patient's functional difficulties and his mental state so that a treatment programme can be formulated.

TREATMENT

It should be remembered that Parkinson's disease is a slowly deteriorating condition and although the patient may improve his performance initially, as a result of physiotherapy, in the long term he may require 'booster' courses of treatment intermittently throughout the course of his disease, as new difficulties arise.

The treatment programme should include some or all of the following:

1. Analysis of functional difficulties and treatment to overcome them, where applicable.
2. Postural awareness.
3. Relaxation training.
4. Advice to relatives.
5. Home exercises.

Analysis of functional difficulties

The core of the treatment programme should consist of goal-oriented therapy to help the patient overcome his individual functional difficulties. The faulty patterns of movement should be analysed and corrected when possible or an alternative way of performing the movement should be chosen and repeatedly practised by the patient until he becomes proficient at it. Auditory and visual cues should be used to reinforce the information. For example, during freezing and festination teaching the patient to place his heels on the ground often corrects the symptoms temporarily. By doing this his centre of gravity returns to a more normal position and he is able to adjust his posture before continuing to walk. In order to facilitate this, the instruction 'HEELS DOWN' reinforces the initial action. The patient may be taught to say this to himself when necessary, or, failing this, his relative or helper should be instructed to use it. Visual cueing may also be used, for example, asking a patient to step over cracks in the paving stones when walking, can reduce the episodes of freezing.

Trick movements such as flexing the leg at the hip and knee or swinging the leg backward may also be used to overcome hesitancy but, as the first step is taken, the heel-toe gait must be emphasised to avoid the immediate recurrence of festination or freezing. It should be remembered that the effect of these trick movements only lasts for a limited time, so a number of them should be taught and the patient encouraged to devise his own.

Over-emphasis of the normal heel-toe gait is necessary to improve the walking pattern and attempt to reduce the occurrence of freezing and festination. Again auditory cueing may help to reinforce this – saying 'HEEL, HEEL' while walking to encourage heel-toe gait, can be helpful.

Postural awareness

Postural awareness training in lying, sitting, standing and walking may also be included in the treatment programme particularly in the early stages of the disease. The position of one part of the body in relation to the adjoining part and to the body as a whole is a useful method to use (Barker, 1981). As the disease progresses patients are often unaware of gross postural disturbances and are therefore unable to correct them, themselves.

Relaxation

Relaxation can be a useful part of treatment particularly if the patient complains of over-anxiety or troublesome dyskinesias. Methods of relaxation with a postural element to reinforce postural awareness are suitable, for example physiological relaxation (Mitchell, 1977).

Advice to relatives

Relatives and helpers should be encouraged to allow the patient to be as independent as possible, even if tasks take longer to complete than previously. This is not always easy, for over the years the relative may have taken on many tasks formally performed by the patient; but this is essential if the patient is to maintain even a minor degree of independence. In such circumstances occupational therapy is useful by providing advice and aids when necessary.

Both patient and his relatives should be advised to alter their daily routine so that activities may be attempted when the patient is feeling well and able to complete them more easily.

As the patient becomes more disabled the relatives may take a more active part in the patient's routine. It is important to teach correct lifting techniques to the relatives although it is rarely necessary for a patient to be lifted. If necessary, the relatives should be taught how to assist the patient when he experiences difficulties, such as when rolling over in bed, standing from sitting. Verbal and visual cueing should also be taught to encourage movement.

Home exercises

Most patients like to practise simple mobilising exercises at home, and once introduced to them will often continue with them. Diaphragmatic breathing exercises to encourage chest expansion should be included. A *written* list of exercises to reinforce hospital treatment sessions is essential.

Many patients, particularly those who are less disabled, respond well to group activities and benefit from the group interaction. The group may be taken in the conventional way, including the treatment suggestions mentioned above, or conductive education may be used (Cotton and Kinsman, 1983).

In *conductive education* the conductor (therapist) acts in a facilitatory capacity. Difficulties common to members of the group are analysed and reduced to their component parts. Each component is practised after the conductor puts into words the intended movement and the patient repeats it and then performs the movement to a count of one. This is followed by a brisk count to five during which the movement is consolidated. The sequence is continued until the total movement is completed.

With more severely disabled patients group work is impracticable and patients should be treated on an individual basis. Domiciliary treatment should also be considered for these patients, if it is available. Some patients find regular hospital visits exhausting both physically and emotionally. Others do not experience the difficulties in the spaciousness of a hospital department that they do in the confines of their homes and these patients may benefit from domiciliary treatment.

As Parkinson's disease is progressive any therapy must be concerned with helping the patient to maximise his physical potential so that the quality of his life can be improved at that time. The difficulties and the goals will constantly change as the disease progresses but prolongation of functional independence is important.

REFERENCES

Barker, S. (1981). *The Alexander Technique*. Bantam Books, London.
Boller, F. and Vignolo, L. (1966). Latent sensory aphasia in hemisphere damaged patients - an experimental study using the token test. *Brain*, **89**, 815-31.
Cotton, E. and Kinsman, R. (1983). *Conductive Education for Adult Hemiplegia*. Churchill Livingstone, Edinburgh.
Haehn, N. M. and Yahr, M. D. (1967). Parkinsonism: onset, progression and mortality. *Neurology*, **17**, 427-42.
Lezak, M. D. (1976). *Neuropsychological Assessment*, pp. 352-6. Oxford University Press, New York.
Marsden, C. D. (1982). The mysterious motor function of the basal ganglia. The Robert Wartenberg Lecture. *Neurology*, **32**, 5, 514-39.
Mitchell, L. (1977). *Simple Relaxation*. John Murray, London.

BIBLIOGRAPHY

Franklyn, S., Perry, A. and Beattie, A. (1983). *Living with Parkinson's Disease*. Available from the Parkinson's Disease Society, 36 Portland Place, London W1N 3DG.
Franklyn, S., Imms, F. J. and Stern, G. (1985). *Physiotherapy and Parkinson's Disease: An Evaluation of Four Treatment Regimes*. Report to the Parkinson's Disease Society, 36 Portland Place, London W1N 3DG.

Chapter 19

Polyneuropathy

by J. M. LEE BA, MCSP, DipTP

Polyneuropathy is a collective term for a syndrome which includes all inflammatory and degenerative diseases involving the peripheral nervous system. The main presenting features include widespread sensory and motor disturbances of the peripheral nerves and it often appears as a symmetrical involvement of the nerves but this is not always so. The syndrome is usually seen in the young or middle-aged adult, men being affected more frequently than women.

Polyneuropathy and polyneuritis are interchangeable terms: strictly speaking polyneuropathy refers to the primary degenerative diseases which begin in the nerve parenchyma and are initiated by toxic, metabolic or vascular causes; whereas polyneuritis covers all primary inflammatory diseases of the connective tissue in peripheral nerves which are due to toxic or allergic substances and infections.

Before looking at the various polyneuropathies an understanding of the organisation and functioning of the peripheral nervous system is essential. The anatomical and physiological descriptions which follow are at a superficial level and serve only to refresh the memory.

Formation of a peripheral nerve

The peripheral nervous system is composed of fibres from both somatic and visceral nervous systems, together with their associated ganglia containing nerve cell bodies, and supportive connective tissue. All the above elements are situated distal to the pia-arachnoid membranes of the spinal cord.

A mixed spinal nerve is made up of parallel bundles of nerve fibres - these fibres are divided into two functional systems: somatic and visceral.

The somatic system consists of afferent and efferent nerve fibres. The afferent fibres conduct impulses from sensory receptors in the skin, joints, muscles and subcutaneous tissues to the central nervous system. These fibres are the long dendritic processes of the sensory nerve cell body which is situated in the dorsal root ganglion. The efferent fibres are axonal processes of nerve somata in the ventral horn of the spinal cord; they are classified as α, β and γ neurones and convey impulses to the skeletal muscles.

The visceral nervous system includes the parasympathetic and sympathetic divisions which innervate glands, viscera and unstriated muscle. The afferent side of this system is in many ways similar to that of the somatic nervous system. The cell body of the afferent fibre being situated in the dorsal root ganglion of the spinal cord and the nuclei of the facial (VII), glossopharyngeal (IX), and vagus (X) cranial nerves.

The efferent pathway is very different from the somatic system. The cell body of the (pre-ganglionic) efferent fibre is found in the lateral grey column of the thoracic and upper lumbar spinal segments. The parasympathetic efferent cell is found in the nuclei of the oculomotor (III), facial, glossopharyngeal, vagus and accessory (XI) cranial nerves and in the lateral grey column of the sacral segments of the cord.

The two divisions of the visceral nervous system normally operate at a subconscious level and are broadly antagonistic in action. The sympathetic nervous system has a more general effect in preparing the body for activity, whereas the parasympathetic has a more localised action on individual viscera, in general producing a more tranquil state of affairs in the body. The afferent pathways of the visceral nervous system are responsible for sensations of nausea, visceral pain, hunger, etc, all of which are perceived as conscious sensations.

Gross structure of a mixed peripheral nerve (Fig. 19/1)

The larger diameter somatic afferent and efferent nerve fibres are wrapped in a layer of lipid material, the myelin sheath. This is formed from the membrane of the Schwann cell. At regular intervals along the nerve a gap occurs between adjacent Schwann cells and the axolemma is exposed. This gap, the node of Ranvier, is essential for saltatory conduction along the nerve fibres. The small diameter somatic sensory and visceral nerve fibres are non-myelinated, that is to say that one or several fibres are loosely

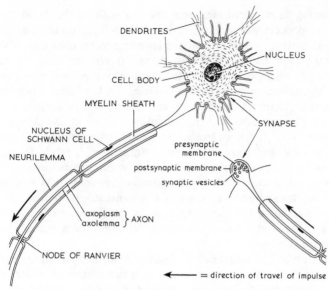

FIG. 19/1 Structure of a neurone

enclosed by Schwann cells and because of this their conduction velocity is considerably reduced.

The outer layer of the Schwann cell was at one time known as the neurilemma sheath but this term is now not in common usage.

Individual nerve fibres are surrounded by a delicate tissue, the endoneurium, which serves as support for not only the nerve fibres but also for the rich vascular system supplying a peripheral nerve; these nerve fibres are gathered together into small fasciculi and supported by perineurium, and the fasciculi in turn are surrounded by a dense connective tissue sheath, the epineurium, which serves as the outer layer of the peripheral nerve trunk.

Transport systems in the nerve fibre

Running the length of the nerve fibre are intracellular microtubules which are more prominent in the axoplasm than in dendrite processes. These microtubules are not surrounded by a membrane as are other cell organelles, e.g. lysosomes, but the walls are composed of repeating sub-units of glycoproteins, resembling those found in cilia and spermatozoa and are thought to have similar contractile properties. The peristaltic-like movement occurring in microtubules from the cell body to the distal end of a nerve process would allow them a role in intracellular transport.

Experiments using radioactive labelling techniques have shown that the axon has fast and slow transport systems from the soma to the periphery of the neurone. The fast transport system carries all organelles, e.g. synaptic vesicles and plasma membrane materials (Group I organelles), at velocities up to 400mm day^{-1}. Group II organelles, e.g. mitochondria, move at the slower rate of 40mm day^{-1}, other cytoskeletal proteins are classified as Group III and IV and move at about 2-8mm day^{-1}, while Group V neurofilamentous and microtubular components move at a velocity of 1mm day^{-1}. The method of movement is similar to saltatory movement – a series of hops and stops; the mechanism postulated includes a myosin-actin type of movement involving cross-bridges which pass the organelles along the microtubules in the axon (Levine et al, 1981).

The ability of neurones to recover from axonal injury varies, those of the peripheral nervous system can regenerate their axons and reform functional synapses but those of the central nervous system cannot. The existence of rapid transport systems for proteins is important in the regrowth of an axon and is thought to be under the control of neuronal genes which regulate the synthesis and transport of proteins. In nerve regeneration the amount of Group I and IV organelles transported markedly increases over normal levels, the stimulus to the soma for this increase is not clear but is hypothesised as being either originating in the axon stump, or by retrograde transport of altered organelles or from the damaged Schwann cell. It is interesting to note that the cell proteins essential for transmission of a nerve impulse are not transported in the axoplasm at their normal rate but at a reduced level.

From this brief revision of nerve cell organisation it can be seen that metabolic disorders which affect the cell body will rapidly result in dysfunction in the ability of the neurones to conduct a nerve impulse and transport molecules which are essential for synaptic transmission and the continued integrity of the distal parts of the nerve process. It may also explain why the first symptoms and signs of a peripheral neuropathy appear in those neurones with the longest line of communication, that is, the feet and lower limbs, closely followed by the hands.

EFFECT OF NERVE DYSFUNCTION ON MUSCLE

The loss of anatomical contact between motor nerve and muscle causes not only biochemical and physiological changes but also profound morphological changes in the muscle cell. Atrophy is most spectacular being due to the loss of myofilaments as catabolism of proteins increases and synthesis decreases.

The greatest atrophy is seen in fast twitch glycolytic fibres compared with the slow twitch oxidative type. The atrophy seen in denervation has been found to be similar to the atrophy observed following excess of glucocorticoids, e.g. in Cushing's disease and when used for anti-inflammatory and immunosuppressive effects. It has been suggested that denervation atrophy may be effected by endogenous glucocorticoids.

The mechanism suggested has been an increase in specific binding sites in the cytosol proteins, which would inhibit the formation of messenger ribonucleic acid (mRNA), which in turn would reduce the rate of translation of proteins and synthesis of cell organelles.

AETIOLOGY OF POLYNEUROPATHIES

There is still argument as to the precise metabolic dysfunction which results in some polyneuropathies but the following classification of causal agents is commonly accepted.

1. Infective condition
   (a) local infections of peripheral nerves:
       e.g. virus – herpes zoster
            bacteria – leprosy, brucellosis
   (b) polyneuritis complicating a current infection:
       e.g. dysentery, influenza, mumps
   (c) infections with organisms whose toxins have an affinity for the peripheral nervous system:
       e.g. diphtheria, tetanus, botulism.
2. Post-infective polyneuropathy
   e.g. Gullain-Barré-Landry syndrome.
3. Toxic substances
       e.g. heavy metals – mercury, lead, arsenic, gold and copper
            organic chemicals – aniline, cyanide, triortho-cresyl-phosphate
            drugs – isoniazid, thalidomide and nitrofurantoin, vincristine.

4. Deficiency, metabolic and blood disorders
    e.g. alcoholism, porphyria, leukaemia, diabetes mellitus, chronic uraemia, liver failure and various vitamin deficiencies.
5. Trauma
    e.g. physical (compression/stretching), electrical (earth shock) or radiation injury to nerves.
6. Connective tissue disease and allied disorders in which abnormalities in metabolism of serum proteins occur
    e.g. polyarteritis nodosa, systemic lupus erythematosus, amyloid disease, sarcoidosis and carcinoma.
7. Genetic disorders
    e.g. hereditary sensory radicular neuropathy (Denny-Brown), hypertrophic interstitial neuritis (Déjèrine-Sottas), peroneal muscular atrophy (Charcot-Marie-Tooth), Refsum's disease.
8. Pure vascular disorders
    e.g. atheroma, collagen disorders, diabetes mellitus, Buerger's disease.
9. Polyneuropathy of unknown origin.

PATHOLOGICAL CHANGES IN PERIPHERAL NEUROPATHY

The pathological changes produced by the causal agent can be divided into two groups – parenchymal and interstitial.

Parenchymal

In parenchymal neuropathies it is the neurone and/or Schwann cell which undergo degeneration. There are three types of lesion:

1. *Axonal degeneration* (sometimes called Gombault's degeneration). The nerve processes and soma atrophy, with associated breakdown in the myelin sheath. Recovery from these changes is slow and incomplete.
2. *Segmental degeneration.* This involves the loss of myelin from sections of the nerve fibre usually in the more proximal parts. The recovery of nerve function is rapid and complete.
3. *Wallerian degeneration.* This occurs when both axon and myelin sheath undergo disorganisation; the demyelination process occurring some time after the destruction of the axon, the nerve soma undergoes chromatolysis. Recovery from Wallerian degeneration is slow and often incomplete.

In all three types of parenchymal pathology nerve conduction is outside normal limits, and due to the loss of conduction capability the muscles supplied will atrophy.

Re-myelination of a nerve fibre is characterised by an increase in the number of nodes of Ranvier, the new nodes formed become sites for the aggregation of sodium channels in the axon membrane so that fairly normal conduction properties can be regained.

Interstitial

In the polyneuropathies of interstitial origin it is primarily collagen changes in the vascular structures which produce the neural changes. The connective tissues supporting the nerve processes can also be involved in producing pathological changes in nerve trunks, e.g. amyloid and tumour tissue.

CLINICAL FEATURES

The clinical picture of peripheral neuropathy comprises a lower motor neurone paralysis, especially in the limbs, the lower one being more involved than the upper limb.

The patient exhibits atrophy, muscle flaccid paralysis, weakness and ataxia, usually complaining of the inability to walk over rough ground – stumbling, even falling, he may present with a chronic ankle sprain due to the balance problems. In the upper limb the patient indicates problems in manipulating small coins, matches, knives, and may drop objects unintentionally.

Foot drop and wrist drop are present and joint contractures and deformity may be seen in hands, feet and spine.

Tendor reflexes are sometimes absent and often sluggish, the latter being due to a reduced nerve conduction velocity and impulse volley dispersal. The ankle jerk disappears before the knee jerk and the plantar response is flexor. Impairment of both cutaneous and proprioceptive sensory modalities are seen initially in the extremities but later progressing proximally. Paraesthesia is a common complaint and if muscle groups or nerve trunks are palpated with a deep pressure pain is often produced.

The loss of proprioception will also contribute to the 'drunken' (ataxic) gait described above. Severe joint disorganisation (Charcot joints) is seen as a result of persistent injury which is not felt due to loss of pain sensibility, resulting in damage and eventually destruction of the joint.

Alterations in nocioception varies from a painless distal sensory loss to a severe burning pain with dysaesthesia and autonomic disturbance. Pain is associated with degeneration (Wallerian or axonal) of unmyelinated and small myelinated fibres, or to partial degeneration and regeneration, and not necessarily due to loss of large diameter myelinated fibres which would lead to 'pain-gate' control dysfunction.

Trophic changes in the skin of the extremities are shown by the red, glossy skin which on palpation seems to have 'double thickness'; later, thickening of the nails is seen. Trophic and sensory changes in their most extreme form are seen in leprosy where loss of digits may occur.

In more serious neuropathies there may be associated myocardial damage, resulting in cardiac arrhythmia and labile blood pressure.

In addition to the above clinical features a history of exposure to toxic chemicals may produce their own symptoms, e.g. the pigmentation in arsenic poisoning.

CLINICAL DIAGNOSIS

First, the existence of a neuropathy needs to be established, then its cause must be determined and treatment prescribed.

The first stage is fairly easy as the clinical history and presenting signs and symptoms may be those associated with a particular neuropathy. The symmetrical and distal distribution of muscle atrophy and weakness together with sensory impairment is characteristic of peripheral neuropathy. But it is more usual for other clinical diagnostic tests to be needed to determine the existence and cause of the disease.

Biochemical tests may be used which will establish the presence of certain metabolic or toxic substances or the absence of nutrients. An electromyograph (EMG) will differentiate between a neuropathy and a myopathy, or a disorder of the neuromuscular junction.

The measurement of nerve conduction velocity can be a help in determining the type of pathological changes occurring in the neurone. It is usual to find in Wallerian degeneration that conduction velocity is reduced by up to 30 per cent. In segmental demyelination conduction velocity is often slowed by more than 40 per cent (Gilliatt, 1966).

The nature of the neuropathy can sometimes be determined by

the biopsy of the sural nerve (the resultant sensory loss is minimal).

MEDICAL MANAGEMENT

The medical management will depend on the speed of onset and the patient's clinical presentation.

In the more severe cases, e.g. Guillain-Barré-Landry, the full services of an intensive care unit may be required whereas in others, e.g. diabetic neuropathy, the patient may receive treatment on an outpatient basis.

The indicator for ventilatory assistance is when the vital capacity is reduced to 800ml and a PaO_2 below 60mmHg. Patients who are thought to be entering respiratory problems should have hourly assessment of vital capacity. As ventilatory help is required for several weeks it is usual for a tracheostomy to be performed and a cuffed tracheal tube inserted. Tracheal toilet and suction is needed to prevent lung infection but antibiotics are not as a rule prescribed unless there is evidence of an infection. Respiratory support is given by an intermittent positive pressure ventilator (IPPV).

Normal nursing care to the bladder, pressure areas, skin care, and mouth toilet is required. In some cases hypotension occurs, usually in the elderly patient, and pressor drugs are required to support blood pressure. The fluid balance of the patient is important so that dehydration does not occur, a nasogastric tube is usually present in patients with bulbar palsy, and depending on the patient's condition may be used to feed them, though intravenous feeding can be used.

Analgesia may be required if pain is a problem and, as pressure can produce pain, a bed cradle is used to relieve the weight of blankets. Careful positioning of the patient's joints is needed to prevent discomfort as well as contractures occurring. In most cases of severe infective neuropathy improvement occurs, the mortality of such patients is approximately 5 per cent if care is given in an intensive unit, compared with about 25 per cent mortality for admission to a general ward. It is important to remember that the patient is conscious and can feel pain, though he may need assistance with breathing and cannot move. Hospital personnel and relatives who have contact with the patient must remember this and not discuss the more depressing aspects of the patient's condition within earshot or treat the patient as non-comprehending.

The patient who is not so severely affected and who can maintain his own airway and is somewhat more independent is in a better position. For these patients rest in bed is often required and is essential if there are signs of cardiac involvement. Analgesia may be required to minimise spontaneous pain and a bed cradle to support the bedclothes. Some medical regimes include a high calorie diet and vitamin therapy especially of the B complex; careful positioning is again necessary to preserve joint integrity.

If toxic substances have been absorbed, removal from the cause will lead to improvement; in some cases, such as lead or arsenic poisoning, chelating agents are given to provide an alternative chemical 'acceptor' for the causal metal agent; the drug used for arsenic neuropathy is dimercaprol.

In polyneuropathy due to vitamin deficiency, e.g. beri-beri, a good diet plus vitamin replacement therapy will facilitate recovery which though slow is usually complete as malnutrition must be prolonged for Wallerian degeneration to have occurred.

Most cases of polyneuropathy, once the cause has been removed, show signs of improvement; in other cases, the disorder persists for some time before improvement begins and yet again in other neuropathies no change is seen.

Chronic pain associated with neuropathy is difficult to manage – but some physiotherapy modalities which have indicated some usefulness include transcutaneous nerve stimulation and acupuncture. Dorsal column stimulation is a highly skilled surgical procedure which requires laminectomy to allow electrode implantation; a more recent development includes percutaneous epidermal stimulation which is not as surgically complex.

PRINCIPAL POLYNEUROPATHIC SYNDROMES

The list of polyneuropathic syndromes is very extensive and it is not possible to cover all of them in this text. The more commonly met polyneuropathies are listed below.

A. Acute Ascending Polyneuropathy
   Guillain-Barré-Landry
   porphyria
   diphtheria
   mononucleosis

B. Sub-acute Sensorimotor Polyneuropathy
  (1) symmetrical
      arsenical
      lead
      thalidomide
      alcoholic
  (2) asymmetrical
      polyarteritis nodosa
      diabetic
C. Chronic Sensorimotor Polyneuropathy
  (1) acquired
      carcinoma
      amyloid
      rheumatoid arthritis
  (2) genetic
      peroneal muscular atrophy (Charcot-Marie-Tooth)
      hypertrophic interstitial neuritis (Déjèrine-Sottas)
      hereditary atactica polyneuriformis (Refsum's)

ACUTE ASCENDING POLYNEUROPATHY

Guillain-Barré-Landry syndrome

This syndrome which affects both sexes at any age, peaking at 20–50, is found worldwide and in all seasons. Its cause is unknown, though current authorities consider it to be due to hypersensitivity or allergy to unknown viruses or allergens. In around 50 per cent of cases the onset of symptoms is preceded by a mild gastro-intestinal or respiratory infection.

Clinically, the syndrome presents as a symmetrical weakness of muscle; there is some wasting, hypotonia and a partial or complete loss of the associated deep tendon reflexes. The motor symptoms start distally and move proximally, with lower limb involvement preceding that of the upper limb, the disease may progress to involve the trunk and cranial muscles. Pain is a variable symptom, though there is usually tenderness on deep pressure, especially to motor points in muscle and nerve trunks. Paraesthesia is often described in the limbs.

Both sensory and motor nerve conduction velocities are reduced. Autonomic functions are sometimes affected, usually cardiac muscle, which may lead to sinus arrhythmias and variable blood pressure.

Visual impairment is rare, though papilloedema is occasionally seen. The hearing is not usually affected and cerebral symptoms rare.

The symptoms may progress for one or several weeks until the disease 'peaks and plateaus out' symptoms gradually regressing in reverse order of onset.

PATHOLOGY

The disease process affects the spinal roots and nerve processes, primarily involving the Schwann cell and this results in segmental demyelination of the nerve process initially, later there is a proliferation of Schwann cells. The axon remains intact through demyelination and can conduct an impulse with a much reduced velocity, later in some patients axonal degeneration may also occur leading to complete conduction block.

There is an associated perivascular lymphocytic inflammatory exudate of the peripheral nervous system, and other organs such as the heart, lungs or kidney may show this. Recovery takes place by axonal regeneration and re-myelination of peripheral axons, though the myelination sheath is thinner and there is an increase in the number of nodes of Ranvier, i.e. internodal distance is less. In the less severe cases nerve conduction velocity returns to within normal limits, however, where axonal damage has occurred, conduction velocities may be permanently abnormal.

PROGNOSIS

In epidemics the mortality is high but usually in a single incidence of this syndrome most patients recover completely. The more favourable ones in 3 to 6 months although more often the time scale is 1 to 2 years.

COMPLICATIONS

In severe cases who need respiratory assistance, infections of the lower respiratory tract can be a hazard. Deep vein thrombosis due to paralysis affecting the limbs and thereby removing the muscle pump effect, and the temporary loss of an effective respiratory system, can also occur. Retention of urine is an uncommon complication.

Cardiac arrhythmias and labile blood pressure have already been mentioned as a possible complication.

TREATMENT

If respiratory assistance is required for the Guillain-Barré-Landry patient ideally it should be managed in an intensive care unit as the chance of life expectancy is enhanced under these conditions.

The normal nursing care for fluid intake, skin and pressure area care is needed. Sometimes ACTH is prescribed for these patients to reduce the inflammatory response but clinical results vary.

PHYSIOTHERAPY MANAGEMENT

A. UNDER INTENSIVE CARE IN THE ACUTE PROGRESSIVE STAGE

During this period of treatment when the patient is to all intents and purposes a tetraplegic with respiratory distress the aims of treatment are to:

maintain a clear airway

prevent lung infection

maintain anatomical joint range

support joints in a functional position to minimise damage or deformity

assist in the prevention of pressure sores

maintain peripheral circulation

provide psychological support for the patient and relatives.

Methods

MAINTENANCE OF A CLEAR AIRWAY: PREVENTION OF LUNG INFECTION

The patient's breathing will be assisted by intermittent positive pressure ventilation (IPPV) via a cuffed tracheostomy tube. This leads to some limitation of the positions in which the patient may be placed to posturally drain areas of lung tissue. Some compromise is necessary and, in the absence of lung infection, two-hourly turning into supine or side lying positions will aid the removal of secretions from all parts of the lung.

A suction catheter is used to remove secretions from the respiratory passages until the cough reflex reappears.

Manual techniques used to assist in maintaining and clearing the airway include vibration with/without over pressure. To enhance expansion a 2- to 4-litre anaesthetic bag can be used for patients with tracheostomy tubes, although care is needed as a reduction in cardiac output can occur as a result of 'bagging'.

Two people are necessary for this technique, one to squeeze the bag, and another to apply chest manipulations.

To simulate a cough, rib-springing techniques are useful, although a faulty technique may produce fractures of the ribs. As chest care is relatively long term for these patients, a 2.5cm thick piece of foam rubber placed under the physiotherapist's hands makes rib-springing more tolerable for the patient.

Once the patient is weaned off the ventilator, respiratory care is a shared responsibility between patient and physiotherapist and adequate expansion in all areas of the lung and effective coughing must be taught to the patient. As neurones recover their function, and muscle once again responds to a nerve impulse, active assisted/active exercises to those muscles may commence. Patients at this stage tire fairly quickly and there are still some 'aches and pains' in the limbs.

TO MAINTAIN NORMAL JOINT MOVEMENT

Gentle passive movements should be given through full range at least three times a day. Multi-joint muscle groups should also be placed on full (normal) stretch. Patients appreciate these simple procedures as they comment (later) on a feeling of tension 'cramp' building up in the limbs, and this sensation is relieved by passive movements.

The hip joint must be fully extended at least daily when the patient is in the lateral position. The shoulder joint range also should be maintained, care being taken that movements occur at the glenohumeral joint and not just the shoulder girdle. The temporomandibular joint should not be forgotten. Ankles, wrists, hands and feet also need accurate passive movement applied; as these areas will be the last to recover, serious loss of joint and muscle extensibility with functional loss and unacceptable cosmetic appearance could be due to ineffective passive movements.

SUPPORT OF JOINTS

Light splintage using Plastazote is required to support the peripheral joints in a comfortable and functional position during the time of flaccid paralysis. Splintage will prevent abnormal movements and untoward damage occurring to the joints. Bed cradles should be used to avoid pressure on the joints from bedclothes.

The general position of the patient in bed will alternate between supine and side-lying positions; sandbags and pillows must be used to stabilise these positions and if splints are used a careful check should be made to avoid damage to other parts of the body from pressure or rubbing by the splint.

PREVENTION OF PRESSURE SORES

The physiotherapist joins the nurse in having a responsibility towards frequent checking of the patient's pressure areas. The patient is normally on a two-hourly turning regime to prevent chest complications and pressure sores.

As the physiotherapist usually times her visit to coincide with these turns she can check the new and old pressure areas. Should a pressure sore develop the physiotherapist may be required to give ultraviolet radiation or ice-cube massage to the sore to enhance the healing process.

MAINTENANCE OF CIRCULATION

The passive movements described above will assist in increasing venous return. Additionally, gentle but firm effleurage massage may be given to the lower limbs, although by some method of communication the patient should indicate if this produces extreme discomfort.

PSYCHOLOGICAL SUPPORT

The patient with this syndrome has *unimpaired* cerebral functions, therefore his perception is unclouded. As treatment is commenced, the patient should be involved in his treatment; he must be told what is to be done to him, very simply and undramatically. Include the patient in conversation if another member of staff is present. Never discuss his prognosis or condition with a colleague within earshot.

The patient's relatives should be briefed on the points above and must be reassured that the prognosis, though slow, is excellent. In this way visiting time is a supportive experience rather than a frustrating and upsetting time for the patient.

B. RECOVERY STAGE

When the patient can maintain his own airway and ventilation and some motor recovery is occurring an assessment of the patient's problems is required to define treatment priorities.

The assessment should be detailed under the following headings:

(a) Respiratory system: rate, depth and pattern of breathing should be noted. Vital capacity and chest expansion recorded.

(b) Joint range on active and passive movement: also noted should be joints which still require splint support.

(c) Motor power of the recovered and recovering muscles.

(d) Sensation: all cutaneous modalities including vibration and two-point discrimination. Proprioception.

(e) Balance in various functional positions together with details of methods of support needed to stabilise a position.

(f) Independence of self-care.

(g) Motivation and general psychological approach to life in general.

Physiotherapy

As patients recover at different rates it is impossible to outline a course of treatment to suit them all. However, certain basic principles should be common to all treatment programmes and these are defined below. Some or all of the principles listed are applicable in a continuing scheme of treatment.

In general during recovery of nerve function, motor improvement occurs more rapidly than sensory and treatment plans should take this into account.

Principles of physiotherapy

MAINTENANCE OF THE AIRWAY AND VENTILATORY CAPACITY

Care of respiratory function is an aim for some time during the recovery phase. Patients can be taught breathing techniques and adequate coughing together with instruction on frequency of practice, i.e. three to four times a day, say, prior to each meal.

MAINTAIN AND IMPROVE JOINT RANGE

The more peripheral joints will require splintage and passive movements for some considerable time. The patient's relatives can be taught care and application of splints and effective and safe passive techniques of movement.

The patient will now be allowed out of bed and in sitting should sit squarely on the buttocks with shoulders level.

STRENGTHEN AND RE-EDUCATE NORMAL MUSCLE FUNCTION

The proximal muscles recover first and to facilitate voluntary contraction of muscle some of the following techniques may be useful:

neuromuscular facilitation techniques

afferent stimulation of skin

free active exercises

equilibrium and righting reactions

progressive resistance exercises

hydrotherapy

suspension

springs/pulleys

simple, progressing to more difficult, circuits for power and endurance.

The patient should have a short programme of 'core' exercises which he must practice for a certain number of repetitions (which are increased daily) and frequency throughout the day. Care should be taken not to tire the patient, as with many neurological patients treatment little and often is the preferred frequency.

RE-EDUCATION OF SENSORY AWARENESS

1. Cutaneous stimulation: the use of different materials, textures, shapes and weights will assist in perceptual re-education.
2. Proprioceptive: the use of equilibrium and balance responses.
3. Use of alternative systems, i.e. vision.

To protect the integrity of the skin the patient or his relatives must be made aware of the importance of skin care both of hygiene and protection (especially the hands) against thermal or mechanical damage.

RESTORATION OF NORMAL FUNCTION

Lower limbs: Various gait aids and orthoses may be required initially to restore a safe walking pattern appropriate to the weakness, inco-ordination and proprioceptive loss.

Upper limbs: Some splintage is often necessary and certain aids to daily living are required to enable the patient to be independent in his personal care, e.g. hygiene, toilet, feeding and dressing.

RESTORATION OF MAXIMAL INDEPENDENCE

In some cases recovery may not be complete and the patient's environment must be restructured to accommodate his disability and his needs.

MOTIVATION

Most patients in the acute stage will not believe that they will recover. It is sometimes, but not always, useful for the patient to see a person who has recovered well from the same illness. Patients often have labile emotions at this stage and need sympathetic understanding and encouragement. The physiotherapist must help the patient and often the relatives to gain the will to join in the treatment and so regain a productive and happy life again.

PORPHYRIC POLYNEUROPATHY

This polyneuropathy is inherited as an autosomal dominant trait which produces a liver defect which results in an excess of porphobilinogen and d-aminolaevulinic acid (precursor to porphyrin) being found in the urine. The onset of the neuropathy is rare before puberty and affects men more than women. The onset can be precipitated by drugs affecting porphyrin metabolism, e.g. barbiturates, oral contraceptives and methyldopa. The clinical presentation is a severe, rapid onset, showing symmetrical motor symptoms beginning in the feet and ascending, and later involving the upper limb and moving centrally. Sensory symptoms are less well marked. Associated with these symptoms are abdominal pains and tenderness with vomiting and constipation. The classical symptom is of urine which becomes port-wine coloured if left to stand.

Cerebral symptoms of confusion, delirium and occasionally convulsions are usually present. Other symptoms include, tachycardia, leucocytosis and fever.

The prognosis of this neuropathy is variable, a disturbance in cerebral function precedes the more severe rather than milder forms. The milder form often regressing and, at the other extreme, a severe form which may progress rapidly to be fatal within days.

Pathology

In most peripheral nerves, typical Wallerian degeneration of nervous tissue is found, along with some segmental demyelination of the remaining nerve fibres.

SUB-ACUTE SENSORIMOTOR POLYNEUROPATHY

Symmetrical polyneuropathies

The use of heavy metals in industrial processes has for many years been subject to legislative controls to minimise the health risk to persons who need to handle these substances. However, occasionally a polyneuropathy is seen which is the result of poisoning by a heavy metal.

One of the most common is lead poisoning; this is increasing in incidence, and is found more often in children whose home or school is close to a motorway or industrial process using lead. The radial nerve is most commonly affected, also the proximal muscles of the arm and shoulder girdle in the upper limb, and the common peroneal nerve in the leg. Arsenical poisoning is more rare and the symmetrical neuropathy is slow to develop. Associated symptoms are intestinal problems, anaemia, a typical brown skin, jaundice and excess of the metal in hair and urine samples.

In all poisoning by heavy metals the symptoms are slow to develop, taking many weeks to reach their peak, and last a variable time. The typical clinical presentation of polyneuropathy is present – pain, paraesthesia, muscle weakness, atrophy and tenderness.

PATHOLOGY

Initially, myelin changes are present but later Wallerian degeneration occurs especially of the larger fibres.

MEDICAL AND PHYSIOTHERAPY MANAGEMENT

Chelating agents are given to remove the heavy metal from the body.

Physiotherapy care depends upon the severity of the disease, and is symptomatic (see p. 447 *et seq.*).

ASYMMETRICAL POLYNEUROPATHIES

The two most commonly encountered in this group are due to polyarteritis nodosa and diabetes mellitus.

Polyarteritis nodosa

In this condition 75 per cent of cases show nutritional changes in nerve tissue due to thrombosis of the vasa nervorum. The clinical finding is either of a diffuse, more or less symmetrical, polyneuropathy or, more often, a mononeuropathy multiplex.

The onset is usually abrupt, pain and numbness being present, together with motor weakness, and sensory loss of cutaneous and proprioceptive modalities.

The medical care may include corticosteroid therapy and symptomatic physiotherapy, but the prognosis is poor in most cases.

Diabetic polyneuropathy

This is a common finding in diabetics over 50 years of age. It appears clinically in two forms, distal symmetrical polyneuropathy and mononeuropathy multiplex.

Distal symmetrical polyneuropathy: This is the most common type exhibited by patients and its clinical features include sphincter weakness, numbness and tingling in the lower limbs, which is worse at night; trophic changes are seen in the distal areas of skin (ulcers may be multiple) and joints. There is usually areflexia of the tendo calcaneus reflex and mild muscle weakness. The resultant weakness and sensory loss leads to an ataxic gait. The symptoms mimic tabes dorsalis, but evidence of raised blood sugar provides the differential diagnosis.

Mononeuropathy multiplex: This form affects older patients who have a mild or undiagnosed diabetic condition; it usually involves nerve trunks supplying the pelvic and upper leg muscles.

The presenting symptoms are frequently a complaint of pain in the lumbar or hip region which is more severe at night, the quality of the pain is described as sharp and lancinating. There is also muscle weakness and atrophy in the affected groups. The deep and superficial sensation is variable in involvement and may only be mildly affected. There are, however, usually sphincter disturbances and urinary incontinence may become a problem.

PATHOLOGY

Changes in the motor end-plate in the form of expansion of the terminal ending are thought to precede the segmental demyelination of peripheral nerves. It is thought that the metabolic activity of the Schwann cell is altered by the disease process, although a causal agent may be ischaemic changes secondary to the disease which occurs in the vasa nervorum.

MEDICAL MANAGEMENT

The treatment of both forms of diabetic neuropathy includes:
1. The stabilisation of the diabetic condition.
2. The inclusion of vitamin supplements to the diet.
3. The management of pain.

PHYSIOTHERAPY

The patient with diabetic neuropathy often presents with other problems, such as osteoarthritis of hip or knee, not associated with the diabetic condition.

The aims of treatment are to:
1. Restore the normal range of joint movement.
2. Increase muscle strength and/or endurance.
3. Improve balance in sitting and standing.
4. Teach the patient a safe walking pattern with aids if necessary.
5. Teach skin and joint care if there is sensory loss.
6. Advise on the fitting and use of orthoses.
7. Advise on alterations or best use of the patient's home environment.
8. Help the patient achieve a satisfactory lifestyle.

CHRONIC SENSORIMOTOR POLYNEUROPATHY

Acquired

A polyneuropathy associated with carcinoma is slow to develop, and may occur prior to the malignancy being found, usually in lung and/or stomach. The symptoms are typical of a neuropathy and a mixed sensori-motor type is more common.

Rheumatoid polyneuropathy develops in some patients, and is usually a painful neuropathy with minimal sensori-motor loss or reflexive changes. Little is known of the link with rheumatoid disease, but it may be due to arterial lesions.

In amyloid polyneuropathy it is usual for both sensory and motor systems to be affected. Amyloid tissue is found in many older individuals and can be considered as part of the ageing process. The symptoms are initially confined to the autonomic nervous system, and the symptoms affecting the somatic nervous system often mimic syringomyelia, though ECG abnormalities in amyloidosis differentiate between the two conditions.

Genetically determined

The main polyneuropathies in this are peroneal muscular atrophy (Charcot-Marie-Tooth disease) and hypertrophic interstitial neuritis.

Peroneal muscular atrophy (PMA): This is due to an autosomal dominant or recessive gene, the onset occurring in late childhood/ early adolescence. It is a neuropathy rather than a myopathy despite its name.

The initial manifestations are a symmetrical weakness and wasting of the peroneal muscles, and later the anterior tibial and intrinsic foot muscles are affected. The muscle weakness spreads to involve the proximal parts of the leg but halts its progress at the distal third of the thigh and the typical picture of 'inverted champagne bottles' is produced.

Involvement of the hands and forearm comes later. There is usually a stocking and glove distribution of sensory loss, and areflexia of the tendon reflexes of affected muscles. The course of the disease is slow and it is not severely disabling.

PATHOLOGY

Changes occur mainly in the cells of the ventral horn and its peripheral processes. The dorsal horn is involved to a lesser degree. Chronic demyelination occurs in nerve trunks, leading to degeneration of the large diameter motor and sensory nerve fibres, leaving connective tissue only. There is degeneration of the posterior columns of the spinal cord.

MEDICAL AND PHYSIOTHERAPY MANAGEMENT

There is no specific medical treatment. Physiotherapy is aimed at relieving symptoms and advice on splinting may also be required. If foot deformities occur, such as pes cavus or talipes equino-varus, orthopaedic surgery may be needed.

Hypertrophic interstitial neuritis: Also known as Déjèrine-Sottas syndrome and is due to an autosomal dominant gene. Symptoms appear in childhood or infancy and slowly progress. The first symptoms are seen distally in the legs, in a symmetrical weakness and wasting of muscle. Pain and paraesthesia are early features of the disease. The symptoms progress to the hands and move centrally to the trunk. There is areflexia of the involved muscles.

It is a slowly progressive disease which is more disabling than PMA and patients frequently deteriorate and have to lead a wheelchair life. Deformities of the feet and hands occur, such as talipes equinovarus, claw foot/hand and, in more severe forms of the disease, a kypho-scoliosis may be found.

PATHOLOGY

There is a proliferation of perineurium tissue in the nerve trunk and this leads to a palpable painless thickening of peripheral nerves. The Schwann cells undergo changes leading to a thinning of the myelin sheath and axonal degeneration.

MANAGEMENT

There is no medical treatment. Physiotherapy is symptomatic with advice on wheelchair living, home adaptation and aids to daily living.

REFERENCES

Gilliatt, R. W. (1966). Nerve conduction in human and experimental neuropathies. *Proceedings of the Royal Society of Medicine*, **59**, 989–93.
Levine, J., Shore, P. and Willard, M. (1981). Gaps and godrin: novel axonally transported proteins. *Trends in Neurosciences*, **4**, 11, 273–6.

BIBLIOGRAPHY

Chusid, J. G. (1982). *Correlative Neuroanatomy and Functional Neurology*, 18th edition. Lange Medical Publications, California.
Gray's Anatomy, 36th edition. (1980). Longman Group Limited, Edinburgh.
Lenman, J. A. R. and Ritchie, A. E. (1983). *Clinical Electromyography*, 3rd edition. Pitman Publishing, London.
Passmore, R. and Robson, J. S. (eds.) (1974). *A Companion to Medical Studies*, volume 3. Blackwell Scientific Publications Limited, Oxford.
Weiss, D. G. (ed.) (1982). *Axoplasm Transport*. Springer-Verlag, Berlin.

ACKNOWLEDGEMENT

The author thanks Mrs E. Bennett for kindly typing the manuscript.

Chapter 20

Motor Neurone Disease

by D.J. OLIVER BSc, MB, BS, MRCGP *and* B. O'GORMAN MCSP
with DAME CICELY SAUNDERS DBE, FRCP

INTRODUCTION

Motor neurone disease (amyotrophic lateral sclerosis, progressive muscular atrophy, progressive bulbar palsy) is characterised by the progressive degeneration of anterior horn cells of the spinal cord causing lower motor neurone lesions; the corticospinal tracts causing upper motor neurone lesions; and certain motor nuclei of the brainstem leading to bulbar palsy.

The aetiology of the disease is unknown but it is found worldwide. The prevalence is 5 per 100 000 and there is a male to female ratio of 1.5:1. It is a disease of later middle life, most patients being between 50 and 70 years, although younger patients may be affected.

The mean duration of survival is 3 years, although some patients live for much longer times. In one large study (Rosen, 1978) the overall five-year survival was 40 per cent. However, the survival depended on the age of the patient as the survival was 62 per cent for patients less than 50 years and only 31 per cent for patients over 50 years, and the presence of bulbar symptoms reduced the five-year survival to 14 per cent.

PRESENTATION

The clinical presentation tends to be insidious and depends on the part of the central nervous system affected. Thus there may be a mixture of spasticity, flaccidity and bulbar signs.

If the lower motor neurone degeneration is predominant the main features are of weakness, wasting and fasciculation of the muscles supplied by the cells undergoing degeneration. Most commonly it first affects the hands, with symptoms of clumsiness and weakness and evidence of wasting of the thenar eminences. The shoulders may also be affected early in the disease. If there is bulbar involvement the tongue becomes wasted and fasciculation is seen and speech and swallowing are affected because of muscle weakness.

Upper motor neurone degeneration also leads to weakness but the muscles become spastic. This may be seen in conjunction with muscle wasting. The bulbar effects are seen as spasticity of the tongue and other muscles with increased reflexes known as a 'pseudo-bulbar' palsy. This leads to dysarthria, dysphagia and impaired control of the emotional responses.

The sphincter control of bladder and bowels are rarely affected and there is no mental deterioration, although anxiety and depression understandably associated with a progressive, seriously disabling disease may be seen.

DIAGNOSIS

The clinical diagnosis is confirmed by electromyography (EMG) and muscle biopsy. On electromyography the motor neurone conduction velocity is normal until late in the disease, but the amplitude is reduced.

On needling, the mechanical stimulation of the needle causes fibrillation potentials, and spontaneous fibrillation and fasciculation potentials are seen when the needle is stationary in relaxed muscle, with greater duration and amplitude of the action potentials. When the muscle contracts there is a marked decrease in the number of spikes.

Other investigations may be necessary to exclude other conditions leading to muscle wasting and bulbar palsy.

SYMPTOMS AND THEIR CONTROL

The pattern of symptoms will depend on the motor neurones involved, and may be a mixture of lower and upper neurone lesions. (The percentages quoted relate to a series of 100 patients (Saunders et al, 1981).)

Weakness

Progressive muscle wasting leads to increasing weakness. Careful positioning and nursing is necessary, in conjunction with physiotherapy, to prevent deformity and maintain possible movement. Particular attention to the support of the neck is essential if the neck muscles are weak (Henke, 1968; Summers, 1981).

Pain

In the series of 100 patients, 40 per cent complained of pain, although sensory nerves are not affected. Pain may be:
1. *Musculoskeletal,* from joints with restricted movements and altered muscle tone. Non-steroidal anti-inflammatory drugs, such as indomethacin suppositories at night only, or twice daily, may be of help and intra-articular injection of steroids and local anaesthetic may be helpful especially if a shoulder is very painful.
2. *Muscle cramps* due to immobility, eased by diazepam or quinine bisulphate at night.
3. *Skin pressure,* as the patient is less able to move. An opiate analgesic may be the most effective treatment, and can be given orally regularly in the day or even only at night.

Dyspnoea

The dysfunction of respiratory muscles caused dyspnoea in 60 per cent of the patients in the series.

A calm and confident approach is necessary as dyspnoea may be exacerbated by anxiety. Careful positioning is important, especially of the neck when there is neck weakness, and morphine, or other opiates, may reduce the feelings of breathlessness. Antibiotics may be considered if there is evidence of infection in the early stages of the disease.

An episode of acute breathlessness may be effectively treated by an injection of an opiate (such as diamorphine 2.5–5mg) with hyoscine 0.4–0.6mg, to reduce secretions and act as a sedative and an amnesic.

Opiate analgesics, when used in carefully selected doses, effectively control distressing symptoms such as pain, dyspnoea, restlessness, cough and, on occasions, feelings of hunger. In the series quoted, 84 per cent of patients received opiates, usually as oral diamorphine or morphine in chloroform water or slow release morphine sulphate (MST Continus), individually titrated. Some 76 per cent of patients received injections of diamorphine, often with chlorpromazine and hyoscine, and this combination remained effective in controlling acute breathlessness or choking and the symptoms of terminal illness. Thus, opiates can be used safely, and the long duration of treatment, over five years in one patient, shows that by controlling distress opiates do not necessarily shorten life but may in fact lengthen life.

Dysphagia

Dysphagia was a troublesome symptom in 58 per cent of patients, and is due to involvement of the motor nuclei of the medulla. There is not only muscle weakness but muscle spasticity and inco-ordination. Careful slow feeding is essential and semi-solids may be taken more easily than liquids. Favourite beverages (from tea to whisky) can be given as ice cubes.

Dribbling salivation can be controlled by atropine tablets or syrup (0.3mg twice daily). Choking is a great fear of patients but is rarely a cause of death (only one patient dying in a choking attack in the series). By careful positioning of the patient and by controlling salivation, choking attacks may be prevented and in an attack, diamorphine (to reduce the cough reflex and lessen anxiety) and hyoscine (to dry up secretions, relax smooth muscles and as an amnesic) should be given as an injection.

In rare cases a nasogastric tube, gastrostomy, oesophagostomy or a cricopharyngeal myotomy may be considered.

Dysarthria

Difficulties with speech were experienced by 75 per cent of patients, and great patience and concentration are necessary to understand the patient. An ice cube may be rubbed around the lips to help stimulate the facial muscles and aid speech in certain patients. Assessment by a speech therapist will allow the most to be made of the remaining speech, and much time may be spent by the carers in aiding communication. Aids for writing and typing may be helpful and very sensitive switches allow a patient with minimal movement to summon help, thus aiding confidence.

Sore eyes

Eye blinking may be reduced as a result of muscle weakness and the eyes may then become sore and later secondarily infected.

Hypromellose eye drops are helpful to lubricate the eyes and antibiotic eye drops may be necessary if infection is present.

Muscle stiffness

The discomfort of stiffened spastic muscles may be reduced by careful positioning. Muscle relaxant drugs such as diazepam, baclofen or dantrolene sodium may be useful, but the side-effects encountered reduce their use. The dose of muscle relaxant may need to be carefully adjusted to allow a balance between spasticity and flaccidity, as relief of spasticity may seem to the patient to be merely increased weakness.

Constipation

Any patient who is inactive, debilitated and taking a diet low in roughage may become constipated. A regular aperient such as co-danthramer prevents this but local rectal measures such as suppositories, enemas or manual evacuation may become necessary in some patients.

Diarrhoea may merely be a reflection of constipation with overflow and this should be excluded. If there is intercurrent disease causing diarrhoea codeine phosphate may be considered.

Anxiety and depression

The mood of patients seriously disabled by a progressive illness will obviously vary. Moreover, communication and the expression of emotion may be restricted by dysarthria, and, due to reduced facial movements, the control of expression may be lost leading to an inability to control laughing or tears. These changes may frighten both the patient and his family and it is important to stress the physiological causes, and that there is no mental deterioration in the illness so that patients are not treated as if they have reduced intelligence.

Anxiety may be reduced by a calm and confident approach by the caring team and by careful control of the other symptoms. Diazepam may be helpful and in an emergency situation of severe panic an injection of diamorphine, chlorpromazine and hyoscine will promptly control the anxiety.

It is often very difficult to differentiate a depressive illness from the natural sadness of a severely disabled patient. Careful listening and explanation are important and tricyclic antidepressants such as imipramine may be helpful.

Insomnia

Insomnia may be due to insecurity, fear and pain. Great attention to detail and regular positioning will aid confidence and, therefore, sleep. Benzodiazepines (such as temazepam), tricyclic antidepressants (such as imipramine) and narcotic analgesics should also be considered.

Tiredness

Activity should be encouraged but not so as to over-extend the patient as tiredness is a common symptom. Corticosteroids may aid appetite and increase the feeling of well-being but, if used for long periods, weakness may be increased and other side-effects encountered.

Pressure sores

In the series only 16 per cent of patients had pressure sores. Prevention by regular turning and skin care is important and treatment of established sores is by the favourite methods of the nursing team.

Urinary problems

Weakness of the abdominal wall musculature may lead to urinary retention in some patients, but urinary incontinence is always due to other pathological processes such as benign prostatic hypertrophy in men. Urinary catheterisation may be necessary in some cases for the convenience of nursing care.

Family care

Listening and support of both patient and his family is an important part of the therapy. They should both be involved in the care and any plans that are made.

PHYSICAL MANAGEMENT

The physical management will depend on the physical symptoms present. The rate of progression, which may be gained from the history, must also be taken into account. Often severe bulbar signs make swallowing and speaking difficult. A speech therapist should be involved at an early stage. If speech is severely affected an alternative means of communication will be needed. Eventually the general weakness is so profound as to confine the patient to bed and/or wheelchair. Many may need admission to a unit caring for the terminally ill or chronic sick, but some families manage to the end in the patient's own home. The overall aim of physical management is the maintenance of independence, however small. The therapist can do much to help in this aspect; as a member of the team looking after such patients she will learn that lines of demarcation of particular skills soon become blurred, and much of her role will be teaching and advising not only the other team members but the patient and his family also.

Exercise

The weakened muscles cannot be strengthened but the joints acted upon by these muscles must be kept free from stiffness. Should the patient's joints become stiff then normal daily activities will become a problem and associated with pain.

Regular exercise is necessary in order to prevent stiffness occurring and to maximise muscle power for as long as possible. If a patient with motor neurone disease has a period of enforced immobility, for whatever reason, it is seldom possible to regain any independence and mobility that has been lost.

Whether patients are affected with an upper motor neurone lesion resulting in spasticity, or a lower motor neurone lesion resulting in flaccidity, or a combination of both, regular exercise is necessary. Spasticity in the legs can be used when standing the patient, and the use of muscle relaxant drugs needs to be carefully monitored as they can decrease this spasm and, therefore, its usefulness.

The patient should be encouraged to move his limbs actively throughout the day in as full a range as possible either using free active exercises or self-assisted active exercises. All limbs affected need to be exercised, together with the head, neck and chest. Once taught, a carer can help the patient perform the exercises, or, if necessary, carry them out for him. When the muscles are still able to contract but are weak, assisted active exercise should be used. Passive exercises are indicated when the limbs cannot be moved at all, by the patient.

Breathing exercises

An attempt should be made to maintain chest expansion by deep breathing and diaphragmatic breathing should be taught. Some patients are prone to cough if swallowing their saliva and liquids are difficult. They may also develop a cough as a result of a cold or 'flu or inhaled food and it is difficult for the cough to be effective. Occasionally gentle shaking of the thorax on expiration, or pressure on the abdomen from a hand, or bending the patient forward so as to increase the intra-abdominal pressure, may aid coughing and clearing of secretions.

Postural drainage is not used to drain secretions from the lungs as it is too traumatic for these patients. Similarly, aspiration of secretions is rarely used, or seldom justified. Accumulation of secretions in the base of the lungs causes relatively little discomfort. However, if the mucus is in the upper areas of the lungs or bronchi it can be extremely distressing for the patient since the main airways become obstructed. At this stage, the use of hyoscine helps to dry secretions while at the same time sedating the patient, so alleviating his distress. In a choking attack the patient *must not be left alone* and, if the attack does not subside naturally, diamorphine and hyoscine can be given (p. 460). The injection has the property of sedation and retrograde amnesia; when the patient awakes he often has little or no recollection of the severity of the attack.

The physiotherapist should tell the doctor of any deterioration in a patient's chest expansion as this is often a sign of the rate of deterioration of the disease. Morning headaches due to a high CO_2 level at night are often another sign of deterioration.

Mobility

It is important to maintain the patient's walking or standing for as long as possible. Careful thought must always be given before keeping a patient in bed. If a patient is unable to stand from sitting unaided, but can still walk, then a chair with an electric seat raise will overcome this problem.

To assist walking, human support can be used, sometimes a stick is sufficient, and occasionally a quadripod or Rollator walking aid is helpful. If the patient is only just able to walk, the surface on which walking is attempted should be considered - it is easier to walk on lino/cork than carpet.

When walking becomes an exercise rather than a means of

getting about, a wheelchair should be considered. A self-propelling model might be possible, if not, then an electric wheelchair will give the patient some independence of movement.

Comfort

It is extremely difficult making patients who are suffering from motor neurone disease comfortable, and the combined resources of the nursing and physiotherapy staff are needed to achieve even some degree of comfort. Families often develop the knack and should be consulted.

Positioning is of prime importance. As the patient's trunk, head and limbs become weaker and emaciated, due to a reduction in the bulk of his musculature, it becomes increasingly difficult to maintain the upright position. This applies whether the patient is standing, sitting in a wheelchair or sitting in bed. It is not sufficient to place more and more pillows behind and around the patient. At all times, whether he is in bed, reclining in a Parker Knoll chair or wheelchair, gravity and its action on the body must be considered. In the upright position the body is kept erect by a balance of muscle groups working in different ways against the constant force of gravity, and without them it would be impossible to maintain the upright position. If, as in motor neurone disease, any or part of these groups of muscles becomes affected, the ultimate maintenance of the body in the erect position becomes increasingly difficult.

If due to weakness of the anti-gravity muscles, especially the head, neck and trunk extensors, the patient begins to stoop forward, gravity will pull the body even further forward and the already weakened muscles will be unable to correct the stoop. As the abdominal muscles and the hip extensors and flexors are also likely to be affected, even maintaining the upright position in sitting can be difficult.

In order to minimise the effect of gravity on the body the patient should be inclined back from the vertical. By doing this, either in bed or in a reclining wheelchair or arm chair, the line of gravity will then pass in front of the head and neck through the thorax. A further advantage to the patient by being placed in the reclining position is the relief of pressure of the thorax on the abdomen. This allows the diaphragm to work more efficiently and so aid breathing, which is often restricted due to involvement of the intercostal muscles with resulting decrease in vital capacity.

Sheepskins can be used, with some form of cushion on which

to sit, such as Ripple, Roho, Spenco or a foam wedge, in conjunction with a small neck or support pillow.

Aids

Aids will be needed, but often they are not accepted readily by the patient who feels that they are a sign of deterioration. For patients with marked bulbar signs, hot plates and heated food dishes make slow eating more palatable. Anti-slip table mats and thickened handles on cutlery, pens and toothbrushes aid independence.

Call systems with a light touch can be operated by head, hands or feet enabling the patient to signal for help. Anti-slip floor mats and the Rototurn aid transfers and the use of Velcro and zips will help dressing. Various communication aids including POSSUM will need to be considered – often being used for environmental control as well as communication.

Collars and splints

Lively or rigid splints and lightweight orthoses can be of use but careful assessment of their value must be made constantly. As has been explained, positioning and inclination back from the vertical so that gravity acts differently on the body are the primary factors in supporting the head and trunk using small pillows attached to the chair or wheelchair. If this fails, collars are sometimes helpful in an attempt to support a drooping head. A collar cut from block foam to act as a wedge on which the chin can rest may help. In extreme cases a head-support which fits over the patient's head like a crash helmet, and being attached to the bed or wheelchair, may help.

Counselling

It is often during the course of treatment that the patient will seek more knowledge or advice about his condition from the therapist. As part of a team the therapist must feel able to seek help from whichever discipline is best suited to deal with the patient's needs. Should it be the physiotherapist, herself, who provides the relevant information she must ensure that not only does the family and patient receive it, but that the rest of the team knows also. While one must not give too much information at one session, or too soon, because it will not be able to be absorbed, it is important that the therapist gives as much support to the family to enable them to cope with this devastating disease. Not all patients with motor neurone disease will be found in special units, and the physiotherapist may not have the back-up of a committed team. In such instances she must apply the principles which are outlined not only in this chapter but throughout this book. She must remember that continual assessment is necessary, and that motor neurone disease follows no rules. What suits one patient may be useless for another. Individual gadgets, aids and appliances are essential.

Some units, where there are a number of motor neurone patients, may arrange regular meetings at which the team can meet the families and enable them to discuss problems together. The physiotherapist can have a useful part in such meetings.

The Motor Neurone Disease Association (see p. 638) publish a number of useful leaflets, both for the patient and the family as well as the professionals involved in care.

REFERENCES

Henke, E. (1968). Motor neurone disease - a patient's view. *British Medical Journal*, **4**, 765-6.

Rosen, A. D. (1978). Amyotrophic lateral sclerosis. *Archives of Neurology*, **35**, 638-42.

Saunders, C., Walsh, T. D. and Smith, M. (1981). Hospice care in motor neuron disease. In *Hospice: The Living Idea*, pp. 126-47, (eds. Saunders, C., Summers, D. H. and Teller, N.). Edward Arnold, London.

Summers, D. H. (1981). The caring team in motor neuron disease. In *Hospice: The Living Idea*, pp. 148-55, (eds. Saunders, C., Summers, D. H. and Teller, N.). Edward Arnold, London.

BIBLIOGRAPHY

Burford, K. and Pentland, B. (1985). Management of motor neurone disease: The physiotherapist's role. *Physiotherapy*, **71**, 9, 402-4.

Chapter 21

Peripheral Nerve Injuries – Clinical

by R. BIRCH FRCS *and* C. GRANT FRCS

STRUCTURE

The conducting elements of peripheral nerves, the axons, are cytoplasmic extensions from neurones in the dorsal root ganglia and in the ventral horn of the spinal cord. Most axons are small, less than 2 micrometres in diameter, they are unmyelinated and groups of them are enveloped by Schwann cells. These axons transmit crude touch, pain and temperature sensation and include the post-ganglionic fibres of the sympathetic nervous system responsible for sudo- and vasomotor control.

Other, larger, axons are surrounded by longitudinal columns of Schwann cells which form a lamellar envelope of myelin (Fig. 21/1). They range from 2–20 micrometres in diameter. These axons convey impulses to the skeletal muscles, and from the specialised sensory receptors in skin, muscle and joint. Feeling, that is the ability to localise stimuli and to recognise objects, depends upon their integrity. Large numbers of axons with their Schwann cells, fibroblasts and blood vessels, are grouped into bundles, or fascicles, surrounded by a cellular membrane, the perineurium. Numbers of these bundles, surrounded by connective tissue condensed on its surface as the epineurium, form the nerve trunk. There is considerable change in the orientation of individual axons in their passage down the limb from the spinal cord, particularly where spinal roots form the brachial and lumbo-sacral plexuses and also by division and reunion of bundles within the nerve trunk. This continuing change in the pattern of distribution of nerve axons has obvious implications for the surgeon as it is clearly impossible to co-apt individual axons or even individual bundles where more than 1 or 2 centimetres of the nerve trunk has been destroyed by injury.

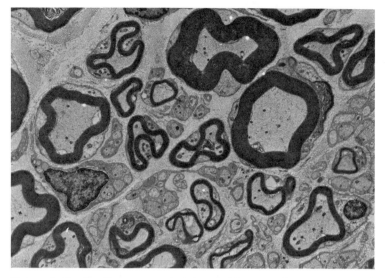

FIG. 21/1 Section from a rat sciatic nerve (electron microscope × 5500). Larger myelinated fibres are seen outnumbered by clusters of unmyelinated nerve fibres

Many nerve trunks pass down limbs within connective tissue sheaths together with major arteries and veins, and bleeding from these may be a serious cause of compression. Other nerve trunks may be vulnerable to injury where they lie in the superficial tissues. At the wrist, the median nerve is covered only by skin and by the palmaris longus tendon, which is not always present, and this is a common site of division. The radial nerve passes behind the humerus in a groove and is not well covered by muscle and may be damaged by external compression. The ulnar nerve, behind the elbow, and the common peroneal nerve at the knee, are superficial and they, too, may be injured. Where nerves pass deeply between muscle planes, and the median nerve in the proximal forearm is a good example of this, they are vulnerable to compression from swelling of the muscles after fracture or bleeding.

Degeneration and regeneration

When a nerve trunk is severed, the distal axons die. The axoplasm fragments and is absorbed by connective tissue cells. This phenomenon is called Wallerian degeneration. There is a great proliferation of Schwann cells and fibroblasts and a progressive deposition of collagen within the nerve trunks. In the proximal stump, there is a great increase in the number of Schwann cells and fibroblasts. The axons send out many filaments. If no attempt is made to repair the nerve, then a neuroma is formed, a mass of cells and regenerating axons. After successful nerve repair, regenerating axons pass across the suture line, but they rarely enter into the pre-existing Schwann tube. The architecture of the nerve never returns to normal after transection and repair; it is closest to normal after a well-executed primary repair. There is considerable disorganisation following delayed repair, particularly where there is tension at the suture line, or following repair by grafting.

CLASSIFICATION AND CAUSES

After recognition of an injury to a peripheral nerve trunk the most important question is 'What is its prognosis?' Can we hope for spontaneous recovery or is operation and repair necessary? Seddon's (1975) classification of nerve injuries remains a most useful guide. He described three categories of injury: first, *neurapraxia*, which is a temporary block to conduction, and interruption of physiological function of the nerve without disturbance of its anatomy and without Wallerian degeneration. In the other two types of nerve injury, *axonotmesis* and *neurotmesis*, there is Wallerian degeneration, although in axonotmesis there is not complete severance of the nerve trunk, whereas there is in neurotmesis.

Neurapraxia

Neurapraxia is a block to conduction mainly affecting the larger myelinated fibres. It is diagnosed by the sparing of some modalities of sensation, by the preservation of nerve conduction distally, and by the absence of fibrillation potentials in paralysed muscles. Full recovery can be anticipated if the cause is removed. Neurapraxia follows concussion or compression of a nerve; it is frequently seen in traction lesions, and in ischaemia, if this is not left untreated for too long. In most cases recovery is rapid and is complete, but in some cases recovery occurs over a prolonged period of time.

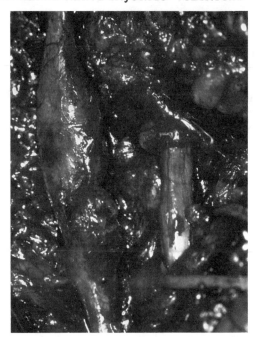

FIG. 21/2 A gunshot wound of the thigh, injury to the division of the sciatic nerve. The tibial nerve (right) went on to good recovery (axonotmesis); the common peroneal nerve (left) required grafting as there was gross internal disruption (neurotmesis)

Axonotmesis

This is the disruption of axons with Wallerian degeneration with preservation of the connective tissue scaffold of the nerves (Fig. 21/2). Spontaneous recovery can be expected if the cause is removed, but the recovery may be incomplete. A typical example is radial nerve palsy following closed fractures of the shaft of the humerus; over 70 per cent of these recover. Clinically, there is little difference between axonotmesis and neurotmesis – in both there is a loss of nerve conduction distally, denervation potentials in the affected muscles are evident.

Neurotmesis

This final stage of nerve injury, where the trunk is completely severed, is usually seen in open wounds; it may also follow violent traction force. Where there is a wound over the course of the nerve, neurotmesis is the most likely diagnosis. Axonotmesis is more likely in closed fractures or dislocations, in many traction lesions, and in ischaemic injuries. Overlap between these categories is common and exploration of the nerve may be necessary to assess the full extent of the injury.

There are many cases of injury to nerves. Transection of a nerve trunk, with little crushing, is a feature of 'clean' wounds from glass or knife. In wounds from missiles, or from compound fractures or dislocations, the nerve is more likely to rupture, with extensive injury along its course. On the whole, nerve trunks are very tough structures and will tolerate a considerable amount of stretching before giving way but they may be tethered by adjacent structures at certain sites and are particularly prone to rupture in closed traction lesions. The brachial plexus, the axillary and radial nerves, and the common peroneal nerve are especially vulnerable in such injuries.

A serious, more insidious nerve injury follows unrelieved ischaemia, either by severance of the major artery to the limb or by compression within a muscular compartment preventing capillary perfusion of nerve and of muscle (Fig. 21/3).

Those responsible for treating patients must be on the alert for nerve injuries in unconscious patients, particularly to the ulnar,

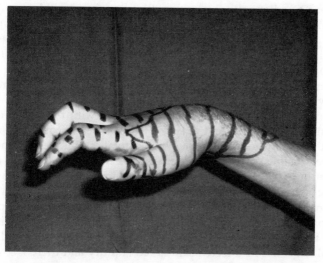

FIG. 21/3 The typical posture of a severe Volkmann's ischaemic contracture. *Note* the sensory loss involving radial, median and ulnar nerves

radial and common peroneal nerves, and be aware of the hazards of badly applied splints, plasters or dressings. Radial nerve palsy was not uncommon when axillary crutches were in vogue and the elbow crutch may lead to permanent disability from compression of the deep branch of the ulnar nerve in the hand, particularly in the elderly patient. Physical agents injure nerves too; the effects of burns or of frostbite are obvious but the pain and deterioration in neural function following radiotherapy may not occur for many years after completion of that treatment. All should remember that the elderly patient, patients whose general health is poor, or those suffering from diabetes mellitus or rheumatoid arthritis are particularly prone to injury from apparently minor compression force and that the resulting disability greatly hinders the treatment and rehabilitation of such patients.

DIAGNOSIS

Delay in diagnosis of nerve injuries is not unusual even where there is a wound over the course of the nerve. The history of injury, the object causing it and the degree of force are all important. A sliver of glass may have severed the median nerve at the wrist, even though the skin wound is less than a centimetre long. Associated injuries of tendon or vessels are important indications of potential nerve injury. Bleeding from axillary or ulnar arteries suggests division of adjacent nerves, and the typical posture of the hand after division of the flexor tendons points to median nerve injury. These observations are most helpful in young children, or the unconscious.

Sensory, sympathetic and motor functions of the nerve demand individual attention. Expensive instruments are not necessary; a nylon whisker, a paper clip and familiarity with the MRC atlas are sufficient. The extent of sensory loss is best recorded by asking the patient to map out the area of total loss of feeling, and of altered feeling, with the uninjured index finger. These areas may be outlined in black and red ink and the limb photographed providing a useful record. There is a considerable variation in the sensory territory of a mixed nerve (Figs. 21/4 and 21/5). A most important sign is loss of sympathetic function following division of a mixed nerve, particularly of the median, the ulnar and the tibial nerves. The affected skin is red and dry and there is loss of turgor of the skin pulp.

Examination of the muscles must be precise or misleading find-

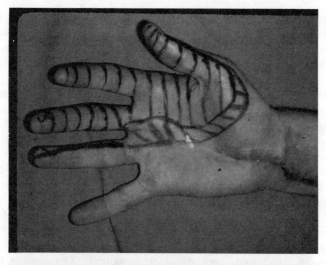

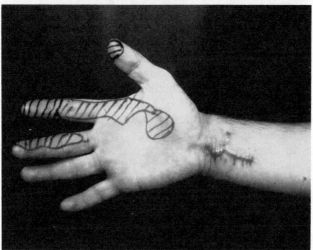

FIGS. 21/4 and 21/5 Sensory loss in patients with transection of the median nerve at the wrist

ings will be recorded. Muscles under examination must be seen and felt to contract. Difficulties may arise because of variation in motor supply; in the hand, the abductor pollicis brevis is almost always innervated by the median nerve and the first dorsal inter-osseous is almost always supplied by the ulnar nerve. Trick move-ments mislead: the apparent flexion of the fingers in a combined high median and ulnar palsy is by a tenodesis effect and is eliminated by grasping the wrist to prevent dorsiflexion. The abductor pollicis brevis will extend the distal joint of the thumb; the examiner must hold the proximal phalanx and keep the thumb in adduction to demonstrate activity in extensor pollicis longus.

The problem in later cases is not only to diagnose nerve injury but to determine the functional loss and judge how this can be improved. Knowledge of the patient's occupation and limb dominance is important. Physical signs in these late cases are clear: the clawing of an ulnar nerve lesion or trophic changes from unnoticed injury of anaesthetic skin are characteristic (Figs. 21/6 and 21/7). Muscle charts are useful and the sensory assessment developed by Wynn Parry and Salter (1976) are the best of their kind in their accuracy and their attention to the function of the limb. Important evidence of recovery following nerve injury is the detection of an advancing Tinel sign. The course of the nerve is gently percussed from distal to proximal. The patient may volunteer a sensation of pins and needles in the nerve territory and if this is found distal to the presumed level of nerve injury then recovery is proceeding. A strong and painful Tinel sign at the level of the nerve injury indicates neuroma formation; conversely, the stronger the advancing Tinel sign, and the weaker it is at the level of injury, the better the prognosis. It is said that nerves regenerate at the rate of 1mm a day or an inch a month, although the rate of advance is quicker in children and is also quicker in more proximal lesions. Electromyography may be helpful in detecting the first signs of muscle re-innervation and this investigation is especially useful following the course of recovery in predominantly motor nerves such as the musculocutaneous or radial nerves.

PROGNOSIS

Many factors determine the final outcome after repair of divided nerve trunks. Some of the most important are beyond the control of those treating the patient and they may be termed inevitable. Age is particularly important; children fare much better than adults, and young children particularly so. The cause of the injury is most important and the outlook for recovery following repair of a cleanly divided nerve is very much better than that in a nerve widely destroyed by missile, burn or sepsis. Unmixed nerves, such as the musculocutaneous or digital, usually recover better

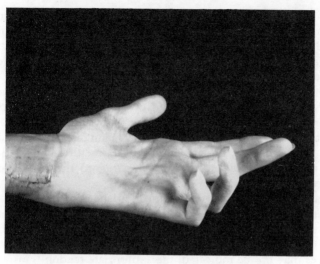

FIG. 21/6 The posture of an ulnar nerve lesion

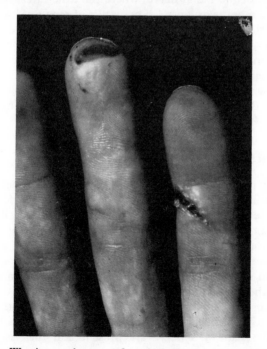

FIG. 21/7 Wasting and sores of anaesthetic skin after median nerve section

than mixed nerves such as median or ulnar. The level of injury is important too; repair of a divided ulnar nerve in the axilla is rarely followed by good function in the small muscles of the hand. Repair of a high lesion of the sciatic nerve is very rarely followed by functional sensation and power in the leg and foot.

Other factors are within the control of those treating the patient and perhaps the most important of those is the delay between injury and repair. The less of this the better and early and correct treatment of associated injuries, the maintenance of a supple, well-perfused limb, the prevention of contractures and fixed flexion deformities are essential preliminaries to the restoration of function.

Patients must be warned about the danger of insensible skin, otherwise they are at risk from burns or other trophic changes and indeed every effort must be made to encourage the continuing use of the impaired part. In some patients operative repair of nerves may not be indicated; the appropriate tendon transfer will restore function more surely and more quickly than repair of a high lesion of the radial nerve, where the time interval is of the order of 18 months or longer. The results of repair of high lesions of the sciatic nerve are generally poor and often attended by pain, and in many patients the better course of treatment is to maintain a supple limb perhaps with the provision of a simple foot-drop splint. Disability may be enhanced by the dependence of patients upon those treating them, and a protracted series of operations and a long drawn-out course of physiotherapy may do more harm than good.

FACTORS BEFORE REPAIR

The hand must feel and grasp and the foot must bear weight without pain. Their limbs must provide stability and afford movement and control. The prognosis for function of the limb after repair of a divided trunk nerve is determined by the overall condition of that limb. It must be supple, the skin must be robust, the perfusion to the limb must be adequate, the skeleton must be stable, and sepsis must be eliminated. To carry out an extensive repair of the median nerve in an arm which is withered, scarred, stiff, and painful is a waste of time. Those attending the patient must see to it that the conditions for proper function following successful repair of a nerve are present and the essential requirements are prevention of stiffness of joints, prevention of deformity, and the prevention of injury to insensitive skin.

The term 'multidisciplinary team' is fashionable, and it is as well to examine their tasks. The most fundamental aspect of general care for the patient and of his integument falls to nurses; it is the task of the physiotherapist to maintain mobility of joints and to enhance the strength of recovering muscles not paralysed. The occupational therapist will assist the patient in the tasks of normal life by the proper selection, manufacture, and application of splints (usually in co-operation with the physiotherapist). Operations may be required to achieve a good field for repair of a nerve; where there is extensive scarring and loss of normal skin, a flap may be necessary; where there is rigid fixed deformity of joints, release at operation may be necessary; and where there is impairment of blood supply, repair of vessels and release of encircling fascia may be indicated. Clawson and Seddon (1960a and b) showed that most patients with high sciatic nerve lesions lived virtually normal lives if fixed deformity of knee, ankle and foot were prevented. However, once equinus deformity develops, pressure sores in the insensitive weight-bearing areas of the skin are inevitable and such changes nullify the potential gain from the most tedious repair of nerves.

Techniques of repair

There is no doubt that in clean wounds, with severance of nerve, vessel, muscle or tendon, the best outcome follows meticulous primary repair of all injured structures. Many injuries are unsuitable for this, particularly those following missile wounds where there is much contamination from severe compound injuries. In cases of sepsis, skin loss, or where there is uncertainty about the extent of damage to the nerve trunk, then delayed repair is the best mode having secured stability of the skeleton and healthy skin cover. Many delayed nerve repairs can be done by direct suture, with successful improvement in function if the postoperative care, particularly splinting, is properly conducted. It is possible to mobilise nerves and it is possible to gain length in some nerves by re-routing them. For example, transposition of the ulnar nerve from the cubital tunnel to the front of the elbow joint, lying deep to the flexor origin, gains 2–3cm. Many other cases require grafting, especially when the initial injury was of traction, leading to rupture, and wide retraction of the nerve stumps, or where there has been extensive destruction of nerve tissue by burn, sepsis or tissue loss. The disadvantage of nerve grafting is that it requires an operation upon a normal limb;

another disadvantage is that the graft must obtain its blood supply from the bed into which it is laid. A good result is rare where that bed is very scarred, although the vascularised ulnar nerve graft has shown to be of some value in the treatment of patients with severe lesions of the brachial plexus.

Postoperative care is of the utmost importance following any mode of nerve repair. The nerve suture should be protected for a sufficient period of time, but there must be only the minimum necessary restriction of function of the limb as a whole. When primary repair of nerves, tendons and vessels have been carried out at the wrist, then immobilisation of the wrist in flexion is necessary for 3 weeks, with restriction but not full immobilisation of the digits. It is wise to prevent full dorsiflexion of the wrist for a further 3 weeks. During this time, movements of the shoulder, the elbow and some degree of movement of the digits should be encouraged. The limb should be kept in elevation to reduce swelling and gentle passive and active flexion of the fingers and thumb reduces adhesion formation. If a delayed direct suture is done, then immobilisation needs to be prolonged. Following such a repair of the sciatic nerve in the thigh, protection of the suture line by flexion of the knee and prevention of flexion of the hip is necessary for a period of 3 months during which the limb is gradually set free. A hinged cast is useful by allowing motion within a restricted range at knee or at elbow (Fig. 21/8). Following a nerve graft the limb should be immobilised as for a primary repair.

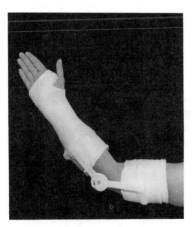 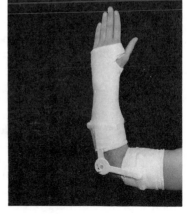

FIG. 21/8 The hinged cast allows flexion of the elbow, while protecting the median nerve repair from tension during extension

PAIN

Some degree of pain is almost always present after nerve injury. In most cases this diminishes with regeneration and return of function. The pain becomes an overwhelming disability for some patients. Several distinct patterns of painful conditions can be defined:

Causalgia

Causalgia is pain of great severity and intensity and it usually follows partial injury of major trunk nerves containing a large number of sympathetic fibres. The patient with causalgia will not tolerate examination of the affected limb and is sensitive to noise, wind, temperature change, or emotional stress. The affected limb is held immobile and is often protected by coverage. Some patients find that a dressing soaked in water reduces the pain.

Causalgia follows injuries of the brachial plexus, the median and ulnar nerves, and the sciatic and tibial nerves. The injury is often a partial one from missile injury, and in some cases there is a foreign body, either a particle of metal or a suture, acting as an irritant.

This syndrome is uncommon, but quite characteristic. The correct treatment is, first, early recognition and then removal of any retained foreign body adjacent to the nerve. In the great majority of cases, sympathectomy is effective in alleviating pain, but it is wise to see the effect of a local anaesthetic block on the cervical sympathetic or lumbar sympathetic chain before proceeding to operation.

Neuroma pain

An exquisitely painful and tender neuroma is a common complication of injury to a cutaneous nerve, particularly the digital nerves in the hand. This condition is very difficult to treat. When an amputation of an injured digit or limb is necessary, then it is wise to bury sectioned nerve stumps in healthy tissues away from pressure-bearing areas. If a sensory nerve is seen to be divided in a wound, and the superficial radial nerve is a particularly common example of this, then it is wise to repair this. Operations are of value in only a minority of established cases, but where a digital neuroma is adherent to skin, then this is certainly worthwhile resecting. In the majority of cases, however, it is important to encourage the patient to use the hand, and to suppress pain by such means as protection of the tender stump, by a trial of the transcutaneous nerve stimulator, or by serial guanethidine blockade which is particularly useful when pain and hypersensitivity extend beyond the territory of the injured nerve (Wynn Parry and Withrington, 1984).

Sudeck's atrophy

This is a common condition, and usually follows fractures or crushing injuries of the wrist and hand. The patient complains of intense burning pain from the outset and in the first few weeks the hand is swollen and red; it may be dry or there may be excessive sweating. If no action is taken, then the patient will not use the hand and ultimately it becomes a stiff, painful and useless appendage. Too many of these patients are labelled as neurotics and it is of the utmost importance to recognise the condition early and to institute vigorous treatment. Tight plasters or tight dressings encircling the limb and causing swelling are an important cause of this distressing syndrome and they should not be used. Sudeck's atrophy is rare following Colles' fractures where the wrist is immobilised in a position of function, where an incomplete plaster with an inelastic bandage is used, and where early vigorous exercises of the digits are encouraged. These injuries are common and if the principles of immobilisation in a position of function with early hand exercises, are followed then the likelihood of this syndrome occurring is reduced.

In more serious fractures or dislocations of the wrist where there is intense swelling, an early decompression of the median nerve in the carpal tunnel is often dramatically effective. Treatment in the established case is extremely difficult; the patient is demoralised and secondary changes of stiffness and disuse in the hand are severe. Manipulation under anaesthesia usually make things worse, and a combination of adequate analgesia and active use of the hand for a prolonged period of time is needed.

The pain from Sudeck's atrophy is perhaps the most common of all pain states described here and, in the author's view, it is nearly always preventable. It is worth emphasising, and repeating, the importance of immobilising the wrist and hand in a position of function, of avoiding swelling and encouraging use of the hand.

Pain in pre-ganglionic injuries of the brachial plexus

Injuries of the brachial plexus are becoming more common. The patients are usually young men, the cause is almost invariably a motor cycle accident, and the dominant limb is usually affected. A large number of these patients suffer irreparable lesions of the spinal nerves forming the brachial plexus with avulsion of those nerves directly from the spinal cord. Some degree of pain is almost invariable after such an injury and where the two lower roots of the brachial plexus have been so injured; that is, the 8th cervical and the 1st thoracic roots, then intense burning pain felt in the anaesthetic hand is so typical as to be diagnostic. Wynn Parry (1981) has made a most extensive study of this and of other pain states. Certain conclusions can be drawn; many patients with avulsion pain note that they are able to cope with it, or that it is less intense, when their minds are occupied. The lesson of this is obvious; the sooner the patient returns to some sort of work the better. To sign these men off as 'sick', to offer them occasional attendance to hospital, or to physiotherapy departments is to enhance their disability and does nothing to diminish it. Frampton (1982) and Wynn Parry have shown how effective the transcutaneous nerve stimulator may be and this technique can be dramatically successful. In a small group of patients, where pain does not respond to conservative measures and where it becomes a problem of such intensity that it alters personality and renders them suicidal, then direct operations on the spinal cord must be considered, hazardous though these are.

RECONSTRUCTION

Transfer of tendons, of muscles, or joint fusions may be indicated to improve function when there has been failure of recovery after nerve repair, where a nerve lesion is irreparable, or where the duration of paralysis is so long that nerve repair cannot be expected to restore useful motor power. As a general rule, the surgeon cannot hope for significant motor function if the delay from injury to repair is around 18 months and in many cases the time interval is very much less. Worthwhile recovery into the intrinsic muscles of the hand is rare, even after primary repair of the ulnar nerve in the axilla; a patient with severe injury to the radial or common peroneal nerves, where the nature of the wound determines delayed repair, gains more certain benefit, within a much shorter period of time, after tendon transfer than following nerve grafting. In ruptures of the suprascapular nerve, from traction lesion, return of powerful and co-ordinated control of the gleno-humeral joint is so rare that fusion of that joint may be the better treatment for certain patients.

If a muscle or a tendon (motor) is to be transferred then it must be of full power and it must be dispensable. Very few patients would be prepared to pay the price of loss of elbow extension to gain elbow flexion from a triceps to biceps transfer. Joints must be mobile, before any transfer. The transferred motor must glide and if the skin and subcutaneous tissues are densely scarred then adhesions will form and the outcome will be disappointing.

Operations to restore opposition of the thumb are of little value if the thumb cannot feel, and are positively useless if the hand is painful. Skilful physiotherapy both before and after such operations is of immense value. The limb must be supple and the motor to be transferred of normal, or near normal power. Reconstructive procedures are the last stage of treatment of a patient and are undertaken once the skeleton is stable; the skin in good condition; when pain has been overcome; and if the problem is of paralysis in the hand, when some degree of sensation has returned.

The shoulder

Brachial plexus injuries are the commonest cause of impairment of shoulder control, either from birth injury afflicting the upper trunk or from closed traction lesions. Internal rotation contracture is the rule in patients who have not maintained mobility. In children this is best overcome by release of subscapularis and the anterior capsule of the shoulder. In adults a generous external rotation osteotomy of the humerus is a more logical choice. Transfer of latissimus dorsi to the outer aspect of the humerus enhances stability of the glenohumeral joint and may give some degree of external rotation (Figs. 21/9, 21/10, 21/11). Restoration of co-ordinated abduction of the shoulder is extremely difficult following these injuries and patients who need a stable and powerful shoulder are best advised to undergo glenohumeral fusion, if the scapula is mobile and if the thoraco-scapular muscles are powerful.

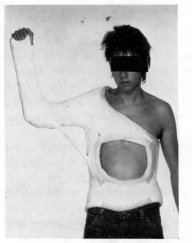 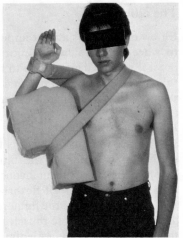

FIG. 21/9 Immobilisation of this type is required for 6 weeks following transfer of latissimus dorsi

FIG. 21/10 Further protection of the repair is needed for 3-4 weeks

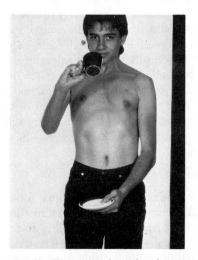

FIG. 21/11 The patient in Figures 21/9 and 21/10 now able to bring his hand to his mouth

The elbow

Elbow extension is a most important function in patients confined to wheelchairs following injuries to the spinal cord. Latissimus dorsi is an excellent muscle to regain powerful elbow extension if this is available, but in patients with tetraplegia at the level of C6, this muscle will be paralysed and the deltoid muscle can be used instead following the technique outlined by Lamb (Moberg and Lamb, 1980).

A more common problem is loss of elbow flexion from injuries to the upper trunk of the brachial plexus or from irreparable lesion of the musculocutaneous nerve. The Steindler procedure, that is, advancement of flexor and extensor origin to the medial and lateral aspects of the humerus, is an effective and fairly simple procedure where those muscles are of full power. A useful test is to see whether these patients can maintain the elbow in flexion by forming a powerful fist with gravity eliminated. However, where the cause is irreparable injury to the upper trunk of the brachial plexus, then there is likely to be paralysis of brachio-radialis, pronator teres and weakness of other extensor and flexor muscles. Alternatively, the pectoralis major or latissimus dorsi muscles may be transferred in extensive operations; the necessary incisions are long, and scarring following transfer of pectoralis major is ugly. However, both muscles are capable of restoring powerful elbow flexion through a considerable range. A particular problem is co-contraction following imperfect regeneration across grafts, or lesions in continuity, of the brachial plexus. Simultaneous contraction of triceps with biceps, or of triceps with latissimus dorsi is common. Biofeedback may be useful in these cases; alternatively transfer of triceps to biceps may be necessary.

Wrist drop

Loss of extension of wrist and of digits following irreparable lesion of the radial nerve or from injury to the middle trunk of the brachial plexus is particularly disabling and successful tendon transfer can dramatically alter a patient's function. If the cause is injury to the radial nerve then pronator teres is available to transfer to the extensor carpi radialis brevis; flexor carpi ulnaris is available for transfer to the extensor digitorum communis and extensor pollicis longus, and palmaris longus is usually available to improve abduction of the thumb by transfer to abductor pollicis longus. This particular tendon transfer is reliable and most

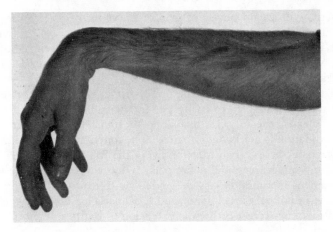

FIG. 21/12 The posture of a radial nerve palsy

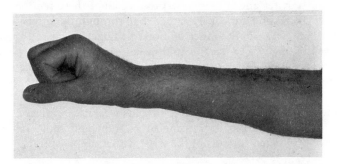

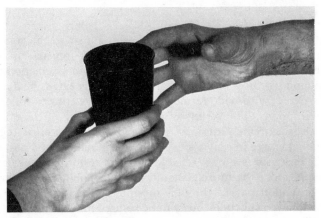

FIGS. 21/13 and 21/14 Extension and flexion after transfer of flexor carpi ulnaris, palmaris longus and pronator teres patients will regain power of grip of the order of 70 per cent of the unaffected forearm and hand. It is wise to support the wrist with a simple splint after the postoperative cast has been removed at 3 weeks to prevent stretching of the transferred muscle. Re-education is usually simple (Figs. 21/12, 21/13, 21/14).

If the cause is injury to the upper trunk, then pronator teres will not be available. In many patients with injuries of the brachial plexus, the muscles available for transfer are weaker and co-ordination is markedly impaired. The functional outcome from the transfer is less than that following the full flexor to extensor tendon transfer for radial nerve palsy. However, considerable improvement in function can be gained by transfer of flexor carpi ulnaris and of palmaris longus, and if palmaris longus is powerful, then this may give worthwhile extension of digits and thumb on its own.

In some cases only flexor digitorum superficialis (FDS) is available for transfer and it seems best to take all of these tendons and to pass them subcutaneously rather than through the interosseous membrane. FDS to the index and middle fingers is passed around the radius and FDS to the middle and ring fingers, is passed around the ulna. Obviously this operation can only be done when flexor digitorum profundus is active and strong. This operation may be indicated when patients have suffered irreparable injury to the C5, 6, 7 nerves and where there is weakness of flexor carpi ulnaris. It is a difficult transfer to re-train and most patients require prolonged support of the wrist with a simple splint.

The leg

Loss of dorsiflexion at the ankle following injury to the common peroneal or sciatic nerves is common. Many injuries to those nerves are caused by missile injuries or occur in association with compound fractures or dislocations and there is extensive damage to the nerve, with wide retraction of the nerve stumps following traction lesions. The results of repair by grafting of these nerve injuries is extremely disappointing and tibialis anterior regains functional power in only a small minority. Transfer of a powerful tibialis posterior is a more reliable means of restoring some degree of dorsiflexion; the muscle should be well mobilised proximally and its tendon passed through the interosseous membrane and then burrowed subcutaneously to be sutured into the tarsal bones. As with other operations where the transferred muscle is passed across an interosseous membrane, mobilisation should be sufficient to allow the muscle belly to pass through the membrane to reduce adhesions. The leg and foot should be immobilised for 6 weeks and then the transfer protected by a foot-drop splint for between 3 and 6 weeks.

Fundamental principles apart, there can be no set routine for an individual patient with a complex injury of nerves. The problems are different with each individual and so is their solution. Although the treatment of patients with complex neurovascular injuries is very demanding, the results in those who are well motivated can be extremely rewarding. The efforts of doctor, nurse, physiotherapist and occupational therapist should be used in an economic and co-ordinated manner, but if the patient is allowed to fall into the trap of dependence and 'disability' then those efforts will be in vain.

REFERENCES

Clawson, D. K. and Seddon, H. J. (1960a). The results of repair of a sciatic nerve. *Journal of Bone and Joint Surgery*, **42B**, 205.

Clawson, D. K. and Seddon, H. J. (1960b). The late consequences of sciatic nerve injury. *Journal of Bone and Joint Surgery*, **42B**, 213.

Frampton, V. M. (1982). Pain control with the aid of transcutaneous nerve stimulation. *Physiotherapy*, **68**, 77–81.

Moberg, E. and Lamb, D. (1980). *The Hand*, **12**, 2, 209–13.

Seddon, H. J. (1975). *Surgical Disorders of the Peripheral Nerves*, pp. 32–3, 2nd edition. Churchill Livingstone, Edinburgh.

Wynn Parry, C. B. (1981). *Rehabilitation of the Hand*, pp. 126–44, 4th edition. Butterworths, London.

Wynn Parry, C. B. and Salter, M. (1976). Sensory re-education after median nerve lesions. *Hand*, **8**, 250.

Wynn Parry, C. B. and Withrington, R. (1984). Painful disorders of peripheral nerves. *Postgraduate Medical Journal*, **60**, 869–75.

BIBLIOGRAPHY

Birch, R. (1984). Traction lesions of the brachial plexus. *British Journal of Hospital Medicine*, **9**, 140–3.

Bonney, G. (1983). Peripheral nerve lesions. In *Postgraduate Textbook of Orthopaedics*, pp. 719–30, (ed. Harris, N. H.). John Wright and Sons, Bristol.

Brooks, D. (1984). Tendon transfer for paralysis and Volkmann's contracture. In *Rob and Smith's Operative Surgery – The Hand*, 4th edition, (eds. Birch, R. and Brooks, D.). Butterworths, London.

Seddon, H. J. (1975). *Surgical Disorders of the Peripheral Nerves*, 2nd edition. Churchill Livingstone, Edinburgh.

Chapter 22

Peripheral Nerve Injuries – Physiotherapy

by M. I. SALTER MBE, MCSP

Physiotherapists play an essential role in the management of peripheral nerve lesions. Regular assessment and advice, support and treatment should be given both initially and at suitable intervals during recovery until a satisfactory result has been effected. This may take many months and in some cases a year or more to achieve.

The treatment involves a team led by the surgeon or rehabilitation specialist and backed by the skill of physiotherapists and occupational therapists. In a peripheral nerve injury the loss of movement and sensation, particularly in the hand and upper limb, may have a profound effect on the patient's personality and outlook and this must be considered when planning treatment. Associated injuries, such as fractures and the division of tendons and arteries, may complicate recovery.

A programme of physiotherapy and occupational therapy for all or half a day for a short period is more effective and economical than less intensive treatment over a longer period. The surgeon and therapists should see the patient together to plan and to integrate treatment. The patient must be given a full explanation of the reasons for treatment so that he can co-operate and work hard both in the department and at home. The social worker should also be involved at an early stage as support may be needed for the patient and his family. Prospects of future employment should be considered and discussed with the resettlement officer if necessary. Unless the patient understands the rationale, is well motivated and is confident, the most skilled therapy is unlikely to be successful.

EFFECTS OF PERIPHERAL NERVE INJURIES

The motor, sensory and autonomic effects should be noted on assessment and treated as necessary with regular reappraisal throughout recovery.

Motor

Interruption of motor nerve conduction produces a lower motor neurone lesion with loss of reflexes, tone, and any active contraction of the muscles. This is followed by atrophy of both muscle and soft tissue. Patients should be made aware that even with intensive treatment this wasting will occur. Deformities are caused by the unopposed action of the muscles, for example the claw hand of the ulnar nerve lesion. The strong pull of the long flexors and extensors of the fingers is unopposed when the intrinsic muscles are paralysed. Clawing therefore results.

Contractures may occur due to the lack of movement, and adhesions may form between tendons and sheaths and also in the joints. Muscles will become fibrosed after a long period of denervation. These complications may be reduced to the minimum by maintaining good circulation together with a full range of passive movement and as much activity as possible.

Sensory

The sensory effects are loss of cutaneous and proprioceptive sensations. The initial size of the anaesthetic area will decrease around its periphery due to adjacent sensory nerves taking over. Loss of temperature sensation means that patients are liable to become burned, and repeated warnings should be given of the dangers of cigarettes, kettles, radiators and hot plates. Fingers slip very easily on to hot objects and even hot soup has been known to cause a burn. Similarly the intense cold from refrigerators and freezers can cause blistering of the skin.

Autonomic

Damage to sympathetic nerves causes a loss of sweating and the skin tends to become dry and scaly, and later thin and shiny. The nails become brittle, and the soft tissues atrophy. The skin is more liable to pressure sores and if trophic lesions occur they are slow to heal. To ensure good healing and re-innervation an adequate circulation must be maintained. As the limb takes on the temperature of its surroundings a warm glove or sock must always be worn during the cold weather.

The area of autonomic change will be found identical to that of the sensory distribution and observation of these changes is therefore usually indicative of sensory change also. Conversely if no autonomic change is evident this may well indicate that some sensation at least should be present.

PHYSIOTHERAPY ASSESSMENT

Subjective and objective data will allow the problems to be identified and an analysis made. A suitable treatment programme can then be planned for each patient. Reappraisals must be regular, and finally a discharge summary recorded.

History

A description of the accident may give helpful information for understanding the mechanics of the injury, especially in a closed injury or a plexus lesion.

The patient is asked how he views his present problems. He may feel that his greatest difficulty, due to both motor and sensory loss, is in performing activities connected with either daily living, employment or leisure. In some patients pain can be severe following nerve damage and yet be non-existent in others. Some may suffer a degree of pain and yet not find it intolerable. Social and economic problems will also add an enormous mental stress in addition to the physical injury, and tend to exacerbate pain if already present.

When pain is a problem the patient is asked to describe it; whether it is burning or shooting, whether it is present continuously, what irritates and what relieves it. He is asked to record the severity on a 10 centimetre self-assessment chart (Fig. 22/1). The 0 symbolises no pain and 10 the worst pain imaginable. It is essential to record this information both before and after treatment in order to assess its effect. The position or distribution of pain can also be recorded on a rubber stamped chart of the limb (Fig. 22/2).

Hyperpathia, an extremely painful response to touch, may be experienced by a small proportion of patients and should also be recorded on the chart.

Name............................   Date..........

.O   10

X = Before treatment   (X) = After treatment

FIG. 22/1 A 10cm line used for recording the patient's own assessment of his pain before and after treatment

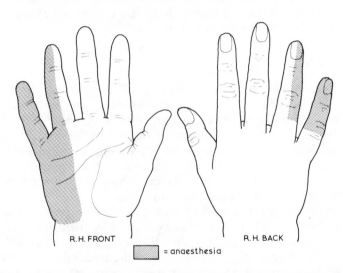

R.H. FRONT   R.H. BACK

[   ] = anaesthesia

FIG. 22/2 An anaesthesia chart showing the area of anaesthesia in a lesion of the ulnar nerve at the level of the wrist

Observation

The posture of the involved limb and also the general demeanour of the patient should be noted. Some patients will make an attempt to use the hand: others may be excessively protective. Most will be obviously worried about the future.

Examination early after injury may show only loss of movement, loss of sensation and temperature changes. Soon the autonomic changes will become evident by the dry scaly skin and alteration of colour. Following this the skin becomes papery thin and shiny. If dipped in warm water the affected part will stay a dense purple-pink colour for several minutes. The patient will complain of his hand remaining cold during cold weather.

Diminished tone accompanied by muscle wasting will result in the gradual appearance of deformities. Wasting does *not* occur in a neurapraxia. If movement of the joints is not maintained contractures will develop. The classical deformities which accompany the different nerve lesions may be altered by the presence of adhesions between skin and tendon. This can be demonstrated by moving the distal joints both actively and passively through full range while watching the scar for signs of adherence.

Movement

Note should be made initially of any active movement of the limb and be followed by a more detailed assessment. This includes the active and passive range of joints proximal to the injury, and the passive range and any muscle activity distal to the lesion.

The range of any stiff joint is measured using a goniometer and both flexion and extension must be recorded. If active movement of the fingers is present the distance of finger tips towards and away from the palm is measured with a ruler.

Muscle power is recorded on the 0–5 Medical Research Council Scale (see p. 127). It is easy to be misled by trick movements (Wynn Parry, 1981) such as the effect of gravity, the rebound following antagonistic contraction, and the tenodesis effect produced by strong contraction of the antagonists at either a more proximal or a more distal joint. For example, in a radial nerve palsy the patient may be observed attempting to extend his wrist by strongly flexing his fingers. The tautening effect that this has on the extensors may be sufficient to extend his wrist passively.

Secondary action of muscles becomes evident when the prime movers are paralysed. Knowledge of origins and insertions of muscles, the diagonals in which they lie and the relationship to the planes of the joints must therefore be detailed. Anomalies of nerve supply should be considered and checked by electrical stimulation of the nerve supplying the neighbouring normal muscles.

Power of the hand should also be recorded using a dynamometer. Gross weakness of the proximal muscles due to nerve damage will inevitably lead to weakness of the hand, and vice versa.

Palpation

The use of the *dorsal* surface of the physiotherapist's fingers for palpation will identify skin changes, lack of response to alteration of temperature and loss of sweating. Several months after the lesion there may be some response to change of temperature and some return of sweating which will indicate that nerve regeneration is taking place.

Thumb and finger webs should be palpated and measured as they are liable to contract. Pulp of the finger tips will be noted to have atrophied.

Palpation around any scarring may identify areas of induration which will need softening. If a crush injury caused the nerve lesions the soft tissues are liable to have become fibrosed following oedema. The normal supple elasticity of the tissues will be lost and the whole hand will feel stiff and woody on manipulation.

Painful areas and possible neuromata should be noted. Tinel's sign is a useful means of testing nerve regeneration (Henderson, 1948). Tapping from distally to proximally over the recovering nerve sets up a sensory discharge and the point of regeneration can be located and measured (see p. 476).

Sensation

Sensory charting will show, initially, the area of anaesthesia (Fig. 22/2) followed, as re-innervation occurs, by hyperaesthesia or pins and needles. As the myelin of the nerve sheath matures this hyper-sensitivity is replaced by a slightly diminished but more normal sensation. Incorrect localisation, due to crossed re-innervation, must also be charted (Wynn Parry, 1981). Testing of cutaneous sensation may be performed by the use of the finger tip or, if greater detail is needed, by the use of different diameter monofilaments (Dellon, 1984). Two-point discrimination, either moving or stationary, is another means by which the result of nerve surgery can be assessed. Electromyography and the use of a sweat meter can also indicate cutaneous and sympathetic re-innervation.

For a more functional approach stereognosis, or the recognition of objects, is a means to test the return of sensation when combined with movement. This will automatically include both cutaneous and proprioceptive function, the latter being a necessity for performance of all manual skills. Objects are handed to the blindfolded patient for identification and timed in seconds (Wynn Parry, 1981) (Fig. 22/3). These tests can only be performed when some sensory recovery has reached the finger tips.

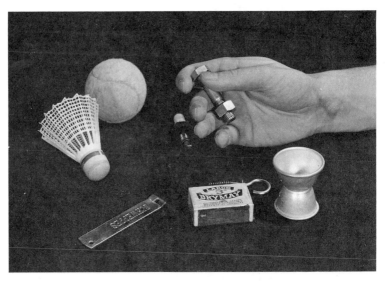

FIG. 22/3 Sensory re-education for a recovering median nerve lesion

Functional assessment

Functional testing, when it becomes possible, should be carried out by the occupational therapist. A self-evaluation by the patient on various activities of daily living, work and leisure interests will identify the difficulties which may need some assistance in solving. Practical testing can then be arranged, and the results may indicate the need for help/advice from the resettlement officer. Difficulties in employment should be considered as early as possible following injury.

PHYSIOTHERAPY

Nerve lesions may or may not require surgery, depending on the cause and severity of injury, but both closed and postoperative lesions will require the attention of a physiotherapist. No two patients are likely to have identical problems therefore individual treatment is a necessity.

Immediate post-injury and postoperative care

To prevent stretch of the sutured nerve ends a plaster of Paris slab is applied after the operation and worn for 2–3 weeks, with adjacent joints positioned to reduce tension. Care must be taken that no passive stretch of the nerve is allowed for 8 weeks.

The limb is supported initially in elevation to prevent oedema, and exercises are given to maintain the range of any free joints during this period of immobilisation. A sling will be necessary for the ambulant patient with paralysis of muscles of the hand and arm, and with autonomic involvement, e.g. a brachial plexus lesion. The sling will support the joints and help control oedema in an otherwise dependent limb. The bed should be elevated for nerve lesions of the leg, and when ambulant the patient should wear a firm elastic bandage or stocking with a well-fitting shoe.

Splintage may be indicated to support distal joints, for example a cock-up splint for the wrist following a radial nerve lesion. Continued stretch of capsule and ligaments can be very painful and allow the development of gross deformities.

Prolonged stretch of muscle is also inhibitory which is undesirable at the re-innervation stage. A drop-foot splint or support is necessary for a lesion of the sciatic and anterior tibial nerve to position the ankle correctly and prevent contractures from occurring.

Pulsed electromagnetic energy, which will help to reduce fibrosis, should be started early following surgery, and continue for 3 weeks.

Stage of paralysis

The main principles of treatment during the stage of paralysis are:
1. Prevent oedema and maintain an adequate circulation for the limb.
2. Control pain.

3. Maintain or regain full passive range of movement.
4. Maintain power of all unaffected muscles.
5. Encourage function.

The first priority must be given to reducing oedema. If the limb is allowed to remain oedematous, fibrin is deposited and the tissues lose their suppleness causing pemanent stiffness.

Whenever possible, activity should be encouraged in elevation as this is the best means to reduce oedema. Massage can be given to small areas, but if the whole hand is swollen pneumotherapy in either single- or double-thickness pressurised bags will effectively reduce the swelling.

The use of cold therapy is contra-indicated for peripheral nerve lesions as the limb remains cold for a long time. Warm water or saline soaks allow the patient to exercise in the water and are preferable to wax baths. Following the soak, massage, using hydrous ointment, will help to improve any dry scaly skin and soften areas round scars. Ultrasound can be given also round the scar to soften scar tissue but must not be given when tendon suturing has been performed recently as it has been found to prevent healing (Roberts et al, 1982).

Pain due to de-afferentation may be present in a small proportion of patients with nerve lesions and must be controlled as early as possible. Transcutaneous nerve stimulation (TNS) will help to reduce pain in most peripheral nerve lesions. In root avulsions or plexus lesions success cannot be guaranteed, but it is usually effective in controlling phantom limb pain following an amputation. Correct placement of the electrodes will be discovered mainly by trial and error. They must be placed on skin with sensation and should be either above and below, or on either side of, the painful area. When pain is present despite large areas of sensory loss the electrodes should be placed over the nerve trunk (Frampton, 1982).

The TNS should be used for several hours to be effective, and it must be tried for at least a week before discarding it as an ineffective treatment. As much activity as possible is encouraged while it is worn. Contra-indications to TNS include its use over the carotid sinus and over broken skin. Its safety during pregnancy has not been established but it should not be used by patients with pacemakers.

Active movements are encouraged as early as possible for all normal muscles both to prevent joint stiffness and to achieve as much sensory input for the limb as is possible. This together with the use of TNS will help to prevent or reduce pain.

When muscles are paralysed passive physiological movements must be given to maintain joint range and web spaces. Accessory movements of roll, spin and slide (*Gray's Anatomy*, 1980) are also used to improve joint stiffness but the range on the sound side must be compared so that the joints are not over mobilised.

Compensatory or trick movements should be taught as they help to maintain function particularly in conjunction with lively splints. These splints may be used to prevent or correct deformities and to increase function. Details are given under the individual nerve lesions.

Stage of recovery

Motor and sensory re-education begins at this stage. As re-innervation occurs a muscle will be found to contract first as a synergist and later as a prime mover. Each muscle should be re-educated individually in outer to middle range first, and into inner range as the power improves. The threshold of the recovering nerve is high, therefore facilitation techniques are important, helping to irradiate and maximise excitation of the re-innervated muscle.

Application of the physiotherapist's hands are particularly essential at this stage as they can give suitable resistance in the correct direction to all parts of the hand. Sensory input ensures the maximum response which will help in recovery of manual skills. There is little point in giving free active exercises for the hand which is normally in constant contact with objects for function. Games of all varieties, the use of rubber bands to strengthen finger movements, and springs to improve power of wrist and upper limb should all be introduced gradually. Specific treatment in the occupational therapy department is important for improving function.

Sensory re-education commences as soon as some sensory re-innervation occurs. Details are given under the median nerve lesion (p. 511).

As the patient's ability to work increases, a functional assessment should be carried out by the occupational therapist. Results of this are valuable in giving guidance about future employment prospects, and the patient is encouraged to return to work as soon as is suitable.

Throughout treatment the physiotherapist must check that the patient is carrying out his own treatment at home, particularly if he is unable to attend the physiotherapy department regularly.

PERIPHERAL NERVE INJURY IN THE UPPER LIMB

The methods already outlined apply to the following injuries, but some specific points will be discussed.

Brachial plexus lesions

As described in the previous chapter injuries to the plexus may be partial or complete, with upper trunk lesions being more frequent than lower. The patient will present with varying effects according to the extent of involvement.

Complete lesions: All the muscles of the upper limb are involved except trapezius and there is complete anaesthesia apart from a small area on the medial side of the arm which has T2 root supply. The limb hangs limply in medial rotation, the head of the humerus may subluxate due to the lack of tone in the deltoid, the elbow is extended and the forearm is pronated. The hand loses its normal contour and becomes blue and swollen when dependent.

A Horner's syndrome with constriction of the pupil and occasionally drooping of the eyelid will indicate a T1 pre-ganglionic lesion. Paralysis of the rhomboids suggests a pre-ganglionic lesion of the C5. Together with paralysis of the remaining upper limb muscles and loss of sensation the prognosis is poor.

Partial lesions: Upper trunk lesions affect the muscles around the shoulder and the flexors of the elbow. Lower trunk lesions affect the long flexors of the wrist and fingers and the small muscles of the hand.

PHYSIOTHERAPY

Motor and sensory charting should be carried out and a regular reappraisal made in the case of post-ganglionic lesions. Passive movements to the affected joints should begin as soon as possible, but delay may be unavoidable if there are un-united fractures. A full range of movement should be given twice a day, and the patient taught to carry this out for himself. Lateral rotation with abduction of the shoulder and supination of the forearm quickly become limited, the thumb web becomes tight and the meta-carpophalangeal joints very stiff if not regularly mobilised. If stiffness occurs it takes weeks of intensive treatment to rectify. Hydrotherapy techniques will help to increase the range of stiff joints, and progressive resisted exercises in water are introduced when recovery occurs. Compensatory movements should be encouraged as they assist in maintaining function.

Pain is experienced by the majority of patients with avulsion lesions of the plexus (Wynn Parry, 1981). TNS will reduce this in a proportion of patients when tried out sufficiently, and most patients will eventually learn to live with a residual degree of pain.

Reconstructive procedures may need to be planned if recovery does not take place. Careful reappraisal by the physiotherapist of muscles, joints and sensation should be made prior to decision by the surgeon to perform any arthrodesis or muscle transfers. Re-education of the latter is usually commenced three weeks after surgery.

Splinting of the flail arm, allowing functional use similar to that provided by an arm prosthesis, must be offered to the patient.

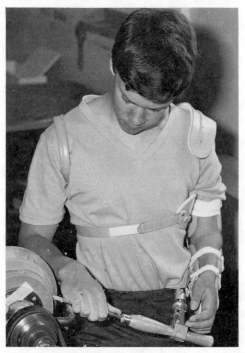

FIG. 22/4 Patient with a brachial plexus lesion wearing a flail arm splint while working with tools at a lathe

The splint can stabilise a flail shoulder and elbow thereby allowing a normal hand to function efficiently. If the hand is paralysed, appliances may be attached to the splint to enable patients to perform activities of work and leisure (Fig. 22/4). Practical use of the splint should be taught in the occupational therapy department.

AXILLARY NERVE LESION

This nerve supplies deltoid and teres minor and may be injured with fractures of the surgical neck of the humerus and in dislocations of the shoulder. There is marked flattening of the contour of the shoulder and an area of sensory loss on the lateral side of the upper part of the arm. Fairly strong elevation can be restored, if the shoulder joint is mobile, by teaching compensatory movements. When lying supine with the elbow flexed, the patient will be able, if the shoulder is externally rotated, to elevate the arm using the long head of biceps. The clavicular head of pectoralis major and serratus anterior help to complete the movement. As the patient's ability improves, the back of the plinth is gradually raised until it is vertical, and he is able to perform the movement without support. Some patients learn this movement by themselves while with others it may take a few weeks of intensive rehabilitation. When re-innervation occurs and deltoid regains strength, the trick movement will disappear.

ULNAR AND MEDIAN NERVE INJURY

The ulnar and median nerves, together with tendons and arteries, are frequently divided at the wrist as the result of putting the hand through a window. The recovery of full function is thus more complicated than with a single and closed nerve lesion, and challenges the skill of the physiotherapist to help achieve a good result.

Both nerves may be involved in elbow injuries, more commonly the ulnar nerve with fractures of the medial epicondyle. A carpal tunnel syndrome may compress the median nerve and need decompressing by dividing the flexor retinaculum.

The ulnar nerve supplies flexor carpi ulnaris, the medial portion of flexor digitorum profundus, the hypothenar muscles, all the interossei, the medial two lumbricals, the deep head of flexor pollicis brevis, and adductor pollicis.

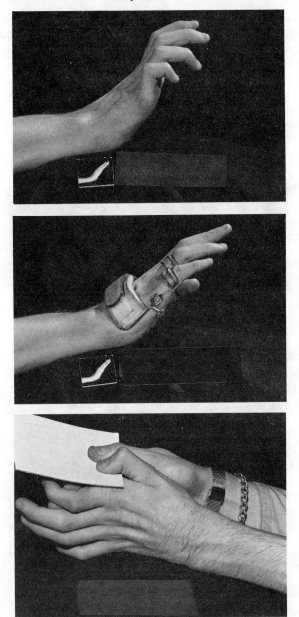

FIG. 22/5 (a) The claw hand deformity of an ulnar nerve lesion; (b) Deformity corrected by a lively splint; (c) Showing trick adduction of the thumb using flexor pollicis longus

The deformity of the ulnar nerve lesion is the claw hand (Fig. 22/5 a.b.c.). There is hyperextension of the metacarpophalangeal joints of the ring and little fingers due to action of extensor digitorum being unopposed by the paralysed medial two lumbricals, and the interossei. There is flexion of the interphalangeal joints of these two fingers, due to the strong pull of the long flexors which are unopposed because of the paralysed intrinsic muscles. The sensory loss to the medial one and a half fingers (Fig. 22/2) does not impair the patient's function severely, though burns may result on the affected fingers and ulnar border of the hand.

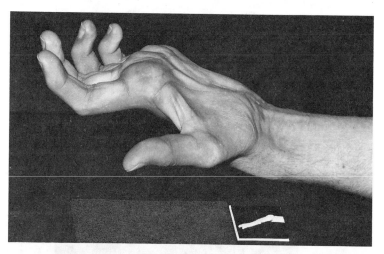

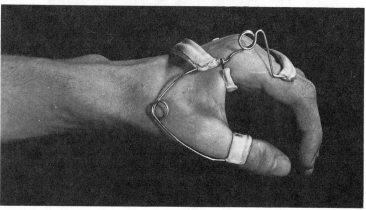

FIG. 22/6 (a) Deformity of a combined median and ulnar nerve lesion; (b) Deformity corrected by a lively splint

The deformity of the median nerve lesion at the wrist is the flat monkey hand (Fig. 22/6 a.b.). The thumb is held alongside the index finger by the action of extensor pollicis longus, unopposed because of the paralysed abductor pollicis brevis and opponens pollicis. The thenar eminence becomes flattened due to atrophy of the underlying muscles. The sensory loss is a severe disability as sensation is lacking over the thumb, index and middle fingers and a large area of the palm. The patient is therefore unable to recognise objects, and the lack of cutaneous sensation and proprioception greatly impairs motor function, especially precision grip. A higher level lesion involving the anterior interosseous nerve leaves the hand in the position of an episcopal blessing. The index and middle fingers are fully extended by the extensor digitorum and without antagonistic tone in the long flexors the clawing will not occur.

A combination of lesion of both nerves is a severe disability needing intensive treatment to ensure maximum return of function. With a high level of lesion of both nerves the deformity is likely to worsen while re-innervation of the long flexors is proceeding. Careful monitoring of joint ranges, provision and checking of the efficiency of lively splints is therefore essential so that contractures are prevented.

Progression of treatment following suture of median and ulnar nerves

If the suture is at the wrist, this joint is usually immobilised in flexion by a plaster splint for 3 weeks. If at the elbow, and an extensive resection has been necessary, a turnbuckle plaster may be applied to maintain the elbow in flexion. After 3 weeks the elbow is gradually extended by use of the turnbuckle, which allows flexion, but controls extension. Full movement is regained within 3 to 5 weeks.

1–3 WEEKS
The limb must be supported comfortably in elevation. Active movements of the unaffected joints of the upper limb are encouraged. Pulsed electromagnetic energy (PEME) should be given daily through the dressings to the affected part.

3–5 WEEKS
The treatment follows the routine described for a peripheral nerve lesion (p. 497). Free active movements are encouraged in

order to retain full joint range and passive physiological movements must be given in the absence of normal voluntary movement. Care must be taken to avoid putting tension on the nerve ends at this stage. The patient must be warned, for instance, not to allow the hand to hang palm uppermost over the table edge thereby stretching the sutured ends. The nails should be cut by the physiotherapist to prevent the patient damaging his anaesthetic skin. If there are unhealed areas, or trophic lesions have occurred, saline soaks are used and the wounds cleaned with a suitable mild disinfectant.

Treatment should be repeated three to four times daily if necessary and should be alternated with periods of occupational therapy. Adequate early treatment is essential and if quite impossible for the patient to attend full time he must be made aware of the importance of carrying on his own treatment at home. Overprotection of the hand at this stage is also liable to produce a poor functional result and pain is more of a possibility.

6–8 WEEKS

Deeper massage with lanolin is given to help free adherent scars and soften indurated areas.

It is essential to differentiate between deformities caused by overaction of the antagonists, those caused by joint stiffness and those caused by tendon adherence. Following laceration of the flexor aspect of the wrist, flexor digitorum superficialis may become adherent to the scar with the result that the proximal interphalangeal joints will be held at 90° flexion. This deformity will disappear if the wrist and metacarpophalangeal joints are flexed, thus relaxing the tension on flexor digitorum superficialis. It reappears at the wrist and metacarpophalangeal joints are extended.

It is safe at this stage to introduce graduated resistance to all movements which will help to free adherence and mobilise any residual stiffness of joints. Facilitation techniques for both may be used in unilateral and bilateral strengthening and relaxation patterns. The flexion, abduction and external rotation pattern in particular will help to improve wrist and finger extension which may be limited following immobilisation in a flexed position.

It is essential that the patient is again using his hand automatically by this stage and not overprotecting it. Constant reminders may be needed, especially if the hand is painful. Pain can usually be decreased, as has already been stated, by the use of TNS. Games, such as table tennis and darts, progressing to badminton, are useful and encourage the patient to use his whole arm, but volley ball, where the hand may be forcibly extended, is not suitable. When finger flexion is very limited handles may need to be padded to provide a firm grasp, and the padding reduced as soon as the flexion improves. Precision movements should be encouraged by playing with such things as cards, matches and Pik-a-Stick.

Lively splints are needed to prevent stretch of ligaments and capsules of joints when full passive mobility has been achieved, and to improve function.

The aim of the ulnar lively splint is to correct the hyperextension of the metacarpophalangeal joints when the patient extends his fingers, and to give support to the proximal phalanges so that the long extensors may extend the interphalangeal joints. The splint should also maintain the palmar arch and allow full flexion and extension of the fingers. Shaped bars are fitted over the dorsum of the hand and over the proximal phalanges of the two medial fingers, with a pad under the palm. A coil of wire, in line with the metacarpophalangeal joints, acts as a spring and maintains these joints in slight flexion while the hand is at rest (Fig. 22/5b).

The aim of the median lively splint is to prevent permanent flattening of the thenar eminence and to place the thumb in a functional position of palmar abduction, rotation and opposition. A pinch grip to the index and middle fingers can then be made by using flexor pollicis longus. This can be achieved by using a long strip of Neoprene, with a stitched loop at one end, which is fitted over the metacarpophalangeal joint of the thumb. The strip is pulled diagonally across the palm to the ulnar border and fastened around the wrist using Velcro. The thumb is thus held in a functional position but it can also extend against the Neoprene.

The splint for the combined median and ulnar lesion works on a similar principle as that for the ulnar. The proximal bar extends over the dorsum of the whole hand and the distal bar over the proximal phalanges of all four fingers. There is a spring wire attached from the lateral side which supports the thumb in a functional position (Figs. 22/6b and 22/7a and b).

8 WEEKS ONWARDS

More vigorous resisted exercises are now introduced. Passive stretching is required if full mobility of the soft tissues has not been regained. The stretch should be slow and steady and combined with relaxation techniques. Serial stretch plasters are necessary in stubborn cases, and this is a skilled technique which must be applied with care and with medical agreement. Plaster of Paris

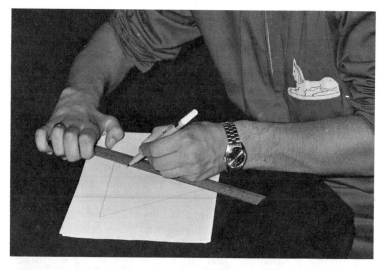

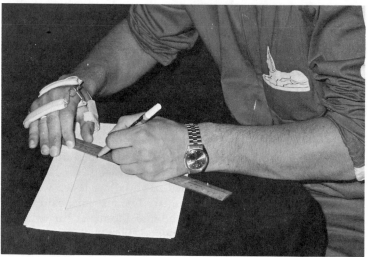

FIG. 22/7 Patient with median and ulnar nerve lesions attempting to hold a ruler (a) without a splint and (b) wearing a lively splint

and Polyform are both found to be suitable materials as they conform well to the contours of the hand, therefore maintaining it in the desired position. The splint is applied by the physiotherapist who treats the patient so that no more than the correct amount of stretch is given. If plaster of Paris is selected, 12 layers 10 cm wide are used with a crescent cut out to allow free movement for the thumb. Petroleum jelly is applied to the skin if it is hairy, to prevent adherence. The layers are soaked in warm water, squeezed out and smoothed well so that no wrinkles remain. They are placed directly on to the skin of the palm and forearm, and held so that the maximum extension of the wrist and fingers is obtained. Care is taken to prevent hyperextension of the metacarpophalangeal joints, and ulnar deviation of wrist and fingers. The position is held until the plaster has set. When dry, the plaster is lined with cottonwool and the forearm placed on the plaster. The fingers are then extended into position and a thin layer of cotton-

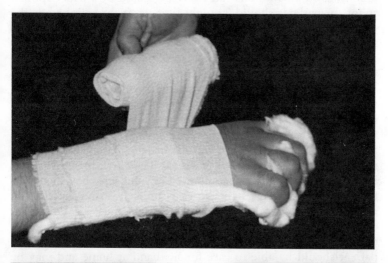

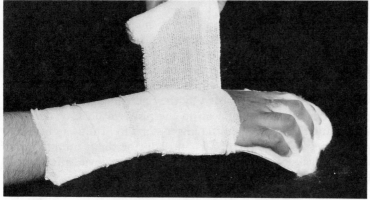

FIG. 22/8 Serial stretch plaster being applied to a patient with median and ulnar nerve lesions with adherence of the flexor tendons at the wrist

wool placed between each to prevent friction. The splint is held in position by a crêpe bandage, keeping the fingertips free so that the circulation may be checked (Fig. 22/8 a and b). The splint should be worn for about one hour only during the day, and a check made by the physiotherapist on its removal. As soon as the range has increased and the fingers can be lifted from the splint a new one should be made. The splint should only be worn at the allotted times so that function is maintained during most of the day. Plasters must be used with extreme care where there is complete anaesthesia especially in combined median and ulnar nerve lesions, as trophic lesions can easily be caused by a badly applied splint. In-patients should, at night time, wear the splint made the previous day, so that any correction obtained during the day is not lost.

Special care must be taken to assess the patient's suitability to wear these splints. He must be sufficiently intelligent to understand the significance of the instructions concerning the circulation and to observe that the limb remains warm and the colour normal. If he is an outpatient he must be able to attend the hospital for the splint to be checked regularly. Contra-indications to the use of stretch plasters include oedema, circulatory impairment, infections and unhealed areas. Their use, when there is intracapsular joint damage, is limited in value and they should be used with great care. If the nerve is unlikely to regenerate, the use of passive stretches and serial plasters must be limited in order to prevent hypermobility of the joints occurring. When the optimum degree of mobility and function has been achieved the patient should be able to care for his hand at home and may be able to return to work.

The doctor checks his progress at intervals and treatment is resumed when re-innervation starts to take place.

In an ulnar nerve lesion, the first muscle to recover is abductor digiti minimi, on average 90 days after a suture of the wrist, and it will contract first as a synergist in opposition to little finger and thumb. It is easy to be misled by the tightening produced by the pull of flexor carpi ulnaris on to the pisiform bone or on to an adherent wrist scar. The little finger starts to drift away from the ring finger as recovery occurs in abductor digiti minimi while there is lack of tone in the antagonistic palmar interosseous muscle.

In a median nerve lesion, flexor pollicis brevis is the first muscle to recover followed shortly by abductor pollicis brevis, the average of the former being 80 days and the latter 90 days.

Before a contraction can be felt, there is usually an improvement in the position of the thumb due to increasing tone.

Intensive rehabilitation is essential and should include individual and group re-education of muscles and functional activities. Facilitation techniques should be used as the threshold of the anterior horn cells is high following a nerve lesion and maximum excitation is necessary to produce a contraction.

Sensory re-education

Sensibility is the interpretation by the brain of the sensory stimuli that it receives and the hand is one of the main sensory organs of the body. It is thought that the differences in sensation are produced not only by the specificity of the receptors but also by the coding of varying combinations and speeds of impulses transmitted along the axons from the peripheral receptors. Good motor function is dependent on feedback of cutaneous and proprioceptive sensations. Wall (1961) points out that a passive stimulus is very rare in normal life and that sensory stimuli usually need motor participation. The function of both is therefore very closely interlinked and sensation combined with active movement needs re-education (Wynn Parry and Salter, 1976).

Any incorrect localisation caused by crossed re-innervation or following neurovascular skin island transfer, can be improved by localisation training. The patient is asked to point, while his eyes are closed, to the place where he is being touched. If incorrect he is told to look so that he may learn to interpret his altered localisation correctly. Gradually he will say that it feels in one position but that he knows it is elsewhere, until he eventually points directly to the spot (Wynn Parry, 1981).

RADIAL NERVE INJURY

The radial nerve is most frequently damaged at the point where it winds round the humerus as a result of fractures or by pressure from callus formation. It may also be damaged in the axilla by pressure from an axillary crutch, or, in the case of 'Friday night palsy', by pressure from the arm of a chair when the arm hangs over the edge for a lengthy period.

Complete interruption of the nerve in or above the axilla causes paralysis of the extensors of elbow, wrist and fingers. If the injury is below the axilla the triceps will not be affected. Although there is inability to extend the wrist or metacarpophalangeal joints, the interphalangeal joints can be extended by the interossei, and the thumb by abductor pollicis brevis, which has an insertion into the extensor expansion of the thumb.

Damage to the posterior interosseous branch will spare the brachioradialis and extensor carpi radialis longus muscles.

A simple cock-up splint is sufficient to support the wrist. Alternatively, a lively splint of wire with a pad supporting the palm and a coil at either side of the wrist will allow the wrist to flex. The hand is returned to a functional position by relaxing the flexor activity. Both these splints will prevent the weight of the hand from producing a painful stretch of the ligaments of the wrist joint.

The patient may find that the addition of a spider splint is useful for finger release in precision movements and for large grasp. This splint consists of four plastic-coated wires, fixed by a cuff round the base of the proximal phalanx of the thumb, spread out and looped under the middle phalanges of the fingers (Fig. 22/9). This allows full flexion of the fingers to take place and holds the metacarpophalangeal joints in slight flexion when the hand is relaxed.

Fingers and thumb should not be suspended in leather loops strung from hooped wire splints as these tend to hyperextend the metacarpophalangeal joints and flatten the thumb. Besides this they are cosmetically unacceptable and exceedingly clumsy when dressing. This type of splint should be reserved for the severe

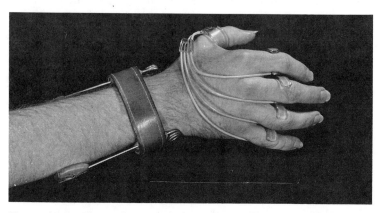

FIG. 22/9 A radial nerve palsy splinted in a lively cock-up splint for the wrist and a spider splint for the fingers allowing the interossei to extend the interphalangeal joints

injury of combined median and ulnar with radial nerve lesion which occurs in limb replacement following traumatic amputation.

RE-EDUCATION FOLLOWING TENDON TRANSFERS

Failure of nerve regeneration may result in loss of movement and function and possibly gross deformity. The disability may be improved by tendon transfers and other reconstructive surgery (Birch, 1984).

Assessment by the therapist will aid the surgeon in making the decision as to which procedure to perform. The present functional problems and future needs should be considered and the muscles graded carefully. The donor muscle must be grade 4 (Oxford scale) as its strength will probably decrease by 1 grade on transfer.

It is an advantage for the patient to recognise the donor muscle contraction and its action pre-operatively, and its alteration of position and action after transfer.

For at least 3 weeks the limb is immobilised in a position which will prevent any stretch on the newly positioned muscle. Gentle active movements are then introduced, working the muscle into inner range, and still preventing any stretch. The range of movement must be monitored to demonstrate an increase in inner range before allowing outer range movement to take place. Wearing of splints or a sling may therefore be necessary for several weeks to protect the muscles.

Usually it is easy for the patient to learn the desired movement. If difficult, there are methods which will facilitate the changed action. The altered position of the donor muscle should be identified and the patient asked to think in his mind of the donor's action, as long as it is not totally antagonistic to the new action. Faradic-type stimulation of the donor muscle may help to give the correct feel of movement and EMG biofeedback can prove most useful in re-education.

PERIPHERAL NERVE INJURY IN THE LOWER LIMB

The sciatic nerve may be severed by wounds of the pelvis or thigh, and quite commonly is damaged either completely or partially by dislocation of the hip. In a complete lesion there is paralysis of the hamstrings and all muscles distal to the knee, and sensory loss also which is extremely disabling. The common peroneal nerve may be damaged by fractures of the neck of the fibula or by pressure from a badly applied plaster cast. A foot drop occurs as there is paralysis of the anterior tibial and peroneal muscles. The sensory loss is over the dorsum of the foot and lateral side of the leg. The patient walks with a high-stepping gait to clear the floor when gravity and the unopposed calf muscles cause the foot to drop into equinovarus. This can be corrected by the use of a foot drop splint made of Vitrathene, Vitralene or Hexcelite fitted inside the shoe.

Passive movements should be given daily to prevent contracture of the calf muscles and clawing of the toes. The patient can carry this out for himself by standing with the affected foot on a low step and pushing his body-weight forward over his foot. A night splint should be made to support the foot at 90° dorsiflexion and in the mid-position between inversion and eversion. The splint should extend for 2.5cm distal to the toes to keep the weight of the bedclothes off the foot, and should be lined carefully to avoid causing pressure sores. If contractures have developed, correction is necessary by passive stretching and the use of serial stretch plasters. Particular care must be taken when using these plasters if there is total anaesthesia of the skin. During the recovery stage facilitation techniques are used for re-education. Balance reactions are effective for stimulating the peronei and anterior tibials and a balance board is also useful. The board may have a rocker underneath or a rounded shape which allows it to roll in all directions. All balance boards are valuable forms of equipment for re-educating proprioception in the lower limb.

As the power of the dorsiflexors increases the splint is removed for increasing periods of time. Postural re-education and correction of gait is important throughout treatment.

Lesions of the posterior tibial branch of the sciatic nerve may occur in supracondylar fractures of the femur. There is paralysis of the calf, posterior tibial and plantar muscles. Contracture of the plantar fascia may follow paralysis of the short muscles of the foot unless kept mobile.

Electrical stimulation

Electrical stimulation is believed to maintain protein metabolism and to preserve the bulk of muscle fibres if carried out regularly. To be effective, though, it must be maintained daily for a considerable period of time. Results from intensive rehabilitation, which maintains the circulation and function, have been so good that routine stimulation has been stopped. Patients with brachial plexus lesions who have received no electrical stimulation have been seen with worth-while recovery in the hand two or three years after injury.

Stimulation is useful for detecting anomalies of nerve supply and for re-education in the stage of recovery if the patient is having difficulty in relearning the feel of movement.

REFERENCES

Birch, R. (1984). Traction lesions of the brachial plexus. *British Journal of Hospital Medicine*, **9**, 140-3.

Dellon, A. L. (1984). Touch sensibility of the hand. *Journal of Hand Surgery*, **9B**, 11.

Frampton, V. M. (1982). Pain control with the aid of transcutaneous nerve stimulation. *Physiotherapy*, **68**, 77-81.

Gray's Anatomy, 36th edition (1980). Chapter on arthrology. Longman, Edinburgh.

Henderson, W. R. (1948). Clinical assessment of peripheral nerve injuries: Tinel's test. *Lancet*, **2**, 801.

Roberts, M., Rutherford, J. H. and Harris, D. (1982). The effect of ultrasound on flexor tendon repairs in the rabbit. *Hand*, **14**, 17.

Wall, P. D. (1961). Two transmission systems for skin sensations. In *Sensory Communication*, pp. 475-96, (ed. Rosenblith, W. A.). MIT Press, Cambridge, Mass.

Wynn Parry, C. B. (1981). *Rehabilitation of the Hand*, 4th edition. Butterworths, London.

Wynn Parry, C. B. and Salter, M. (1976). Sensory re-education after median nerve lesions. *Hand*, **8**, 250.

BIBLIOGRAPHY

Barr, N. R. (1975). *The Hand: Principles and Techniques of Simple Splint-making in Rehabilitation*. Butterworths, London.

Caillet, R. (1982). *Hand Pain and Impairment*, 3rd edition. F. A. Davis Co, Philadelphia.

Maitland, G. (1977). *Peripheral Manipulation*, 2nd edition. Butterworths, London.

Omer, G. E. and Spinner, M. (1980). *Peripheral Nerve Problems*. W. B. Saunders Co, Philadelphia.

Tubiana, R. (1984). *Examination of the Hand and Upper Limb*. W. B. Saunders Co, Philadelphia.

Wynn Parry, C. B. (1981). *Rehabilitation of the Hand*, 4th edition. Butterworths, London.

Papers

Frampton, V. M. (1984). Management of brachial plexus lesions. *Physiotherapy*, **70**, 388.
Raji, A. R. M. and Bowden, R. E. M. (1983). Effects of high-peak pulsed electromagnetic field on the degeneration and regeneration of the common peroneal nerve in rats. *Journal of Bone and Joint Surgery*, **65B**, 478.

ACKNOWLEDGEMENT

The author acknowledges the help and encouragement received from Dr C. B. Wynn Parry MBE, DM, FRCP, FRCS. She thanks Mr Norman Chandler for assistance with the photographs. She is grateful to the Director-General, Medical Services, RAF, for permission to publish this chapter on peripheral nerve injuries.

Chapter 23

Cerebral Palsy – Clinical

by G. T. McCARTHY MB, FRCP, DCH

Cerebral palsy is a term used to describe a broad spectrum of motor disability which is non-progressive and is caused by damage to the brain at or around birth. Although the damage is non-progressive, the clinical picture changes as the nervous system develops and the child grows. There are usually associated handicaps.

The prevalence of cerebral palsy is the number of cases present during a specified time, and is usually calculated as age-specific prevalence rate (Alberman, 1984). A reasonable estimate of the prevalence of cerebral palsy at school age is 2 per 1000 live births in industrialised nations (Paneth et al, 1981). The incidence of a condition is the number of new cases occurring during a defined time-period in a population at risk. Because there is a high mortality among the very low birth-weight babies, incidence figures tend to be misleading.

CAUSES OF CEREBRAL PALSY

Prematurity

The chapter on normal development (Chapter 3) describes some of the ways that the immature brain can be damaged. Preterm infants are much more likely to be brain-damaged both at delivery by trauma, and after because of their immature respiratory and cardiovascular systems making them more likely to develop hypoxia and low blood pressure.

They are also more likely to develop low blood sugar and jaundice. Immaturity of the liver makes haemorrhage more likely to occur and be severe.

Asphyxia

Severe asphyxia is still an important cause of cerebral palsy even in mature infants, and may be caused by accidents at birth, knotted umbilical cord, cord around the neck or prolapsed cord. Antepartum haemorrhage may be associated with severe asphyxia. Multiple deliveries may be associated with delay and asphyxia of the second or third infant, especially with malpresentation.

Trauma

Birth trauma occurs in the following ways:
(a) Disproportion – the baby's head or shoulders are too large to pass safely through the birth canal.
(b) Forceps delivery – especially high forceps with rotation of the head in the birth canal.
(c) Breech delivery – especially occurring through a partially dilated cervix, and without forceps applied to protect the head.
(d) Rapid delivery – especially of a preterm infant with a very soft skull.
The trauma is usually caused by distortion of the head, and tearing of the tentorium.

Severe jaundice

This occurs much less frequently since Rhesus incompatibility can be prevented by immunising mothers at risk. The preterm baby who is also having breathing problems is now most at risk. A high level of unconjugated bilirubin in the blood damages the basal ganglia causing athetoid cerebral palsy and high tone deafness.

Hypoglycaemia

Low blood sugar for a long period can cause severe brain damage and epilepsy. The cerebellum seems vulnerable causing ataxia, and there are often visual problems. Besides preterm infants, infants who are light-for-dates and infants of diabetic mothers are particularly vulnerable.

Intra-uterine virus infection

Rubella virus infection and cytomegalovirus infection are two viruses that can cause severe brain damage and associated deafness and visual problems including cataracts.

Neonatal meningitis

Early meningitis is usually associated with severe residual brain damage.

Genetic causes

These are becoming relatively more common as perinatal care improves, and should be considered particularly in ataxic and some athetoid syndromes.

Vascular causes

Occlusion of the internal carotid or middle cerebral artery may occur before or after birth and cause hemiplegia.

CLASSIFICATION OF DISTRIBUTION

The position and extent of the damage determines the final clinical picture.
1. One side of the body affected – hemiplegia.
2. All four limbs affected, upper more than lower – quadriplegia.
3. All four limbs affected, one side more than the other – bilateral hemiplegia.
4. The legs mainly affected, but arms less so – diplegia.
5. One limb only affected – monoplegia (very rare).

TYPES OF CEREBRAL PALSY

Spastic

Spasticity is a disorder of tone characterised by an initial increased resistance to stretch which may then lessen abruptly. It is caused by damage to the upper motor neurone in the cortex or along the pathways which terminate in the spinal cord, and is characterised by increased deep tendon reflexes and extensor plantar responses.

Spastic muscles are continuously contracting, and there is

apparent weakness of their antagonists leading to abnormal positions of the joints on which they act. Deformities of joints develop which may become fixed contractures with time.

Dystonic choreo-athetosis

Involuntary movements (choreo-athetosis) are so frequently combined with dystonic posturing that they are conveniently classified together. The damage is centred on the basal ganglia. Choreo-athetosis is most frequently found with damage to the caudate nucleus, and dystonia with damage to the globus pallidus.

Athetosis is defined as irrepressible slow writhing movements, the result of imperfectly co-ordinated activity of agonist and antagonists, which are exacerbated by attempting voluntary movement.

Choreic movements are rapid involuntary jerks present at rest which are increased by voluntary movement.

Dystonia is a disorder of muscle tone expressed as postural abnormality, intermittent contractile spasms and complex action dystonias where purposeful movements are deformed.

Voluntary movements are partially or totally disrupted anywhere in the body, including the lips and tongue. The baby is usually markedly hypotonic, developing abnormal movements during the second year. Muscle tension develops as a mechanism to control posture in the adult, but characteristically there are marked variations in tone.

Ataxia

Ataxia is caused by damage to the cerebellum or its pathways. The signs are of hypotonia, disturbance of balance, inco-ordination, intention tremor, dysarthria and sometimes nystagmus. This is a relatively rare form of cerebral palsy and may be part of a dysmorphic syndrome or be associated with intra-uterine infection. Mental handicap is common.

COMMON ASSOCIATED PROBLEMS

Because damage to the brain is likely to be generalised, other neurological problems may also be present and should be looked for.

Visual problems
Optic nerve damage – atrophy leading to visual handicap.
Damage to visual pathways or visual cortex leading to cortical blindness.
Squints. Retinopathy of prematurity.

Hearing problems
Nerve deafness. High frequency loss in kernicterus.
Cortical damage, bilateral.

Speech
Disorders of articulation as in bulbar palsy associated with quadriplegia, or movement disorders affecting speech as in athetosis or ataxia.
Central damage to language centres is rare.

Mental handicap
Damage preventing development of memory. Loss of association fibres linking parts of the brain causing learning problems.

Epilepsy
Scars of the brain may be epileptic foci. All types of epilepsy can occur and be related to learning problems. Many children with cerebral palsy have infrequent seizures and medication should be considered carefully.

Emotional problems
Early bonding problems may occur, with extreme irritability, poor sleep and feeding patterns. The spastic child may be hypersensitive and very anxious. Later depression may occur in severely affected children.

NATURAL HISTORY OF CEREBRAL PALSY

For many years it was felt that early diagnosis of infants with cerebral palsy was impossible. The increasing sophistication of techniques available to keep small preterm infants alive has stimulated precise observation and development of neurological evaluation of these tiny babies. Dubowitz and Dubowitz (1981) have shown that it is possible to observe neurological abnormality, and in their study of 250 premature infants they do not have a single instance of an abnormal infant at 6, 9 or 12-month follow-up who was considered to be completely normal at 36 or 40 weeks postmenstrual age. However, their experience has shown that the *initial severity* of neurological signs is not the indicator of future prognosis, but their *persistence or speed of resolution*. The signs which most consistently correlate with future abnormality are persistent asymmetry, increased tone and diminished mobility of the legs.

After the initial insult there may be a silent period before a baby presents with a motor handicap. However, careful evaluation of its behaviour, neonatal reflexes and tone will usually reveal abnormality. Early common problems are feeding difficulties, poor sleep pattern and increased time in state 6 (Table 3/1, p. 41) behaviour of screaming inconsolably, especially in babies with an increased startle response. This provokes problems in bonding as the baby is not producing normal attachment behaviour.

Visual problems may also inhibit normal gaze following and smiling responses and interfere with the development of balance.

The *persistence* of the neonatal reflexes or *pathological responses* are also indicators of abnormality (p. 42).

(a) Persistently closed hands and a strong grasp reflex.
(b) Asymmetry of the Moro reflex or its persistence past 4 months.
(c) Excessive startle responses.
(d) Obligatory ATNR on turning the baby's head.
(e) Absence of walking and placing reflexes.
(f) The symmetric tonic neck reflex(STNR) is always abnormal. On passively extending the head there is increased extensor tone in the arms and flexor tone in the legs. Flexion of the neck has the opposite effect.
(g) The tonic labyrinthine response is never seen in the normal baby. It is evoked by changing the position of the head in space. In supine a massed extensor pattern develops, in prone the opposite occurs.

Delay in the usual developmental milestones is a common reason for referral for assessment. Early assessment must include hearing and vision, and early intervention if speech delay occurs. Interdisciplinary management is important involving occupational therapists and speech therapists as part of the team approach, and recognising the importance of the support which can be given by the health visitor (Cork, 1984).

A home visit is important in the early stages, and it is helpful to go through the daily routine with the mother so that she is able to see when she might be stimulating the baby as part of everyday experience (Charon, 1984).

COUNSELLING

Early counselling of parents is important and difficult. Once given the diagnosis of cerebral palsy they want to know what this means for their child. Making a prognosis for walking, talking and mental ability is often difficult in the early stages and requires experience and time. One of the most difficult prognostications is the degree of deformity which may develop, particularly at teenage. Spinal deformity may become a major problem, and the possibility may not be obvious in the young child.

DRUGS

The use of drugs in cerebral palsy may be helpful at times, but any prolonged use should usually be unnecessary.

Diazepam may be helpful in relaxing the very tense baby who sleeps badly and startles readily. A single dose at night is usually the most effective way of giving it to prevent the possible side-effects of drowsiness. It is important to give very small doses at first as there is considerable variation in response.

Baclofen is an anti-spastic drug most effective in cases of spinal spasticity. It can be helpful in very severely handicapped children who are almost impossible to relax. However, it has side-effects which may be unpleasant, like headaches, enuresis, lowering of blood pressure and a psychotic state. It can be useful for relaxation in specific circumstances, such as starting to use an ankle-foot orthosis (AFO), and should be introduced slowly.

EDUCATION

Children with moderate or severe cerebral palsy often have associated learning problems. These may be associated with sensory handicaps. Full assessment by an educational psychologist experienced in handling children with cerebral palsy is necessary. The severely affected athetoid child may only be able to communicate intelligence by eye-pointing, and a combined assessment with a speech therapist may be necessary.

REFERENCES

Alberman, E. (1984). Describing the cerebral palsies: methods of classifying and counting. In *The Epidemiology of the Cerebral Palsies*, (eds. Stanley, F. and Alberman, E), CDM No. 87. Spastics International Medical Publications. William Heinemann Medical Books Limited, London.

Charon, P. (1984). In *The Physically Handicapped Child: An Interdisciplinary Approach to Management*, p. 38, (ed. McCarthy, G. T.). Faber and Faber, London.

Cork, M. (1984). In *The Physically Handicapped Child: An Interdisciplinary Approach to Management*, p. 35, (ed. McCarthy, G. T.). Faber and Faber, London.

Dubowitz, V. and Dubowitz, L. M. S. (1981). *The Neurological Assessment of the Preterm and Full-term Newborn Infant*, CDM No. 79. Spastics International Medical Publications. William Heinemann Medical Books Limited, London.

Paneth, N., Kiely, J. L., Susser, M. and Stein, Z. (1981). Cerebral palsy and newborn care, III: estimated prevalence rates of cerebral palsy under differing rates of mortality and impairment of low birth-weight infants. *Developmental Medicine and Child Neurology*, **23,** 801-17.

Chapter 24

Cerebral Palsy – Management

by C. SHUMWAY BSc(Mass), RPT, MCSP, PG Dip

The definition of cerebral palsy (cited in Christenson and Melchior (1967)) as a 'persistent but not unchanging disorder of movement and posture' is as appropriate today as it was over 25 years ago although controversy continues over differentiation into sub-groups as well as over treatment. The words 'but not unchanging' were added to the original definition as it became evident that, although the lesion itself is static, the resulting clinical manifestations are seen to change considerably over time. The damage occurs to an immature central nervous system which then matures in the presence of that damage; as more is demanded of the child, the less he is able to cope and the more disabled he may appear.

The clinical signs associated with cerebral palsy vary in type as well as topography and hence lead to two means of classification.

Classification by type is neither uniform nor clearcut, and a mixture of types is often found in one child. The commonly accepted categories of spastic, athetoid, and ataxic have been described in Chapter 23.

Topographical classifications are an attempt to describe what is seen clinically according to the part or parts of the body involved. They have been described in the previous chapter as hemiplegia, quadriplegia, bilateral hemiplegia, diplegia, and monoplegia. These terms are not precise, and terms used vary from centre to centre. Often, limbs that not included in the classification are actually involved. Also, the trunk, head and neck are ignored in the classifications, but are nearly always involved to some extent and, in the long term, their involvement is frequently of more significance than that of the limbs.

The diagnosis derived from these two classifications gives very little indication of the child's physical state or ability. A cerebral palsied child may be one who is totally dependent and posturally disorganised, or one who is able to talk, walk, and even to run, with little hindrance. Consequently, as a specific diagnosis does not imply a certain level of ability, the aims of physiotherapy can only be defined following appropriate assessment.

Analysis of the child's functional deficit is dependent upon an understanding of the actual phenomena resulting from the lesion. These phenomena can be divided into two groups, the principal motor disorders which will be discussed, and the associated disorders (see Chapter 23).

PRINCIPAL MOTOR DISORDERS

These are the disorders of posture and movement which justify the diagnosis of cerebral palsy, and which differentiate cerebral palsy from cases of mental subnormality without motor abnormality (Foley, 1977). These can be sub-divided into positive signs and negative signs.

Positive signs

These are abnormal, or primitive, clinical signs which are often used as diagnostic tests. Although they are usually less significant in determining the child's ability than are the negative signs, and they might be regarded as only symptoms of the child's inability, it is important to understand them and to recognise their existence. Included are reflexes and reactions, and disorders of muscle tone.

Reflexes and reactions can be either those that are seen in normal newborn babies (persistent perinatal reflexes/reactions), or those seen only as a result of brain damage (abnormal or primitive reflexes). Those most often referred to include the asymmetric tonic neck reflex (ATNR), the symmetrical tonic neck reflex (STNR), the tonic labyrinthine reflex (TLR), and the Moro or startle reflex (see Chapter 3). Also included are associated reactions which result from the inability to isolate the effort of a movement, examples of which are irradiation and grimacing. Any combination of these reflexes and reactions can be present in one child. However, recognition of their presence is not an end in itself, but should be regarded as a sign of deficient postural mechanisms.

As stated previously, the disorder of muscle tone is the characteristic that defines the cerebral palsied child by type of abnormality. A combination of tone abnormality is often seen, in which case the classification is made according to which predominates. The situation is further complicated by the fact that two types of tone can be differentiated: intrinsic and postural. *Intrinsic tone* is specified by the state of reactivity of the stretch reflex, and in the normal child can only be elicited with the tendon tap. *Postural tone* is the 'state of continuous and unfatiguable contraction of postural muscles that is needed to overcome gravity and maintain posture' (Foley, 1977) and, as such, is decreased if the postural mechanism is impaired as is often the case in cerebral palsy. Therefore, it is not uncommon for a 'spastic' child – one whose deep tendon reflexes are increased – to feel floppy due to impaired postural mechanisms. The child who is very floppy in the early years often develops positive signs of athetosis as he grows older.

Negative signs

Negative signs result from the absence of normal functions, including the stretch reflex, so muscular hypotonia is one negative sign, as are paralysis and inco-ordination. The most important negative signs in cerebral palsy are, however, those due to deficiency of one, some, or all of the postural reactions (Martin, 1967). Included are:

(1) Antigravity mechanisms: those that support the body against gravity.
(2) Mechanisms for postural fixation:
    (a) Head and trunk erecting mechanisms.
    (b) Counterpoise reactions which prevent the body falling by resisting external and internal forces causing it to pivot about its base as, for example, during limb movement.
    (c) Tilting reactions of head, trunk and limbs as a result of instability of the base of support.
(3) Protective, or staggering, reactions: those that protect the upright posture following horizontal displacement of the body. Parachute reactions are included.
(4) Righting reactions: those sequences of movement that enable the body to gain or regain the upright position while maintaining balance in the process.
(5) Locomotive reactions: those necessary for the initiation of stepping, turning, and the maintenance of gait.
(6) Ocular postural responses: these aid the other postural reactions.

ASSESSMENT/MANAGEMENT/TREATMENT

The great variety of approaches to the treatment and management of cerebral palsy only serves to emphasise the enormous complexity of the problems and the fact that, at present, there are few definite answers. The problems encountered are multifactorial and it is probably impossible to deal with each one fully. The chosen treatment and management techniques will therefore inevitably be a compromise, influenced by factors of time, the child's age and situation, and the abilities of others involved. The therapist must assess the *overall* benefits to the child of various treatment approaches and decide which, if any, are significantly worthwhile and therefore appropriate at that time. The methods, techniques and their emphasis will inevitably change as the child grows older, not only in response to physical development, but also due to changing environment and expectations. It is essential that the therapist dealing with cerebral palsy gains guided experience, preferably in a centre where the various disciplines can assess, treat and discuss the problems together as a team. Often, it is the physiotherapist who is involved with a patient on a regular basis and it is important that she can deal not only with his physiotherapeutic needs, but is aware also of the wider sphere of problems and can request the appropriate advice or involvement from other specialties, such as occupational therapy, speech therapy, psychology, and orthopaedic surgery. This is becoming even more important as the policy of many countries is toward integration and community-based care, resulting in therapists frequently working on their own.

ASSESSMENT

It is logical and essential that an assessment of the child gives a baseline that will point to appropriate treatment and management aims and techniques. Re-assessment should be a continuing part of treatment which allows for improvement or deterioration to be noted, thus enabling treatment to be more effective. The fundamental problems to be considered are those of deficient ability and developing deformity. The therapist should also ascertain information regarding problems as seen by the parents, other 'carers' and the child himself, including handling and sleeping problems.

Ability

The standard, normal child development charts are useful to alert the clinician regarding a child's developmental delay and therefore the need for treatment, as well as to note the important relationships between the various developing abilities, for example the dependence of eye movements on head control and of hand movements on the postural ability of the trunk. Although they provide general guidelines to treatment progression, the levels are usually too gross to indicate the essential underlying postural abilities. Also, the normal child does not perfect one ability before going on to the next, for instance he pulls to standing before perfecting sitting. It is, therefore, incorrect to follow the developmental sequence strictly in treatment.

In order to break down gross motor abilities into their postural components, the therapist must understand some basic biomechanical principles.

1. In order for a part or parts of the body to form a base of support, the body must be so orientated that the line of the centre of gravity falls within the area defined by this base. If the line of the centre of gravity does not fall within the base of support the body will fall.
2. In order to maintain the line of gravity within the base, and therefore maintain balance, the normal body is equipped with mechanisms which automatically counterbalance any movement. These are the postural reactions and the anticipatory postural responses (Traub et al, 1980). If these mechanisms are impaired, the movement is impaired.
3. These postural adjustments are centered in the trunk.

In assessing the child's ability it is helpful to look at the following factors relative to each of the positions of lying (prone, supine, side lying), sitting (floor, chair), and standing.

1. The ability of the child to be placed in each position. Does his body conform easily to the supporting surface, or do parts of his body rebel against it? Is he able to anchor his base of support, for example when he is pulled to sitting?
2. The distribution of weight when the child is placed in each position. Note if there is more weight on one side of the body than the other, or if the child's centre of gravity appears to be unusually high, resulting in 'floating legs' and poor ability to raise the head against gravity.
3. The ability of the child to maintain the position while he

moves, which means that he must counterbalance the movements without changing his base of support. Note if the movements are free, or restricted due to inability to anchor the base and therefore fear of falling. If they are restricted, note what sort of support the child needs in order to free the movements.

4. The ability of the child to move out of a position, for example, to change his base of support as in rolling or getting from a chair to the floor.

5. The ability of the child to attain a position; for example to establish organised lying, to get from lying to sitting, or to get from sitting to standing.

With regard to these levels, it is important to recognise that the ability to be *placed* in a position is a definite level of ability. There are many cerebral palsied children who are unable to be placed; their bodies are disorganised, usually asymmetrical, and are therefore very difficult to handle. If they do not become 'placeable', they will develop severe deformities.

Every movement begins and ends in a position. It is the ability developed within the position which allows controlled movements out of it to occur. All children should be assessed in each of the positions of lying, sitting and standing, as many of them, although they may be fairly able, still have deficiencies of posture and movement in lower positions.

Deformity

It is well known that the cerebral palsied are generally limited to so-called 'preferred postures', and that it is very common for deformity to develop and progress. Over the years this has been attributed to a number of factors, but the basic concept is that if the body spends prolonged periods of time in a position, it will gradually deform into that position (Dunn, 1976; Fulford and Brown, 1976; Robson, 1968). This is seen in cases of plagiocephaly. The positional preferences typically seen in *spastic* cerebral palsies are for 'mid-positions' of the body. In the arm, this generally consists of shoulder protraction or retraction, adduction and internal rotation, elbow flexion, forearm pronation, and wrist and finger flexion. In the leg, one sees hip semi-flexion, internal rotation and adduction, knee semi-flexion, ankle plantar flexion, and foot pronation or supination. *Athetoid or dystonic* posturing usually incorporates extremes of movement such as total flexion or extension.

It is important for the therapist to understand the natural history of deformity: postural deformity usually precedes fixed deformity, which usually precedes structural deformity (Scrutton, 1978). It is essential that a postural deformity be noted early as it is at this stage that measures must be taken in order to prevent its natural progression. Once a deformity has become fixed or is structural, it must either be accommodated in handling and positioning, or dealt with surgically.

In connection with the typical postures mentioned above, the deformities that develop are closely linked with the child's abilities, or lack of ability. If the child is unable to establish a base of support, distribute his weight through his base, and maintain his base while he moves, he will use whatever he can in order to keep himself from falling. For example, the child who is unable to anchor his bottom sufficiently when sitting on a chair will often excessively flex his knees in an attempt to 'hook' on to the chair. The child who, when sitting or standing, tends to fall backward will often round his shoulders and poke his head forward, resulting in an increased kyphosis. In order to initiate walking the child who is unable to bring his weight forward in standing might instead launch himself forward by plantar-flexing. It is for this reason that treatment aimed at prevention/reduction of deformity must be directed also toward the deficient ability that is contributing to the deformity.

One of the most important complexes to note is the windswept deformity of the hips. Most children with cerebral palsy are asymmetrical to some extent, bearing more weight on one side of the body than the other. The resulting deformities can be seen in lying, as well as in sitting and standing, and include the following:

> windswept hips: one flexed, abducted, and externally rotated, the other flexed, adducted, and internally rotated and in danger of posterior dislocation
>
> knee flexion
>
> ankle and foot deformities, often mirror images of each other
>
> pelvic obliquity
>
> scoliosis
>
> preferred head turning
>
> preferred hand usage.

In passively measuring the ranges of motion around the hip, each leg should be measured individually in relation to the pelvis, especially when measuring abduction. Both the adductors and the medial hamstrings can contribute to limited abduction. In order to differentiate, hip abduction should be measured with the knee in extension to demonstrate the effect of both muscle groups, and with the knee in flexion to demonstrate the effect of the adductors only.

Traditionally, in order to prevent or ameliorate deformity, passive movements were performed by the physiotherapist and taught to the parents. Such a routine may be helpful in monitoring joint ranges, but it is now felt that the gradual, prolonged stretch obtained during early, persistent postural management in the form of treatment plus correct handling and positioning, is much more likely to be effective.

Weakness

As the child lacks the ability to use certain movement patterns, the muscles involved can eventually become weak due to disuse. In treatment it is pointless to solely emphasise strengthening of these various muscle groups without at the same time ensuring that the child has the range of motion required for the movement, and is developing the ability to actually use these muscles.

As a result of her assessment, the therapist should be able to define the child's present level of postural ability, and existing or potential deformity. She should then be able to define:

1. The abilities to be promoted in treatment and handling.
2. The positions and handling required to prevent or ameliorate deformity.
3. The support required in various positions which will allow the child to function optimally.

MANAGEMENT

It is difficult to differentiate between treatment and management, although most experienced physiotherapists in the field of cerebral palsy probably agree that periodic treatment sessions only are inadequate. The therapist must become involved with the parents, care staff and others and train them to physically manage the child appropriately throughout the day and night. However, this is not to say that specific, well-chosen treatment techniques performed by the skilled therapist are not an essential part of treatment as well. The aims of all management and handling techniques are:

1. To promote the child's assets and abilities, and, if possible, to stimulate normal patterns of movement.

2. To prevent or reduce deformity.
3. To discourage positions, movements and behaviours that make handling difficult, such as extending and thrusting backwards.

Techniques included are lifting and carrying, positioning, positioning for function and movement between positions.

Lifting and carrying

The adult should first decide how the child will be carried (Fig. 24/1). She should approach him from the front, explain what she is going to do and organise his body (arms and legs especially) so both she and he feel secure. She should then lift, keeping a straight back and a wide base of support, bending the knees, and holding the child as close to her as possible. Enough support should be provided so that the child is safe, but not so much that he is passive.

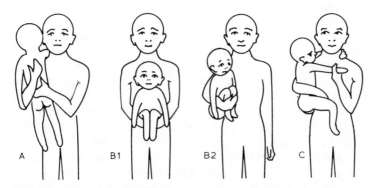

FIG. 24/1 Methods of carrying the cerebral palsied child

A. For flexed children.
B. For extended or thrusting children. The adult's hands may be under or in front of the child's knees in either method of carrying.
C. For children with tight hip adductors, hemiplegia and more able children. *Note* the position of the hemiplegic right arm, held by the adult in the extended position. For a *left* hemiplegia carry on the left hip

Positioning

It is important that a cerebral palsied child experiences a variety of positions throughout the day. Most of the children, regardless of level of ability, will eventually be spending a good deal of the day in sitting. To counteract the detrimental effects of time spent in this flexed position, each child must also spend time in 'straight' positions, either lying or standing, preferably both. Each of the positions discussed below is both posturally and functionally beneficial *and* detrimental, and it is up to the therapist to determine which ones suitably complement each other and are therefore appropriate.

LYING

In *supine*, many cerebral palsied children are completely unable to function, and in this position they may be most asymmetrical. If the supine position must be used, a pillow placed under the head and shoulders often promotes symmetry and the ability to get the hands together. In *prone*, the children are often more symmetrical, but they usually need to be raised off the floor, such as on a wedge, in order to use their hands and heads. A sandbag or strap placed across the child's bottom may be needed to help the child maintain the position. Some children are very difficult to place in the prone position and do not tolerate it well. Others utilise the position to strengthen and improve their ability to extend and thrust, which should be discouraged. *Side lying* is a position in which the child can be quite symmetrical; both hands are within his vision and are more likely to be used together. However, care must be taken that he does not fall partially into prone or supine lying, and therefore into a windswept deformity. Positions for sleeping can be difficult: children who have windswept hips tend to sleep in this position and often are woken by discomfort. A comfortable, non-detrimental position can only be found by trial and error. It may involve changing from supine to prone or side lying, or tilting the bed/mattress slightly to tip the child's weight on to his relatively unweighted side. Leg gaiters, if tolerated, can help in maintaining a relatively symmetrical position.

SITTING

Long sitting, with the knees slightly flexed or straight, is the position in which a normal baby learns to establish his bottom and legs as his base of support. He first flexes his trunk right forward over his legs, and then gradually brings his trunk more upright as his base becomes more established (see Chapter 3). It is not until he is able to rotate his trunk and reach freely outside his stable base that he develops a straight back, and then a lumbar lordosis, in sitting. It is at this time that he develops the ability to stand with support and may be starting to take his first step, signifying that his body has 'split in two': one half anchoring, supporting and adjusting, while the other half counter-balances and moves. The postural education that takes place in long sitting is obviously important. This is also a position in which the hamstrings and hip adductors can be stretched. If the child is unable to sit flat on the floor without his pelvis rotating posteriorly, he can be placed so that his bottom is slightly raised, such as on a very low stool, telephone book, or in sitting downhill on a wedge.

Some children choose to side-sit. If they do this more easily to one side than the other, there is probably a related problem of windswept hips, and the child should be encouraged to sit symmetrically, or on the other side for part of the time.

More able children will sit cross-legged (tailor-sitting) readily, less able children find it difficult. It is for some a comfortable, acceptable alternative to long sitting. The only contra-indication might be a child whose legs 'frog' (hips externally rotate and abduct) excessively, when the hips might be in danger of anterior dislocation.

W-sitting (between heels) has long been frowned upon by therapists. This is due to its possible reinforcement of the flexed, adducted and internally rotated position of the hips. It may contribute also to tibial torsion and foot deformity. However, for many cerebral palsied children it is an easily assumed and stable position for play, and such children must already have the necessary range of motion at the hip joints. Probably the major worry is when a child is placed into the position, or adopts it himself, but has great difficulty getting out of it and is there for a prolonged period.

If the child sits on the floor for prolonged periods in a position felt to be detrimental and there is not an acceptable, floor-level alternative, it might be best to promote chair-sitting. For children able to sit on a chair freely without falling, consideration must be given to (a) the stability of the chair; (b) its height – the child's feet should reach the floor, or a foot platform; and (c) the height of the work surface. If the child's bottom tends to slide about, and he is otherwise stable, a Dycem mat placed under his bottom might be sufficient to anchor it.

STANDING

Hip deformity is a common orthopaedic problem in cerebral

palsy. The correct formation of the acetabulum and femoral head and neck, which results in a stable hip, is apparently dependent upon early weight-bearing in a correct position. Therefore, standing 'appears to hold the key to combating the problem of the hip joint deformity' (Scrutton and Gilbertson, 1975).

Other benefits of standing include:

(1) Prevention of flexion deformity at the trunk, hips and knees and equinus deformity at the ankles.
(2) Development of weight-bearing surfaces of the feet.
(3) A child is often more able to use his head, arms and hands in standing than in other positions.
(4) Sensory feedback in standing is important both proprioceptively and perceptually.
(5) The child benefits socially from being at the same height as his standing peers.
(6) The cardiovascular, digestive, respiratory and excretory functions are stimulated.

In general, any cerebral palsied child who is not standing well by the age of 12–18 months should be stood regularly. The hips should be extended and slightly externally rotated and abducted. Knees should be straight and feet should be plantigrade. Care must be taken to prevent the child from standing in a windswept position; the use of asymmetrical straps to pull the pelvis and, possibly, the thorax to the middle is often effective. The upright standing position is usually preferable to 'prone' standing, when the entire body is angled forward and supported on a platform. This is because many children, when placed in prone standing either *flex* their trunks and pull down strongly with their arms, and therefore inch their way up the prone board, removing any weight from their feet; or totally *hyperextend*. However, a prone stander may be the best choice if (a) the child is very flexed and the main aim is to straighten him out, or (b) he has developed severe deformities and the effect of gravity in upright standing only serves to pull him down into his deformities. In this case, the main aim is straightness and amelioration of deformity, with weight-bearing a secondary aim.

If a child hyperextends when stood in upright standing, a position in which the hips are slightly flexed (5° to 10°) is often effective in overcoming this tendency. The position should be similar to that naturally adopted by a normal person when standing symmetrically and leaning forward slightly on to an elbow-height work surface.

A child who has flexion deformities of his knees, or deformities of his feet, can be positioned in upright kneeling, usually by minor adaptation to a standing frame.

Positioning for function

The physiotherapist is often asked by other therapists and colleagues to advise on appropriate positioning for various functional activities. For example, improved exhalation and breath control for speech can often be obtained in prone lying or standing. A position in which the child can produce a reliable, repeatable response may be required for auditory, visual or psychological testing. Positioning for the optimal use of head and eyes may be needed educationally. With the increasing use of electronic aids for communication, play, and mobility, positioning for the most appropriate means of access to switches is a frequent and important consideration. Positions for dressing should encourage maximum participation from the child. The appropriate positions will vary from child to child and according to the activities required, but it is important to convey the idea that a variety of positions should be considered.

Movement between positions

The everyday handling of a child will inevitably include movement from one position to another. This is an opportune time to promote some of his abilities without disrupting daily life.

ROLLING

The ability of the child to roll from supine to side lying should depict his ability to shift weight from side to side. However, some children hyperextend their necks, arch their backs and flip themselves on to their sides, which serves only to strengthen their ability to totally extend, and should therefore be discouraged. When rolling to side lying, the child should be encouraged to turn his head and tuck in his chin. Once he has rolled to prone, an adult can encourage him to turn his head and free his trapped arm by fixing his bottom with one hand and retracting his shoulder on the same side as his trapped arm with the other.

LYING TO SITTING

When a cerebral palsied child is pulled from supine to sitting, two of his basic abilities should be encouraged: (1) fixing the bottom so that it does not slide; and (2) raising the head. However, many children either arch or round their backs and strongly adduct their legs. For these less able children, various means of promoting their abilities can be tried, including: (1) supporting the child proximally and protracting the shoulders as the child is lifted; (2) starting with the child's head and shoulders raised by a pillow or something similar, so gravity has less effect; or (3) starting from the sitting position and working gradually down to lying. Care must be taken that fixing the neck in hyperextension, poking the chin and hunching the shoulders are not mistaken for head control. An asymmetrical child will often anchor one side of his bottom better than the other, and will favour coming to sitting over one side only. When brought to sitting over the other side, being unable to anchor his bottom, he will spin around. For children who cannot be brought from supine to sitting without excessive effort or abnormal, asymmetrical activity, it is often best to roll them to side lying prior to bringing them to sitting. For more able children, the adult might encourage the child to assist with lying to sitting by pulling him gently up with one arm and waiting for the other arm to be used spontaneously to lean on and push.

SITTING TO STANDING

When a normal individual rises from sitting to standing, his base changes from his bottom/thighs/feet to just his feet. In order to

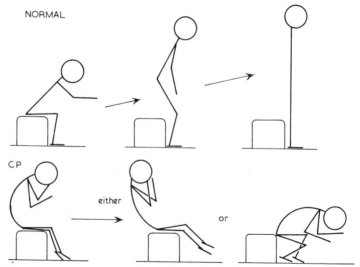

FIG. 24/2 Sitting to standing. *Normal*: the line of gravity is always through the base. *Cerebral palsy*: either pushes back or the bottom slides off the chair and the legs collapse

(a)

(b)

(c)

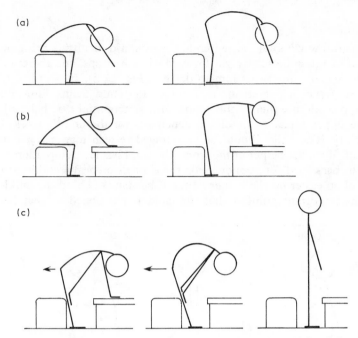

FIG. 24/3 Progression of exercises for sitting to standing: (a) head down, supported at upper arms/shoulders; (b) leaning with flat hands on a second stool; (c) one hand to knee, then both hands to the knees and stand. *Note* that the bottom is brought back to preserve the line of gravity through the base

keep from falling, he must bring his feet back and lean his trunk well forward ('nose over toes') prior to rising. The cerebral palsied child often either fails to organise his feet and trunk correctly before attempting to rise and therefore pushes himself over backward; or, in attempting to get his 'nose over his toes', he is unable to anchor his bottom and slides forward off the chair in a heap (Fig. 24/2). Most children with cerebral palsy, if given assistance in organising their bodies and given balance support (usually at the upper arms or shoulders), have some ability to rise and bear their weight in standing. This ability can be a great help in the day-to-day management of the less able child, especially as he grows older and heavier, and should therefore be encouraged whenever practical. Figure 24/3 shows some of the activities aimed at improving the ability to rise from sitting to standing and to balance in standing.

WALKING

Again, the cerebral palsied child's common difficulty is bringing and maintaining his weight forward while he steps, and therefore the helper must assist him to do this (Fig. 24/4). It is probably best if the helper stands in front of the child facing him and supports him either at the hands (arm gaiters might be helpful), the upper arms, or shoulders depending on the child's level of ability. The child should be encouraged to lean forward, *not* to pull. With the helper at the front, the child has less temptation to lean backward for support. For some small or heavy children it is often easier on the helper's back if he stands behind the child. The important point is that the child is positioned so that his

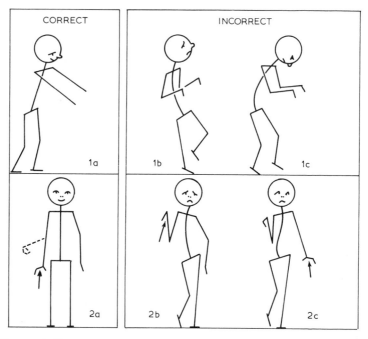

FIG. 24/4 Walking. 1a Correct method with support in front: arms extended; weight forward; support at elbows or hands. 1b and c Incorrect: (b) do not allow the body to lean back; (c) do not support from the front with flexed arms

2a Correct method with support at one side: support at elbow and hold hand; support extended elbow and hand; with a hemiplegic, support the affected arm and keep it forward. 2b and c Incorrect: (b) do not support hemiplegic arm in a flexed position; (c) do not support only the good arm

weight falls through or in front of his feet and *not* behind them. With a hemiplegic child, support should be given to the affected arm/hand in an attempt to increase the child's awareness of it and to prevent the affected side of the body from lagging behind. In more able diplegic children, support at the hips only will reduce the child's abnormal tendency to use his upper trunk for shifting his weight.

TREATMENT

Treatment techniques cannot be prescribed: different techniques or variations work for different children. The therapist should attempt to define answers to the following questions:

What is the child's level of ability?

What is preventing him from reaching the next level?

What should I aim for?

What techniques of treatment, handling, and positioning should I use?

How do I know they are working?

How do I know I have reached a goal?

What do I need to do to maintain this level?

Individual treatment sessions should consist of a logical, effective sequence of activities, each of which plays a role in improving the child's abilities and in preventing progression of deformity. The sequence will often consist of the following:

Mobilisation activities: The area of the body which most often requires some sort of initial mobilisation is the trunk, specifically the low back, pelvis, and shoulder/thoracic area (Fig. 24/5). It is the trunk which is fundamentally responsible for establishment of a position, anchoring through the base of support, and adjustment

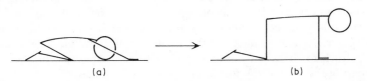

(a)   (b)

FIG. 24/5 Suitable activity for mobilisation of the low back, pelvis and shoulders. (a) Knees and feet together, bottom resting on heels, arms well above head, head down. (b) Resist at the sacrum, asking child to push bottom up. He should not initiate with his head. Arm gaiters are often useful during this activity

to counter-balance movements of the appendages. When these abilities are deficient, as in cerebral palsy, the trunk is stiffened and, instead, the limbs are used in an attempt to balance. Therefore, before we can ask the child to use his trunk for postural anchoring and adjustment, we must help him gain the mobility required. Once mobilisation of the child's trunk allows him mechanically to be placed in various positions, further mobilisation of the trunk and the extremities can be carried out as part of the remaining treatment activities.

Activities to facilitate the postural abilities needed to be placed in or to maintain a position: These include the ability to shift weight on to the side of the body which normally bears less weight, and the ability to shift weight in to the lower half of the body. Improvement of these two abilities should result in the child being more able to establish a symmetrical base of support in various positions.

Activities to challenge the child's postural abilities once a position is established: These might range from (1) asking the child to lift his head and follow an object with his eyes without losing his position; to (2) tipping him out of his base of support and asking him to regain his position; or (3) asking him to stretch to reach something outside his base of support without falling.

Activities to improve the child's ability to move from one position to another with control: This might, for example, include rolling from supine to side lying and back again, or moving from sitting to standing (Fig. 24/3).

This should be regarded as only a guideline, not as a strict sequence. Many of the activities overlap and one activity can achieve a number of goals. For example, while working on sideways balance reactions in the trunk in long sitting, the therapist can also consider the aims of increased mobilisation of the trunk, the ability to get weight forward over the base, stretching of hamstrings and adductors, the ability to shift weight from one buttock to the other, and the ability to re-locate one buttock as part of the base of support after it has been displaced.

Principles of treatment

In spite of there being various approaches to the treatment and management of cerebral palsy, there are certain general principles that would be generally agreed and are helpful in understanding occurrences throughout the changing course of the disorder.

1. Treatment should begin as early as possible.

2. The children do not progress steadily. Numerous factors, including growth and ill-health, can result in regression.

3. A major part of treatment is aimed at encouraging muscles to grow in accordance with lengthening bones, and limbs to grow symmetrically. Treatment should, therefore, continue at least throughout the growth years.

4. Every treatment should result in some change. It is helpful to have a specific test in mind to evaluate treatment effectiveness. For example, if a child sits asymmetrically and the therapist is working in lying or standing to improve his ability to shift his weight, she should place him back in sitting to see if he has improved.

5. Each child should experience a variety of positions throughout the day; verticality and symmetry are important aspects of this.

6. Fear should not be dismissed as lack of confidence; more often than not it is a sign of deficient balance.

7. Establish aims which are realistic; this is important in maintaining your own enthusiasm.

8. Movement depends upon the ability to establish a base of support, to anchor through that base and to adjust weight to counterbalance. The child needs points of reference from which to move.

9. Gaiters (splints) to maintain elbows/knees in extension are useful (Fig. 24/6):
   - as an extra pair of hands during treatment/management;
   - as a means of providing an added base of support, for example use of arm gaiters in conjunction with a grab bar;
   - to help organise the child's body;
   - during treatment, to 'channel' balance activity into the trunk.

   However, they should not be used as a matter of course, but only if better results are achieved.

10. Note what the child can do without touching him. The things we do instinctively to help him are probably just the abilities that we want to actively encourage in him.

11. Always note the position and activity of the whole body during a movement.

12. Interrelate with other therapists so you can incorporate their aims into your treatment and vice versa.

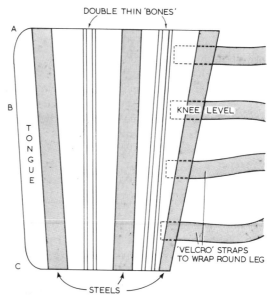

FIG. 24/6 Pattern for gaiters. Measurements are taken at A, B, C. A = circumference at the upper third of the thigh; B = circumference at the knee; C = circumference at the lower third of the leg. A–C = length

13. Benefits of group treatment include improved socialisation and motivation among the children as well as provision of a practical forum for interdisciplinary work.

THE MULTIPLY HANDICAPPED, VISUALLY IMPAIRED CHILD

A congenital visual handicap results in problems in all areas including language, sensory development, motor development, and bonding with parents. These problems must not be overlooked in the posturally impaired child who also has visual impairment. Techniques for dealing with these problems are quite straightforward but are not, however, immediately obvious (see Levitt, 1984).

THE BABY AND YOUNG CHILD

When seeing a baby or young child for the first time, the therapist should see him with his parents, and take special care in

approaching him. The first session may well consist of only discussion with the parents and observation of the child on the parent's lap or while playing in the room. To begin with, treatment
in the home may be more acceptable and beneficial to the parents
and child. The therapist can gradually introduce the child to a
nursery/play school setting. Assessment of the young child cannot
follow a strict regime, and co-operation with verbal instruction
cannot be expected. The therapist must learn to manipulate play
and adapt her interaction with the child in order to get the information and activity she requires. Early treatment may consist
mainly of advising the parents on handling. At the appropriate
time, the therapist may also need to encourage the parents not to
baby or over-protect their child. The therapist may well feel she
needs advice from other professionals, but she must also be aware
of the confusion caused by the involvement of too many people.
The appointment of a 'key person' through whom all information
and communication is filtered is often effective.

THE OLDER CHILD/ADULT

If mentally able, the older child should be given some responsibility for decisions regarding treatment aims and methods. The
therapist must be sensitive to the attitudes of his peers, and it
may be best to avoid treating him at school. Communication with
appropriate school staff, however, is essential. Some orthotic
devices may become cosmetically unacceptable, but it may be
possible to compromise with suitable alternatives.

Potential problems, such as increasing spinal deformity with
pain, obesity, dysphagia and incontinence, must be anticipated.
As the child is growing taller and heavier, his parents are ageing
and less able to cope. Home adaptations or alternative accommodation might be required. Power wheelchairs and electronic
aids should be investigated if they have not been already. The
therapist may also become involved in discussions regarding the
patient's sexual needs, and his desire to move away from home or
drive a car.

ORTHOPAEDIC SURGERY IN CEREBRAL PALSY

Orthopaedic surgery in cerebral palsy has no effect on the central
neurological problem, and can only affect the mechanics of movement dictated by it. It should not be viewed as an alternative to

physiotherapy or as a final treatment after physiotherapy has failed, but should form part of the overall management of the child and be carried out when appropriate. General aims of surgery in cerebral palsy are to improve function, alleviate pain, improve cosmesis and/or ease of care and dressing. Any surgical procedure is disruptive and must not be undertaken lightly. There should be strong indications that a significant benefit will be achieved. The intermittent use of corrective plasters on children's feet can often be very effective in maintaining the range of soft tissues, as well as providing a good base of support for improved sitting and standing activities. They can also delay the need for surgery, and give some indication as to the likely effectiveness of a proposed surgical procedure (Cusick and Sussman, 1982). For similar reasons long-leg cylinders applied with the knee in full extension can be useful.

The physiotherapist should provide input regarding pros and cons of surgery. Pre-operatively she should assess range of motion, both passively and in functional positions; strength of relevant muscle groups; and functional ability. Pre- and postoperative management must be well planned and the parents must be prepared. Consideration must be given to positioning of the child postoperatively while in plaster, both while sleeping and for daily activities. If special splints, boots, orthoses, or seating will be needed postoperatively, they should be ordered and obtained at the appropriate time. There are generally two difficult periods of time postoperatively: immediately post-surgery when the child may be in pain and discomfort; and following removal of immobilisation casts, when the limbs often spasm painfully. Mobilisation of the joints must be carried out gradually and carefully. Treatment will also aim to improve postural ability, maintain joint range, strengthen appropriate muscle groups, and support unstable joints.

ORTHOTICS

Many cerebral palsied children require special footwear which will support unstable ankles, or correct, or maintain, deformity. The position of the feet in sitting and standing has a great influence on the position and ability of the rest of the body, and it is important that appropriate footwear is provided. Leather footwear will eventually deform to the feet and must be replaced as necessary. The addition of a heel-retaining strap will help to keep the heel well back in the boot. Support or correction of hindfoot varus or valgus can be accomplished by using an inside or outside iron with a T-strap, or by using a polypropylene ankle-foot orthosis (AFO), which provides more intimate support and is less likely to deform. Some deformities make getting boots on difficult and periodic use of corrective casting (as described previously) can be helpful.

EQUIPMENT

Nowadays, there is a plethora of equipment available. It is not intended to elaborate, but certain points will be made relating to positioning and mobility aids. The Bibliography on page 550 lists some titles which are concerned with aids and equipment.

Seating

Sitting is a position in which many children will spend a good deal of the time and appropriate support is important. Ideally, a number of seats should be available for one child. Seating should not be viewed as something separate from treatment, but should reinforce and reflect the child's ability. A seat should be changed not only when the child physically outgrows it, but also when his level of ability changes. The therapist must, therefore, be involved in prescribing the type and amount of support required. As an example, a very disorganised and/or deformed child should have a seat which will intimately support him, such as a moulded seat or even a hammock seat. Modular or ply-and-padding seating systems are usually appropriate for more able children who are able to be easily placed in sitting but require full support in order to function effectively. In assessing seating needs, the relative height of floors, seats and working surfaces are important (Nelham, 1981, 1984).

Standing

Various devices provide support in standing; they either support in an upright, vertical position, or are inclined forward or backward to varying degrees.

Prone crawlers and sit-on trucks

Some prone crawlers support only the child's trunk in prone and leave the head, arms and legs free for weight-bearing, propulsion and play. They are often more effective if the support can be angled down at the back to prevent the child from falling forward onto his nose and to aid purchase between the knees and the floor. Other prone crawlers leave only the head and arms free and support the rest of the body in one horizontal plane with the legs held in abduction.

Many of the sit-on toys on wheels which are propelled by the feet are useful for some cerebral palsied children.

Walking aids

There is a range of walking aids for various levels of ability. The child who, if given support at the shoulders or upper trunk, can support some of his weight against gravity and step might be able to use a Cheyne nursery walker (Fig. 24/7). Rollators and push

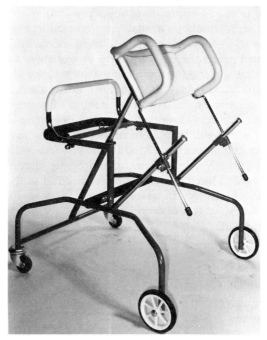

Fig. 24/7 The Cheyne walker

toys are suitable for children with more trunk control, and more able children may be able to progress to sticks; some will progress from quadripods to tripods to canes. For some, Canadian crutches (see p. 359) with loose arm bands are more suitable.

Wheeled mobility

Although the position in a buggy is not ideal, it is usually safe and easy for the parent to use. For children who extend and have difficulty anchoring their bottoms, a Cheyne insert which introduces additional hip flexion is often effective. With older and larger children, wheelchairs with appropriate support can be posturally effective and easier to push over rough ground than buggies. However, the hammock effect of the seat can aggravate problems of asymmetry and instability and should be removed by the use of a shaped cushion or a cushion on top of a flat baseboard. For children requiring total, intimate support, a moulded seat or a shapeable matrix seat can be made to fit into a wheelchair.

Powered mobility

It is becoming evident that provision of powered mobility early on has dramatic benefits in terms of motivation, perception, and socialisation. With new technology, a variety of switches is being developed to allow access to powered chairs. Before switches are investigated for a particular child, it is essential that correct positioning and support are first provided.

REFERENCES

Christenson, E. and Melchior, J. C. (eds.) (1967). *Cerebral Palsy – A Clinical and Neuropathological Study*, CDM No. 25. Spastics International Medical Publications. William Heinemann Medical Books Limited, London.

Cusick, B. and Sussman, M. D. (1982). Short-leg casts: their role in the management of cerebral palsy. *Physical and Occupational Therapy in Pediatrics*, **2**, 2/3, 93–110.

Dunn, P. M. (1976). Congenital postural deformities. *British Medical Bulletin*, **32**, 1, 71–6.

Foley, J. (1977). Cerebral palsy: physical aspects. In *Neurodevelopmental Problems in Early Childhood*, pp. 269–82, (eds. Drillien, C. M. and Drummond, M. B.). Blackwell Scientific Publications Limited, Oxford.

Fulford, G. E. and Brown, J. K. (1976). Position as a cause of deformity in children with cerebral palsy. *Developmental Medicine and Child Neurology*, **18**, 305–14.

Levitt, S. (1984). *Paediatric Developmental Therapy*. Blackwell Scientific Publications Limited, Oxford.

Martin, J. P. (1967). *The Basal Ganglia and Posture*. Pitman Medical, London.

Nelham, R. L. (1981). Seating for the chairbound disabled person. A survey of seating equipment in the United Kingdom. *Journal of Biomedical Engineering*, **3**, 4, 267–73.

Nelham, R. L. (1984). Principles and practice in the manufacture of seating for the handicapped. *Physiotherapy*, **70**, 2, 54–8.

Robson, P. (1968). Persisting head turning in the early months: some effects in the early years. *Developmental Medicine and Child Neurology*, **10**, 82–92.

Scrutton, D. and Gilbertson, M. (1975). The physiotherapist's role in the treatment of cerebral palsy. In *Orthopaedic Aspects of Cerebral Palsy*, CDM No. 52/53. Spastics International Medical Publications. William Heinemann Medical Books Limited, London.

Scrutton, D. (1978). Developmental deformity and the profoundly retarded child. In *Care of the Handicapped Child*, CDM No. 67. Spastics International Medical Publications. William Heinemann Medical Books Limited, London.

Traub, M. M., Rothwell, J. C. and Marsden, C. D. (1980). Anticipatory postural reflexes in Parkinson's disease and other akinetic-rigid syndromes and in cerebellar ataxia. *Brain*, **103**, 393–412.

BIBLIOGRAPHY

Bobath, K. (1980). *A Neurophysiological Basis for the Treatment of Cerebral Palsy*, CDM No. 75. Spastics International Medical Publications. William Heinemann Medical Books Limited, London.

Cotton, E. *Conductive Education and Cerebral Palsy*. The Spastics Society, London.

Egel, P. F. (1948). *Technique of Treatment for the Cerebral Palsy Child*. Henry Kimpton, London.

Finnie, N. (1974). *Handling the Young Cerebral Palsied Child at Home*, 2nd edition. William Heinemann Medical Books Limited, London.

Foley, J. (1983). The athetoid syndrome. A review of a personal series. *Neurology, Neurosurgery and Psychiatry*, **46**, 289–98.

Hare, N. (1984). *Ideas Developed at the Cheyne Centre, 1969–1983*. Friends of the Cheyne Centre for Spastic Children, 63 Cheyne Walk, London.

Kanda, T., Yuge, M., Yamori, Y., Suzuki, J. and Fukase, H. (1984). Early physiotherapy in the treatment of spastic diplegia. *Developmental Medicine and Child Neurology*, **26**, 438–44.

Keshner, E. A. (1981). Re-evaluating the theoretical model underlying the neurodevelopmental theory. *Physical Therapy*, **61**, 7, 1035–40.

Levitt, S. (1984). *Treatment of Cerebral Palsy and Motor Delay*, 2nd edition. Blackwell Scientific Publications Limited, Oxford.

Munton, J. S. (1982). An overview of research on seating. *Engineering in Medicine*, **11**, 3, 107–10.

Pritchett, J. W. (1983). The untreated unstable hip in cerebral palsy. *Clinical Orthopaedics and Related Research*, **173**, 169–72.

Scrutton, D. (1966). Prevention and management of incorrect spinal posture in cerebral palsy. *Developmental Medicine and Child Neurology*, **8**, 322–6.

Scrutton, D. (1976). The physical management of children with hemiplegia. *Physiotherapy*, **62**, 9, 285–93.

Scrutton, D. (ed.) (1984). *Management of the Motor Disorders of Children with Cerebral Palsy*, CDM No. 90. Spastics International Medical Publications. Blackwell Scientific Publications Limited, Oxford.

Cheyne Centre for Spastic Children tape-slide of *Plaster Boots*. Available from Camera Talks, 31 North Row, London W1R 1DJ.

For those interested in the provision of orthoses the following chapters in *Cash's Textbook of Orthopaedics and Rheumatology for Physiotherapists* edited by Patricia A. Downie (1984), published by Faber and Faber, London are helpful:

Chapter 1 *The Mechanics of Lower Limb Orthoses* by John Stallard
Chapter 2 *Biomechanics of Gait* by G. K. Rose
Chapter 3 *Applied Gait Assessment* by P. B. Butler
Chapter 4 *Footwear* by G. K. Rose

ACKNOWLEDGEMENTS

Figures 24/1, 24/4 and 24/6 are adapted from illustrations in *Ideas Developed at the Cheyne Centre 1969–1983* by Noreen Hare. Figure 24/7 is reproduced from *The Physically Handicapped Child: An Interdisciplinary Approach to Management*, edited by G. T. McCarthy, by permission of the publishers, Faber and Faber.

The author gratefully acknowledges the inspiration and guidance of Miss N. Hare MCSP and Dr J. Foley FRCP in the management and treatment of patients with cerebral palsy.

Chapter 25

Spina Bifida and Hydrocephalus

by G. T. McCARTHY MB, FRCP, DCH
and O. R. NETTLES MCSP, ONC

Spina bifida is one of the neural tube defects. These are the group of developmental abnormalities that occur when the neural tube fails to fuse anywhere along its length.

The commonest position of the lesion is in the thoraco-lumbar region of the spine, then lumbo-sacral, thoracic and cervical regions. If the forebrain fails to develop, anencephaly occurs – a condition incompatible with life. An encephalocele lesion may occur anywhere along the midline of the skull, commonly in the occipital region.

The spinal lesion may involve nervous tissue, meninges and bone producing a myelomeningocele. If the defect only involves bone and meninges it is called a meningocele. This is relatively uncommon and may be associated with skin lesions, hair or a naevus.

Spina bifida occulta is a hidden lesion which may only involve a bony defect, but may be associated with abnormalities of the spinal cord, which may be split or tethered or associated with a lipoma causing progressive neurological signs as the child grows.

INCIDENCE

It has been noticed that the prevalence of neural tube defects began to decline in England and Wales after 1972. Between 1972 and 1981 the national notification rate fell from 1.47 per 1000 live and stillbirths to 0.39 for anencephaly, and from 1.88 to 1.04 per 1000 for spina bifida (Leck, 1983).

There is known to be a genetic element in neural tube defects. The Welsh and Irish have a higher incidence than the English, and Europeans a higher incidence than Asians. The risk of recurrence after one affected child is 1 in 20, with a similar risk of the affected person passing the defect on. After two affected children the risk rises to 1 in 10, and after three to 1 in 4. A recent multicentre trial using multivitamins and folic acid periconceptually suggests that prevention of neural tube defects is possible (Smithells et al, 1981; Seller, 1982).

Before the design of the shunt to control hydrocephalus, 90 per cent of all known cases of spina bifida died. Between 1959 and 1969 all affected infants were treated in Sheffield resulting in a unique record of the outcome (Lorber, 1971, 1972). This was followed by a policy of selective treatment (Lorber and Salfield, 1981). A careful study of the results leads to the outline of four prognostic criteria:

1. The degree of paralysis: The greater the paralysis the worse the prognosis, not only in terms of mobility, but also IQ, associated spinal deformity and severe renal complications.
2. Excessive head circumference: If the infant's head circumference at birth is at or above the 90th centile and disproportionate to the weight, the degree of hydrocephalus is usually gross with poor prognosis in terms of IQ.
3. Kyphosis: Kyphosis present at birth has a very poor outlook in terms of later severe deformity, paralysis and incontinence.
4. Associated gross congenital abnormalities or major birth injury: The presence of gross congenital abnormalities such as heart disease or severe birth injury is of the gravest prognostic significance.

HYDROCEPHALUS

Hydrocephalus occurs when there is an increase in cerebrospinal fluid (CSF) circulating in and around the brain. Normally the fluid is produced by the choroid plexuses situated in the cerebral ventricles and circulates through the ventricular system and around the base of the brain to the surface where it is absorbed by the arachnoid granulations into the sagittal sinus. It also circulates around the spinal cord and down the central canal (Fig. 25/1).

If there is a block in the pathway, particularly at the aqueduct or around the base of the brain, the CSF cannot be reabsorbed and pressure begins to build up. In the baby the head is able to grow easily as the sutures of the skull and fontanelles are very flexible (Fig. 25/2).

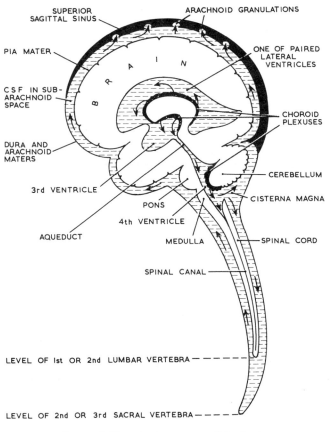

FIG. 25/1 Ventricular system of the brain

Hydrocephalus develops in 80 per cent of children with spina bifida. It may be present at birth, but usually develops after closure of the spinal lesion, when the head circumference rapidly rises. This is caused by a change in the fluid dynamics acting on the Arnold-Chiari malformation which is usually present. The medulla and part of the cerebellum are displaced into the foramen magnum causing a block of the fourth ventricle which is usually incomplete (Fig. 25/3).

Treatment

Until 1956 no effective treatment for hydrocephalus was available, but some time before this a child, whose father, John Holter, was

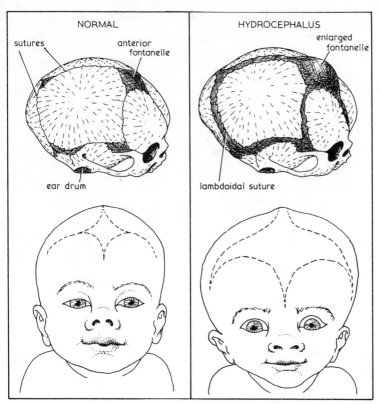

NORMAL

sutures anterior fontanelle

ear drum

HYDROCEPHALUS

enlarged fontanelle

lambdoidal suture

FIG. 25/2 Enlarged fontanelles and separated sutures

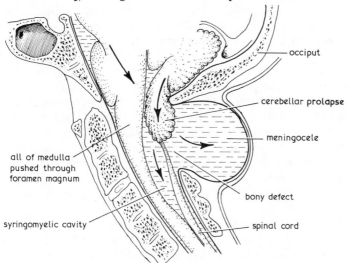

occiput

cerebellar prolapse

meningocele

all of medulla pushed through foramen magnum

bony defect

syringomyelic cavity

spinal cord

FIG. 25/3 Type 3 Arnold-Chiari malformation

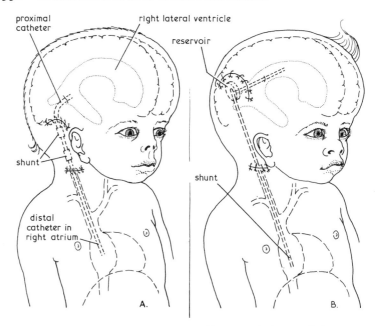

FIG. 25/4 Shunt systems for treatment of hydrocephalus; (a) Spitz-Holter; (b) Pudenz

an engineer, was born in America with this complaint. John Holter and a neurosurgeon, Eugene Spitz, perfected the Spitz-Holter shunt (Fig. 25/4a) which is designed to drain excess CSF from the ventricles into the right atrium of the heart. Other valve systems have been devised, notably the Pudenz shunt (Fig. 25/4b), and more recently shunts which can be switched on and off. Many surgeons use the peritoneal sac, instead of the circulation, to absorb the CSF. The need for lengthening the lower catheter occurs less often, but the catheter may become blocked by adhesions.

The most serious complication of shunt surgery is infection which may involve the brain, causing ventriculitis and severe brain damage. The infection may also cause endocarditis, infected pulmonary emboli, and a type of nephritis. If the lower end is situated in the peritoneum, peritonitis may develop, causing the catheter to block.

The valve system may malfunction or block suddenly or insidiously. In the latter case the child may become irritable or slower in performance, and teachers and therapists often notice these changes first.

Common neurological problems occurring with hydrocephalus are:

1. Spasticity of one or both arms.
2. Cerebellar signs, with clumsiness or inco-ordination and poor balance.
3. Dissociated sensory loss and weakness in the arms and hands associated with syringomyelia.

SPINA BIFIDA CYSTICA (APERTA) (Fig. 25/5)

Meningocele (Fig. 25/5a): The meninges form a sac lined by arachnoid membrane and dura containing cerebrospinal fluid (CSF) and, rarely, a small amount of nervous tissue. It is relatively uncommon (4 per cent of cases of spina bifida cystica) and may be associated with cutaneous lesions. The skin over the sac is usually intact.

Myelomeningocele (Fig. 25/5b): The neural tube is closed and covered by a membrane centrally and skin peripherally, but the spinal cord and all the nerve roots are outside the vertebral canal. In many cases there are associated anomalies of the cord with dilatation of the central canal, lipomata and other associated neural defects, such as split cord or tethering of nerve roots. In rachischeisis there is no sac and the spinal cord is flattened and lies wide open on the surface (Fig. 25/5c).

Assessment of the neonate with spina bifida aperta

Whether or not a policy of selection is carried out, all babies with spina bifida should be examined by a paediatrician or paediatric surgeon experienced in assessing such babies and in their long-term management.

NEUROLOGICAL EXAMINATION

The purpose of the examination is to determine, as far as possible, the level at which normal cord function ceases, and to assess the presence and degree of hydrocephalus.

Skull: The skull should be examined and the sutures and fontanelles palpated for evidence of distension and increased pressure. Measurement of the occipital frontal circumference (OFC) should be carried out and charted, and examination of the optic fundi also carried out, and eye movements noted by stimulation of the optokinetic responses.

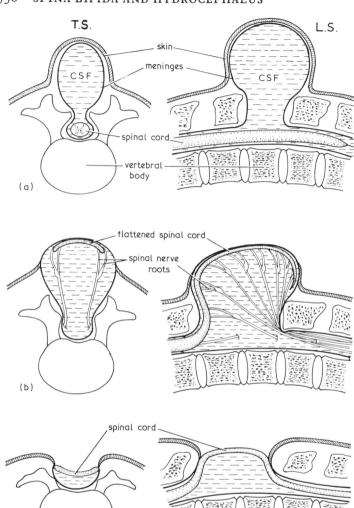

FIG. 25/5 (a) Meningocele; (b) Myelomeningocele; (c) Rachischeisis

Cranial nerves: The cranial nerves may be assessed by observation of the movement of the face, tongue and palate and by watching the baby suck. Occasionally bulbar problems can arise in the newborn period, especially immediately after back closure if hydrocephalus begins to develop rapidly.

Spine: The spine should be palpated along its length as sometimes there are multiple lesions which are not always obvious. The length and width of the lesion should be measured and the position on the spine noted.

Limbs: The presence of active movements of the limbs should be looked for by stimulating the legs and eliciting neonatal reflexes. The power of the muscles may be assessed by making them operate both with and without gravity and with and without resistance, and it is useful to make a muscle chart. Deformities such as talipes and congenital dislocation of the hip should be looked for.

Bowel and bladder: Sphincter tone and bladder function should be assessed, and anal reflex tested by stroking with an orange stick. A patulous anus and dribbling incontinence are associated with a lesion at the level of S2, 3 and 4. Retention of urine is associated with a lesion at S1.

Sensory level: It is difficult to elicit a sensory level in a baby. If he is asleep, it may be possible to produce a level by stimulation with a pin, starting at the lower sacral territory perianal region, buttocks, thighs and legs and moving upwards over successive dermatomes of the anterior surface and on to the abdomen.

Radiological examination of the skull and spine and hips should be carried out, and bacteriological swabs taken from the sac and umbilicus.

TYPES OF LESION

At birth, two types of lesion are recognisable (Stark and Baker, 1967).

Type 1 (one-third of patients): There is complete loss of the spinal cord function below a certain segmental level, which results in sensory loss and absent reflexes. These infants have characteristic deformities of muscle imbalance, the deformity depending on the level of the lesion.

Type 2 (two-thirds of patients): Associated with interruption of the corticospinal tracts. There is preservation of purely reflex activity in isolated distal segments.

There are three sub-groups:

1. Below the level of spinal cord involvement there is a segment with flaccid paralysis and sensory and reflex loss and, below this, isolated cord function with reflex activity and spasticity. Toe clonus may be striking.

2. A flaccid segment is almost absent and, therefore, there is virtually complete spinal cord transection with only reflex activity below the level of the lesion (Stark and Drummond, 1971). On the basis of evidence of clinical and electrodiagnostic studies, it is likely that paralysis in myelomeningocele is due to a lesion of the upper motor neurone (UMN) rather than the lower motor neurone (LMN). In high lesions the UMN lesion tends to occur above the plaque. In low lesions it may occur elsewhere, e.g. within the plaque itself. The UMN lesion may be a primary developmental anomaly, but is more likely to be related to secondary changes occurring before, during or shortly after birth.

3. Incomplete transection of the long tracts occurs, so the child has a spastic paraplegia with some preservation of voluntary movement and sensation. There is also a small group of patients (5 per cent) with a hemi-myelomeningocele in whom one leg is more or less normal, but the other leg is affected by a Type 1 or 2 lesion.

Neonatal physiotherapy

As well as the paediatrician, paediatric or neurosurgeon, orthopaedic surgeon and experienced nursing staff, the spina bifida team also includes a physiotherapist who has a very important role to play from the day the baby is born until be becomes independent.

As soon as the baby is admitted the physiotherapist is called upon to make a physical assessment of the child and this early assessment, if correctly done, can give a fairly accurate indication of the future physical ability of the child. The movement of the legs in some babies appears to improve after the back is repaired, but movement can also be lost after back closure. When an assessment is made after about one year it nearly always relates very closely to the neonatal one.

This assessment – both of movement and sensation – is almost always done with the child in an incubator. It may be done by the paediatrician or it may be the responsibility of the physiotherapist. The baby may have had to travel a long distance to the hospital and been subjected to a lot of examination and handling, so it is vital for the operator to work quickly and efficiently. She needs to be experienced and to have some knowledge of the developmental progress of a normal newborn child for comparison in order to detect the abnormal.

To carry out the assessment the examiner first records her general impressions – abnormal position of limbs, deformities present, movement (if any) and so on. Reflexes are tested as far as possible and then groups of muscles as individual muscle testing is impossible in one so small in the time available (Holgate, 1970). A sensory chart is then completed and to do this the protopathic or deeper feeling is tested with a safety-pin, as testing the epicritic feeling or light touch as with cottonwool is unsatisfactory at this stage. The most reliable test of feeling is whether the baby cries when pricked with the pin. This obviously shows that he has felt it. If the limb moves when pricked, the movement may be an uncontrolled reflex action and is not evidence of sensation.

While the baby is still in hospital, providing he is well enough, the physiotherapist turns her attention to any deformities that may be present. Most common of these is talipes equinovarus and treatment will be according to the wishes of the consultant concerned.

Talipes equinovarus: This may be strapped with zinc oxide or elastic strapping, or treated by splinting. Whichever is used the physiotherapist must remember that the baby has impaired sensation, poor circulation and probably limbs that are in a poor condition generally so that she must be even more careful than usual in applying corrective measures. The limb should be coated with Tinct. Benzoin Co. BPC (to get better adhesion and prevent sores) and a length of 2.5cm strapping attached down the inside of the leg below the knee, around the heel to hold it in the correct position and up the lateral side of the leg to the knee but not over it. The second piece of strapping is to correct the forefront of the foot. It is attached to the dorsum of the foot at the level of the fifth metatarsophalangeal joint, carried across the top of the foot along the line of the joints, under the sole and again up the lateral side of the leg. This is under tension so that the deformity is corrected as far as possible. Some prefer this length of strapping to be started on the plantar side of the fifth metatarsophalangeal joint before being carried across the dorsum, but by using this method there is more danger of constricting the circulation. Short lengths of strapping are then passed around the leg (not under tension) to keep the first two in position. One length around the calf may be enough but a second piece near the ankle may also be necessary. A continuous piece of strapping used as a bandage is not advised in cases of spina bifida because of the poor skin condition and danger to the circulation. Once in position the feet must be watched for any interference in the circulation.

Different consultants like different methods of strapping for talipes equinovarus, but the principle is the same – to strap the foot into eversion and dorsiflexion to correct the varus and equinus (i.e. inversion and plantar flexion) of the feet. Occasionally the feet may lie in a calcaneo-valgus position (in eversion and dorsiflexion) when the strapping or splinting, if used, is into plantar flexion and inversion. In either case the physiotherapist will be called upon to stretch the feet.

As the child grows the foot deformities will be reviewed by the orthopaedic surgeon. Early surgery is rarely indicated unless the deformity is impossible to hold by strapping. A simple tenotomy of the deforming tendon will usually allow further effective correction by conservative means to continue (Fixsen, 1984).

The calcaneo-valgus foot may require surgery if the deformity is severe. Division of overactive dorsiflexors is often helpful. Stabilisation of the subtalar joint by a Grice graft – fusion of the subtalar joint using a small fibular graft – can be helpful once the bones have reached a reasonable size.

The knee: Both flexion and hyperextension may be present at birth. In the first two years passive stretching and splintage should be used to try to mobilise the knee and get as good a passive range of movement as possible.

The hip: Dislocation, subluxation and dysplasia are common. Nowhere has the attitude to orthopaedic treatment changed so much in the last few years (Fixsen, 1984). It is vital to remember that the dislocation is neurological in origin. In the 1960s an aggressive approach to reducing and stabilisation of hips by surgery was strongly advocated. However, this led to large numbers of stiff and sometimes painful hips, which were of no benefit or even a positive disadvantage to the children. Nowadays, if both hips are dislocated, they should nearly always be left alone unless the child has a pure lower motor neurone lesion and is going to be an active community walker, probably without aids at all.

A single dislocated hip should be reduced if the child is going to be a good walker, but not otherwise. If the child has a dislocated hip at birth which is not reducible, it should be left alone until it is clear that he is going to be a good walker. If a hip is dislocated but reducible at birth, a simple abduction broomstick-type splint can be used.

Sometimes a closed adductor tenotomy is all that is required followed by passive stretching.

When the baby is sent home a new but equally important team of workers look after the child and his family. This will include the family doctor and probably a clinical medical officer, the health visitor, district nurse, social services department and a physiotherapist. Later this team will be extended to include a teacher at the child's school.

The physiotherapist is an essential part of this team – she may be the one to act as liaison between the team and the hospital concerned, and her work will include far more than pure physiotherapy. It will be 'healing by physical means' in the truest sense by becoming an adviser in the physical management of the child.

Most spina bifida children are treated in paediatric hospitals with a large catchment area and frequent visits to the outpatient department may be impossible; the physiotherapist becomes a vital link here as she sees the child and parents regularly for treatment. With tact and understanding she can help the family to accept the baby as he is – a normal child born with a disability.

Acceptance by the family from the beginning and their future attitude to the child are very often dependent on the attitudes of the professional people who advise them. If the physiotherapist, while not showing undue optimism, can accentuate what the child *can* do and do her best to improve what is difficult and minimise what is impossible, then not only the family but also the child himself is likely to have a practical outlook for the future.

Physiotherapy

Physiotherapy already started while the child was in hospital should be continued at home for many reasons – to treat any deformities present and to prevent others developing; to encourage what movement there may be in the limbs and to strengthen the muscles producing it; to exercise limbs that the child cannot exercise himself and by so doing improve the circulation; to encourage the child to keep up with his peers in his milestones, i.e. rolling over, crawling, sitting up, and in later stages to teach him to walk in whatever orthoses are necessary.

The experienced physiotherapist will be aware of any particular treatment advocated by the hospital concerned, and a frequent exchange of ideas and information is helpful, but the principles are the same in all cases.

Treatment of any deformities started in hospital will be continued and all joints will be exercised in their full range to prevent contractures. In general the flexor muscles are stronger than the extensors and this especially applies to the hips, even though the difference may be only slight. Hip flexion is often present and with the consent of the orthopaedic surgeon, hip extension stretching should be routine – as well as teaching the mother to place the baby in a prone position during playtime, preferably on the floor. It is hip flexion that causes the marked lordosis that is characteristic of older children with spina bifida.

Any movement present must be noted and encouraged, and if there is any sensation in the legs this can be used to stimulate movement by tickling or touching. There may be little or no sensation present and, until the baby can respond to toys, most of the movement will be passive. These passive movements must be given in as full a range as possible to all joints starting with the toes, then the tarsal joints, ankles, knees and hips. This not only helps to keep them supple but it gives the circulation the pumping action that normal babies provide by their kicking. Mothers must be taught how to carry out these movements and advised to do them each time they change the baby's nappy.

Arm movements can be started as soon as the baby responds and exercises to strengthen the shoulder girdle gradually introduced. This is necessary because most patients with spina bifida will need to rely on sticks or crutches to help them to walk and a strong shoulder girdle is very necessary.

A knowledge of the developmental progress and milestones of a normal child is necessary to be able to assess when a disabled child is ready to be encouraged to attempt another skill such as rolling over, sitting up and even his own brand of crawling (see Chapter 3). The physiotherapist must be alert to his development and start instructing him in the next step just before he is ready for it. The mother is encouraged to prop him up as soon as he shows an interest in his surroundings. In the past, children have become more disabled simply because, having been told that their child is disabled, the parents have not realised and have not been told that their child needs all the challenges and stimuli he can get to develop his potential to the full in the same way as any other baby.

Play therapy forms a very important part of the general physiotherapy. As soon as the baby begins to respond, brightly coloured toys and those that make a noise are excellent to encourage any movement – squeaky toys to press on; coloured balls to push

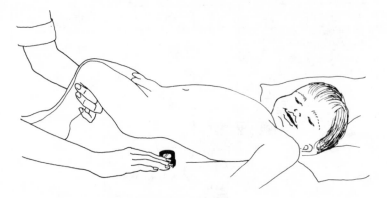

FIG. 25/6 'Bridging' to encourage gluteal contractions

away; 'bridging' to allow a toy motor car to go under is useful for encouraging gluteal contractions (Fig. 25/6); all these activities have a useful place in treatment.

As the child gets older, bigger toys can be introduced – nursery slides to pull *up* rather than slide down, to strengthen the shoulders, and small trampolines to teach the child to sit on an unsteady surface and later to stand on it.

The ingenuity of the physiotherapist will be taxed to the full to make the treatment interesting and so get the child's full co-operation because routine exercises are boring to small children and they rarely respond.

Resisted exercises can be devised to encourage action in muscles which are innervated, i.e. putting baby's feet with knees and hips flexed on one's chest and saying 'push me away' is useful in some sacral lesions where hip and knee action is present, but weak.

If spasticity is present, treatment is given following that used for cerebral palsy (Chapter 24).

Ambulation (Cartwright, 1984)

When the child is ready to stand, usually between 18 months and 2 years, an assessment needs to be made of the degree of support required from the orthosis. At first, more support may be necessary, and can be removed gradually as the child becomes stronger and more confident. Table 25/1 shows the usual degree of support needed according to the neurological level of the lesion. Figure 25/7 shows the relevant muscle innervation.

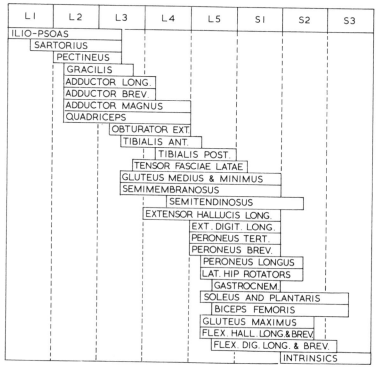

FIG. 25/7 Muscle innervation chart

TABLE 25/1   Ambulation support according to the neurological
level

Level of paralysis	Equipment required
Above L1	Thoraco-lumbar-sacral orthosis (TLSO) with knee-ankle-foot orthoses (KAFOs) Hip guidance orthosis (Rose et al, 1981)
Below L2	TLSO with KAFOs or lumbar-sacral orthosis (LSO) LSO with KAFOs
Below L3-4	LSO with KAFOs or KAFOs
Below L5	KAFOs or AFOs
Below S1	AFOs

ORTHOSES (Figs. 25/8 and 25/9)

If they are to be used successfully, orthoses must become as much part of the child's daily living routine as his clothing. It has been clearly shown that children who require orthoses with pelvic support or higher are very unlikely to use them as adults. They almost invariably prefer to use a wheelchair, and it is important to be realistic about the aims in these children. There are positive gains to standing and walking, even for a short time in childhood. Circulation is improved as the child starts to move and kidney function is also facilitated. A change of posture is important so that standing, even without walking, is worth while in a small child, and a standing table may be used for him to play on or to be used as a desk in the schoolroom when he is older.

The child with the high lesion requires a pelvic or thoracic band for support, and he usually needs a Rollator walker initially; he learns to move by a swivel movement, changing weight from one leg to the other. He may then go on to a 'jump-to' gait, either using the Rollator walker or parallel bars. The length of time taken to progress to using quadripod sticks, independent sticks or

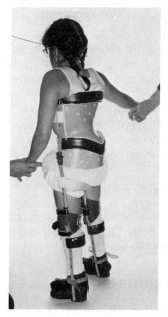

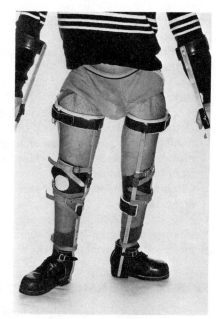

FIG. 25/8 TLSO with KAFOs   FIG. 25/9 KAFOs

crutches varies tremendously according to the child's self-confidence and personality, and also to the enthusiasm and encouragement given to the child by the parents. A swing-through gait using crutches allows for rapid movement and is achieved by many children, even with high lesions. Some very active children may damage their ankle and knee joints by over-enthusiastic walking, especially using a swing-through gait. Parents need to be informed and realistic about the aims of walking and the use of orthoses, and encourage the child to continue at home under the supervision of a physiotherapist.

The hip guidance orthosis (hgo) was developed for children with high lesions with a relatively poor prognosis for long-term walking (Rose et al, 1981) (see p.362).

In the more severely handicapped child, a wheelchair will be used and seating must be looked at regularly as the child grows. Transfers and press-ups must be practised daily and the child taught to transfer from one position to another when on his feet or in a wheelchair.

Before starting primary education, the therapist (occupational therapist (OT) or physiotherapist) and the parents will need to visit the chosen school to look at access to toilets, classroom and playground and talk to the teachers and school helpers. A supportive role is then established so that when difficulties arise the therapist will be contacted.

Parents need advice and encouragement in the management of the orthosis:

1. Toes may become curled inside a boot and produce pressure sores.
2. A regular check of boot size needs to be made.
3. Orthoses, jackets and boots can rub sores very quickly, and regular inspection of the anaesthetic areas must become a routine. Red areas will develop and need to be distinguished from true pressure sores.
4. Clothing must be pulled down to prevent pressure under the orthosis.
5. Nappies are difficult to apply, especially when the child is wearing a thoraco-lumbar-sacral orthosis (TLSO), and nappies need to be well out of the way of orthoses.

SPINAL DEFORMITY IN SPINA BIFIDA

Spinal deformity commonly develops in high or severe spina bifida lesions. It arises for a number of reasons and may be present at birth, when the prognosis is very poor. All the curves are progressive, particularly at adolescence.

Structural abnormality of the vertebrae:
The vertebrae may be malformed – hemivertebrae are not uncommon, and there may be fusion of part of the vertebra leading to abnormal growth and increasing curvature. In cases with wide open spina bifida there is loss of posterior stability and kyphosis occurs.

Paralytic curves:
These are related to muscle imbalance and become worse with growth. Many are associated with deformity in the anterior-posterior plane causing lordo-scoliosis or kypho-scoliosis.

Often curves are caused by a mixture of structural abnormality and paralysis, and are complicated by pelvic obliquity (Fig. 25/10).

Treatment

Bracing: The general indications for bracing are: a small curve under 45° which remains flexible, and remaining growth potential.

Braces will not affect the progression of a structural curve, or a large curve over 50° which has become stiff, or where growth has ceased. Nevertheless in certain situations a brace is the only realistic method of control in the severely handicapped, and in these cases the rationale for its use must be clearly understood by the parents, child and the staff caring for the child.

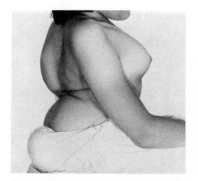 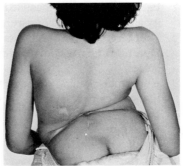

FIG. 25/10 A mixed structural and paralytic curve – lordo-scoliosis made worse by pelvic obliquity. (a) lateral; (b) posterior

Surgical techniques:

(a) In some instances minor surgery may prevent serious progression. This is particularly useful in congenital curves with a localised area of uneven growth, and should be done early.

(b) Spinal corrective procedures are usually carried out between 10 and 13 years. Both anterior and posterior surgery is usually required – distracting the spine with a Harrington rod and fusing the spine posteriorly (Morley, 1984).

Postoperative treatment: Immediately postoperatively no brace is worn. At about 2 weeks the child is allowed to sit in a brace which is worn at all times except when lying flat. This is maintained until the fusion is solid, usually between 10 and 12 months.

MANAGEMENT OF ANAESTHETIC SKIN

From birth the mother has to be vigilant in the care of anaesthetic skin. Friction from crawling, hot liquids and pressure from shoes and appliances may cause problems. Poor skin and tissue cover over a prominent kyphos may easily be damaged by pressure and lead to ulceration. Regular inspection of the anaesthetic areas must be carried out by the mother while the child is young, and as soon as the child is able to take responsibility he must learn to examine himself, using a mirror for the back and bottom. Bathtime is a good time for this.

Pressure sores

Pressure sores almost inevitably develop in some children. The factors involved are:

1. Excessive pressure localised to a small area, caused by deformity and asymmetrical posture.
2. Poor circulation of both blood and lymph.
3. Optimum micro-climate-wet skin, contaminated with urine or faeces.
4. Abnormal skeletal structures, e.g. prominent kyphosis, scar tissue over excess callus formation following orthopaedic surgery.
5. Scar tissue associated with poor subcutaneous tissue following closure of back lesion.

All of these factors are exacerbated by the absence of sensation which normally stimulates alteration of posture before tissue necrosis occurs.

PREVENTION

Buttocks: Good basic hygiene, with a daily bath, combined with control of incontinence is the first consideration. The sitting posture is also of great importance, and the use of a cushion carefully chosen to minimise the danger of excessive pressure localised to a small area. In addition the child should be encouraged to lift the pelvis off the seat several times each hour.

Lower limbs: Great care should be taken in the fitting of orthoses and in providing extra padding for postoperative plasters. Paralytic toes should be uncurled before the shoe is laced up.

Spine: Pressure areas related to spinal deformities can be protected by the use of Stomahesive applied directly to the skin.

Lumbar sympathectomy in some cases improves circulation in the legs.

MANAGEMENT

Conservative: The essential is to provide effective relief of pressure. In the buttock area this can sometimes be achieved by the use of a chip-foam cushion with a cut-out area over the vital point, but it will often be necessary to avoid sitting until sound healing has occurred; the use of a self-propelled prone trolley can be a useful aid in such circumstances. For the legs plaster of Paris or Baycast splints – changed weekly – can be a most effective aid in relieving pressure.

Local preparations: Initially, when necrosis and infection are present, the twice-daily application of eusol and paraffin emulsion is most effective. Once the area is clean, sterile petroleum jelly gauze impregnated with chlorhexidine (Bactigras) provides a mild stimulus to the formation of granulation tissue; excess granulation will need the application of silver nitrate.

Once the ulcer is well healed, careful massage with grease can mobilise adherent scars, so reducing the risk of recurrence.

Minor surgery: The healing process can be accelerated by the excision of necrotic tissue and fibrotic areas. Traumatising the edge of an indolent ulcer will stimulate the inflammatory reaction and so promote healing.

Plastic surgery: While most pressure sores arise from without, others are due to shearing forces. The latter can cause a deep breakdown of tissue, with the formation of bursae which can be very extensive. Final ulceration through the skin will then lead to communication into the bursa. Surgical excision of the bursa, combined with a rotation flap, is then required.

MANAGEMENT OF NEUROGENIC BLADDER AND BOWEL

Most spina bifida children with paralysis of the legs will have some degree of neurogenic bladder and bowel. This will lead to incontinence and may become the greatest barrier to normal life.

In the past few years there has been a change in management of the bladder problems. It is helpful to carry out urodynamic studies on the bladder which show how the bladder functions. There are several patterns of abnormality:

1. The hyper-reflexic bladder with poor sphincter tone which continuously empties but is safe.
2. The moderately reflexic bladder with inco-ordination between bladder and sphincter – 'detrusor-sphincter dyssynergia'. This may result in the bladder incompletely emptying, causing a rise in pressure in the bladder and reflux up the ureters.
3. In some cases the sphincter does not relax fully and the bladder contracts against the closed sphincter, and becomes dilated and trabeculated and a source of infection. This type of bladder is very dangerous and may seriously damage the kidneys very rapidly if unrecognised.

Methods of management of incontinence

1. Clean intermittent catheterisation is a means of management which has been introduced in the past few years. Sometimes drugs need to be added to give a good result. Most children can learn to catheterise themselves independently, and there does not appear to be any increase in infection in this group. The pressure problems are allayed, and improvement in the upper urinary tracts has occurred in many cases.
2. Boys who have safe urodynamics may prefer to wear a urinary appliance such as a sheath or a pubic pressure urinal.
3. Not all cases can be managed by intermittent catheterisation and an indwelling catheter is sometimes used successfully.
4. Urinary diversion used to be a common method of managing incontinence in girls and also in treating cases where renal damage was occurring from back pressure. A loop of ileum or

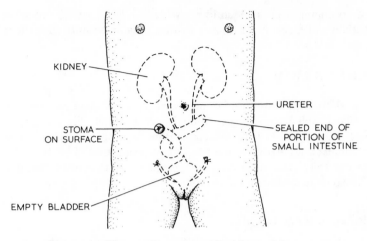

KIDNEY

URETER

STOMA
ON SURFACE

SEALED END OF
PORTION OF
SMALL INTESTINE

EMPTY BLADDER

FIG. 25/11 Uretero-ileostomy or ileal loop with stoma

colon is isolated and one end brought out on to the abdomen and the ureters inserted. The ileal loop acts as a conduit or drainage sac (Fig. 25/11). Unfortunately it has been shown that the ileal loop may become atonic and produce back pressure on the kidneys. Some cases are being reversed with augmentation of the bladder to allow intermittent catheterisation.

5. Artificial sphincters: In the past few years the implantation of an artificial sphincter has become possible which allows the bladder to be emptied regularly with continence between.

Bowel control

Some 90 per cent of people with spina bifida have a neurogenic bowel with problems of control. Anal tone is frequently weak at birth, but gradually increases with age. In some cases the sphincter tone may be completely absent. It is important that the bowel is trained as far as possible and is not allowed to become overdistended. In children with some sphincter tone, toilet training can usually be achieved by a regular time of evacuation schedule which is continued indefinitely.

Type 2 lesion: In children with no sphincter tone there may be frequent soiling with the smallest rectal contraction. In this situation frequent defaecation and careful dietary management is necessary to try to maintain a firm stool. It is helpful to empty the bowel before exercise and swimming. Unfortunately this type of sphincter occurs in children with low lesions who are more active, and faecal incontinence can be a major disability for them.

EDUCATION

Children with spina bifida and hydrocephalus often have educational problems relating to their hydrocephalus. They need full educational assessment which is done by the educational psychologist who institutes the 'statement procedure'. This is related to the 1981 Education Act and provides a statement of the individual child's educational needs.

Independence training

As more children with spina bifida are reaching adult life it has been shown that they often need special training to achieve independence, particularly if they are home-based. The Association of Spina Bifida and Hydrocephalus runs independence training courses for young people. Many boarding schools also have expertise in helping young people in this way.

THE ADULT WITH SPINA BIFIDA

A large number of young people with spina bifida and all its complications are now reaching adult life. Their medical problems make the adjustments we all have to make on reaching maturity even more difficult. Some will always require sheltered care because of the severity of their handicaps, but they will have the same hopes and aspirations as anyone else.

Sadly, there will be continuing morbidity and mortality from the complications. In a recent survey of adult spina bifida sufferers attending a clinic in Sheffield, (Rickwood et al, 1984) there was a 1 per cent mortality per year in the 205 cases followed up since 1976.

The continuing bladder and kidney problems are a major cause of illness and disability. Pressure sores tend to become a problem in adults, and seating with correct cushions is essential. The valve systems may also malfunction even after many years.

In the women pregnancy is possible but hazardous in the presence of urinary diversions, spinal deformity and renal impairment.

The young men need advice on their sexual performance which may be given by an experienced urologist, or in a spinal injuries centre.

The continued medical follow-up of these young people is a cause for concern. In some areas regional clinics are operating to give multidisciplinary care, but there is no coherent plan for the country as a whole.

In spite of all their problems many young people are living independently and working or studying. They intend to make the most of the present that they and their parents have worked so hard to achieve.

REFERENCES

Cartwright, R. (1984). Spina bifida and hydrocephalus. In *The Physically Handicapped Child*, pp. 92–7, (ed. McCarthy, G. T.). Faber and Faber, London.

Fixsen, J. A. (1984). Spina bifida and hydrocephalus. In *The Physically Handicapped Child*, pp. 86–90, (ed. McCarthy, G. T.). Faber and Faber, London.

Holgate, L. (1970). *Physiotherapy for Spina Bifida*. Available from Queen Mary's Hospital, Carshalton, Surrey.

Leck, I. (1983). Epidemiological clues to the causation of neural tube defects. In *Prevention of Spina Bifida and Other Neural Tube Defects* (ed. Dobbing, J.). Academic Press, London.

Lorber, J. (1971). Results of treatment of myelomeningocele. An analysis of 524 unselected cases. *Developmental Medicine and Child Neurology*, **13**, 279.

Lorber, J. (1972). Spina bifida cystica. Results of treatment of 270 consecutive cases with criteria for selection for the future. *Archives of Disease in Childhood*, **47**, 854.

Lorber, J. and Salfield, S. A. W. (1981). Results of selective treatment of spina bifida cystica. *Archives of Disease in Childhood*, **56**, 822–30.

Morley, T. R. (1984). Spina bifida and hydrocephalus. In *The Physically Handicapped Child*, pp. 186–200, (ed. McCarthy, G. T.). Faber and Faber, London.

Rickwood, A. M. K., Hodgson, J., Lonton, A. P. and Thomas, D. G. (1984). Medical and surgical complications in adolescent and young adult patients with spina bifida. *Health Trends*, **4**, 16, 91–5.

Rose, G. K., Stallard, J. and Sankarantutty, M. (1981). Clinical evaluation of spina bifida patients using hip-guidance orthoses. *Developmental Medicine and Child Neurology*, **23**, 30–40.

Seller, M. J. (1982). *Paediatric Research: A Genetic Approach. Neural Tube Defects – Cause and Prevention*. Spastics International Medical Publications. William Heinemann Medical Books Limited, London.

Smithells, R. W. et al (1981). Apparent prevention of neural tube defects by periconceptual vitamin supplementation. *Archives of Disease in Childhood*, **56**, 911–18.

Stark, G. D. and Baker, C. W. (1967). The neurological involvement of the lower limbs in myelomeningocele. *Developmental Medicine and Child Neurology*, **9**, 732.

Stark, G. D. and Drummond, M. (1971). The spinal cord lesion in myelomeningocele. *Developmental Medicine and Child Neurology*, **13** (Supp.25), 1.

BIBLIOGRAPHY

Nettles, O. R. (1979). *Counselling Parents of Children with Handicaps*. Tappenden Print Company Limited, Crawley, Sussex.

The following booklets are available from the Association for Spina Bifida and Hydrocephalus (ASBAH (address, p. 638). A price list will be sent on request (please enclose a stamped addressed envelope).
The Effects of Hydrocephalus on Vocational and Non-vocational Training. A research project by L. Holgate (1982).
Further Education and Vocational Training of Young People with Spina Bifida and Hydrocephalus. A report of a project by R. Gueliford and H. Benner (1982).
The Nursery Years by S. Haskell and M. Paull.
The Handwriting of Spina Bifida Children by J. Cambridge and E. M. Anderson.
Children with Spina Bifida at School.
Sex for Young People with Spina Bifida and Cerebral Palsy.
The ASBAH fact sheets are available in many languages.
The following booklets are available from the Scottish Spina Bifida Association (address p. 638).
The Spina Bifida Baby by O. R. Nettles (1982).
Growing Up with Spina Bifida by O. R. Nettles (1979).
Keeping Fit by J. M. Temple.
Self-help with Spina Bifida by E. Wilson and E. Taylor.

ACKNOWLEDGEMENT

Mrs O. R. Nettles wishes to thank all her friends and colleagues in the Association of Paediatric Chartered Physiotherapists who have so willingly helped in the revision of this chapter.

Chapter 26

Muscular Dystrophy – Clinical

by G. P. HOSKING MB, MRCP, DCH

The term 'muscular dystrophy' was first introduced during the last century, principally within the context of disordered structure of muscles seen on microscopic examination; only later to be applied by convention to a number of differing disorders. What these disorders have in common are, first, a hereditary nature and, second, a primary involvement of voluntary muscles and with this a tendency towards a progressive deterioration because of a gradual destruction or necrosis of muscle.

In the early stages of a muscular dystrophy there is a characteristic involvement of muscle in highly selective patterns. It is these patterns, together with the rate of progression and the mode of inheritance, that serve as the most effective basis for the separation of the different forms of muscular dystrophy and their resultant classification.

The structural abnormalities seen on muscle biopsies show considerable overlap between the different dystrophy, and by themselves are an unreliable means of differentiating one form from another.

The most common form of muscular dystrophy – and the most severe – is that which was described by Duchenne (Duchenne, 1868) and subsequently referred to as either Duchenne type muscular dystrophy (DMD) or the pseudohypertrophic form of muscular dystrophy.

CAUSATION

Over the years there have been a number of theories concerning the pathogenesis of the muscular dystrophies as a whole, and DMD in particular. Perhaps one of the earliest was the so-called 'neurogenic theory'. This postulated that the primary problem was in the nerve supply to the muscles rather than in the muscles themselves (McComas et al, 1970), and this has been suggested by some as the explanation for the high association of intellectual impairment in DMD boys. In spite of some strong evidence to support the neurogenic hypothesis in the late 1960s and early 1970s, the main body of opinion is now against this as being the underlying fault. Another theory of causation has been the 'vascular theory', in which it was suggested that the problem in the muscles was secondary to an impairment in their blood supply (Hathaway et al, 1970). Some elegant experiments were conducted which lent support to this hypothesis. But overall the weight of evidence now seems to be against the vascular theory. Currently, what appears to be the most likely explanation for the changes seen in the muscles of dystrophy patients is a primary disorder of the muscle membrane – the 'membrane theory'. The impairment of membrane function is not confined to the muscle membrane but also exists in the membranes of other tissues. Abnormalities may be found in the red and white blood cells of boys with DMD, although this is not always a consistent finding. This apparent impairment of membrane function has been thought to explain why a number of studies have revealed a high intracellular accumulation of calcium – the membrane is said to be 'leaky' (Rowland, 1976; Emery and Burt, 1980).

PRINCIPLES OF DIAGNOSIS

The diagnosis of muscular dystrophy depends upon a combination of a family history and clinical observations of the functional impairment due to muscle weakness, coupled with a careful examination of individual muscle groups to determine the patterns of selective involvement.

The clinical evaluation of a patient with a suspected muscular dystrophy is usually accompanied by some specific investigations:

Creatinine phosphokinase (CPK): CPK is an enzyme present in high concentrations in skeletal muscle and some other tissues. Damage to a muscle, whether as the result of a primary muscle disorder or secondary to some other disease or trauma, may give rise to a leak of CPK into the bloodstream and higher than usual levels in the blood. The highest levels are usually in primary muscle disorders with particularly high levels being found in DMD.

Electrophysiological examination – electromyography (EMG): Examination of the electrical activity of an active muscle may be carried out using a needle electrode and the recording of muscle action potentials is made on an electronic recording apparatus. In the neuromuscular disorders abnormal action potentials will be found and the different types of abnormalities help to differentiate neuropathic from myopathic conditions.

Muscle biopsy: Muscle biopsies are carried out in the majority of patients in whom a neuromuscular disorder is strongly suspected, especially in possible dystrophies. Samples can be obtained either by means of a small surgical technique or a special muscle biopsy needle. Either procedure can be undertaken under local anaesthetic. Careful handling of the small muscle samples is needed and specialised techniques for staining these are essential. This is a procedure that should not be undertaken by laboratories unfamiliar with processing muscle biopsies.

Other investigations: Abnormalities in the electrocardiograph (ECG) are found in a number of patients with neuromuscular disorders and this form of examination is often undertaken.

In some neuromuscular disorders there will be an identifiable metabolic dysfunction so that appropriate investigations will be undertaken. This is unlikely to be necessary if the disorder in question is thought to be a muscular dystrophy.

DIAGNOSTIC DIFFICULTIES

There are a large number of muscular dystrophies, varying not only in their prevalence, but their genetic patterns, age of onset, early selective involvement of muscle groups and the rate of progression. At times it may be difficult to decide whether an individual has a form of muscular dystrophy or one of the spinal muscular atrophies. The distinction between a dystrophy and a spinal muscular atrophy requires a combination of careful clinical examination and specific investigations. Even then at times it may be difficult to decide which is the underlying disease.

DUCHENNE MUSCULAR DYSTROPHY (DMD)

Duchenne dystrophy is not only the most severe of the muscular dystrophies but also the most common, and this chapter will confine itself to discussing the clinical features and course of this disease.

The incidence of DMD is 1 in 3000-3500 male births. It is sex-linked and therefore occurs only in boys, although transmitted by 'carrier' females. In two-thirds of boys the disease is inherited from a carrier, who most usually will not exhibit any neuromuscular symptoms.

Early history

There are no abnormalities in early infancy but 50 per cent of boys with DMD are not walking at 18 months. While in the early months of walking no major concerns may be expressed it soon becomes apparent that the young boy with DMD is less active than his peers. He walks more slowly, falls more frequently, does not run - or run normally - and climbs stairs only with difficulty.

More frequently than not mothers of young DMD boys are 'reassured', the boys being 'diagnosed' as either flat-footed, clumsy or lazy. Not infrequently the mother may be diagnosed as over-anxious or inexperienced.

With time, certainly by the age of 4 years, the slightly lordotic stance and the waddling gait, combined with the perceived locomotor difficulties serve to increase diagnostic suspicions that there may be a significant muscle weakness. The diagnosis of DMD is often not suspected by a doctor until between 4 and 5 years, this being very often two or more years after parental concern was first expressed.

Clinical findings

The informal observations of a young boy with DMD should commence with watching him walk. Even when under the age of 3 years the gait will be generally clumsy, slow and, by 4 to 5 years, the lumbar lordosis and waddling gait will at least begin to be apparent. A boy will be unable to jump up even a very small step and attempts at running will at best produce a 'fast walk'. Climbing stairs will be slow and laborious with always the assistance of the arms to pull himself up. In getting up from the floor this will always start with the boy going into prone and, depending on age, using his hands to some extent to assist in standing up. At any time from about 4 to 5 years onwards the typical Gowers' manœuvre will be seen (Fig. 26/1).

In a number of boys even informal observations may raise the suspicion of at least a degree of intellectual impairment (see p. 585). This at times may be such as to divert attention away from the motor deficits.

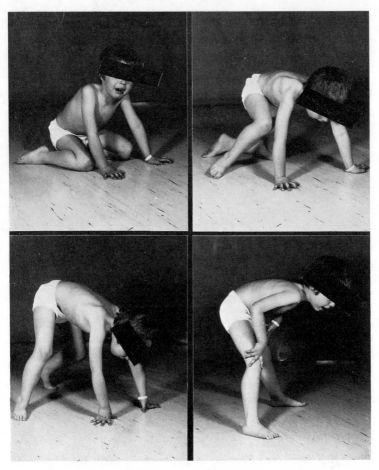

FIG. 26/1 Gowers' sign in a boy with muscular dystrophy

Examination will reveal hypotonia at the shoulders, apparent when attempting to lift the boy with axillary traction, early hypertrophy of some muscles – particularly the calves, lateral vasti, deltoids, the extensor muscles of the forearm and the temporalis muscles, and weakness initially in the brachioradialis, costal head of the pectoralis major, latissimus dorsi, biceps, triceps, ilio psoas, hip extensors, medial vasti of quadriceps and rectus femoris.

With the progression of the disease there tends to be better power retained in the distal muscles than in the proximal, in the hamstrings than quadriceps, in deltoids than biceps or triceps, in wrist flexors than extensors, in neck extensors than flexors and

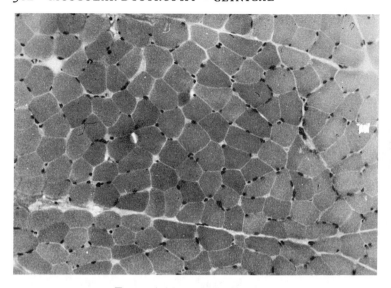

FIG. 26/2 Normal muscle biopsy

in inverters and plantar flexors of the feet than in everters and dorsiflexors (Gardner-Medwin, 1980). The hypertrophic muscles become 'pseudohypertrophic' with time due to infiltration by fat and fibrous tissue.

Tendon reflexes may eventually be lost, although those of the ankle tend to be preserved.

Investigations

The CPK will be extremely high, even in early infancy before the clinical features of DMD emerge. With increasing age the levels will drop, but never to normal.

The EMG will give a characteristic myopathic picture with an abundance of small short duration polyphasic muscle action potentials.

The muscle biopsy will show extensive abnormalities with great variation in the size of the fibres, the nuclei of the fibres migrated towards the centre of the fibres, and accompanied by widespread fat and fibrous tissue infiltration (Figs. 26/2 and 26/3). It is this increased fat and fibrous tissue which gives the impression of increased muscle bulk (pseudohypertrophy).

The ECG is very frequently abnormal in boys with DMD even though cardiac disease as such is rare except terminally.

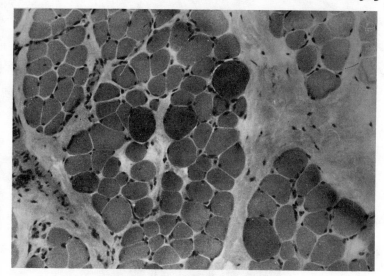

FIG. 26/3 Muscle biopsy showing typical histology findings in Duchenne muscular dystrophy

Clinical course

In a significant minority of boys with DMD there may be little in the way of functional deterioration between 4 and 6 years. Some may even show an improvement in their locomotor function. But for the majority there is from the time of diagnosis a relentless deterioration.

A lordosis (Fig. 26/4) and the Gowers' manoeuvre are obvious and fully developed in practically all boys by the age of 6 years. Frequency of falls will increase and getting up from the floor (and chairs) will be a more laborious exercise until the ability to do so is completely lost. Few can manage stairs much after the age of 8 years.

Towards the end of the ambulatory phase of DMD contractures start to develop resulting partly from the posture the boys have to adopt. These may often be asymmetrical and are prominent in the calves and the tensor fasciae latae.

The age at which the ability to walk is completely lost will vary between 7 years at the earliest and 12 to 14 at the latest. Very often 'going off the feet' will seem to be precipitated by a specific illness or a period (even short) of immobility.

Soon after losing the ability to walk boys with DMD will begin

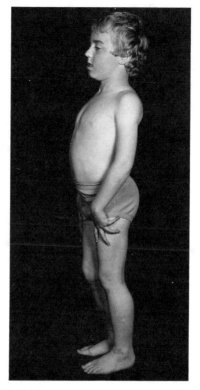

FIG. 26/4 Typical lordotic posture seen in Duchenne muscular dystrophy

to have significant impairment of upper limb function to the extent that electrically powered wheelchairs are needed (see p. 598).

By the early teens muscle weakness is extreme and extensive. Dependency will develop for dressing, bathing and toileting and turning in bed at night.

Joint contractures develop at the hips, knees, elbows and wrists and in the majority the lumbar lordosis is replaced by a kyphoscoliosis.

Respiratory insufficiency gradually develops throughout the course of the disease and by the teenage years chest infections aggravated by the presence of ˄ scoliosis, become a serious threat to survival.

Death will ultimately occur any time from the mid-teens to, in extreme cases, the mid-twenties, most usually from an overwhelming respiratory infection.

There is no specific treatment for DMD, although physical management can help maintain independence for as long as possible. This will be fully discussed in Chapter 27.

Associated problems

Intellect: The mean IQ in DMD is between 70–85 with some boys having very low intelligence, others impairment in relation to verbal skills, but some with normal or above normal intelligence. The intelligence does not deteriorate with age (Worden and Vignos, 1962).

Skeletal abnormalities: Reference has already been made to the development of a variety of joint contractures. Some of the most important are the development of a scoliosis and deformities around the feet and ankles. In addition to contractures, fractures of grossly osteoporotic bones may readily occur.

Bowels: Constipation for many becomes a major problem once they are no longer ambulant. This may become severe enough to cause not only discomfort but overflow incontinence.

Bladder function: Urinary incontinence is not a specific feature of DMD but it does occur either because attendants do not respond quickly enough to requests for assistance (or the boys do not ask early enough) or in conjunction with severe constipation.

Vomiting: Uncontrolled vomiting may occasionally occur in the wheelchair bound boy due to pressure of the superior mesenteric vessels on the third part of the duodenum. This occurs most commonly in boys who retain their lumbar lordosis. Surgery may be necessary

Obesity: Obesity is very common in the chairbound boy with DMD and is virtually impossible (or inappropriate) to treat at this stage. The only treatment is prevention.

Pressure sores: Pressure sores may develop, particularly in the obese chairbound boy.

Emotional difficulties: (a) *In the family*. The diagnosis of DMD comes to parents as an enormous shock, certainly as soon as the full implication of the diagnosis is realised. Paradoxically, for some, it comes as a bizarre relief after the years of being 're-assured' that no problem exists.

The acceptance of the diagnosis becomes impossible for some, and the stage when the boys are no longer able to walk serves only to emphasise for all the inexorable progression of the disease. Intra-family relationships are put to a very great strain and it is often fathers who find the progression of the disease most hard to accept. Marital break-up is common, with the mother being left to meet the heavy physical and emotional demands of a severely handicapped teenager. The eventual death of the young man with DMD does not necessarily, after years of caring, bring with it the emotional and physical relief that others might have expected (Firth et al, 1983).

(b) *In the boy/young man.* While the implications of the diagnosis of DMD are (or should be) fully discussed with the parents, this seldom happens for the boy himself. He is left to work out by himself – which he inevitably does – what his fate is to be. The death of a schoolfriend or an older affected brother leaves him in no doubt. Equally, as much as this realisation, is the one that he is different to other boys or young men of his age. He will have a poor body image so that he is reluctant to be undressed in front of relative strangers, he is unable to live out any of his (normal) sexual fantasies, he will not be able to masturbate, and in both school and home he will be dependent more often than not on a female to attend to his most basic daily needs. It is frequently remarked that the DMD teenager lacks 'motivation': the reasons for this very valid observation must be obvious.

Genetic counselling

As already stated, in two-thirds of boys with DMD the mother will be a carrier. In half this may be obvious on the basis of the family history which demonstrates a pattern of an X-linked in-heritance. In the remainder, estimates of the risks of the mother being a carrier should be undertaken through a combination of CPK estimates, (the CPK being elevated in between 60 to 80 per cent of carriers) and an examination of the family pedigree. Great care is needed to ascertain the risks of not only the mother being a carrier, but any of her sisters and her daughters. The services of a geneticist are invariably required.

In a small number of mothers who are carriers there will be some clinical evidence of muscle weakness. These mothers are referred to as 'manifest carriers' and in them the CPK will always be high.

In more recent times the identification of a carrier for DMD (or the exclusion of this possibility) has apparently been advanced by the development of DNA gene probes. These very new techniques are extremely promising but as yet have not reached the point of direct clinical application in genetic counselling (Harper, 1984).

Screening

There is currently no reliable means of antenatal diagnosis for DMD. In the case of a carrier mother the current practice has been to offer to terminate any pregnancy with a male fetus, still leaving 50 per cent of female fetuses as carriers.

It is, however, possible to detect even in early infancy a male infant with DMD using CPK analysis on dried blood–spot samples. This has given rise to considerable controversy over the wisdom and ethics of such screening for a condition with as yet no specific treatment, notwithstanding the advantages for genetic counselling (Firth, 1983)

An alternative screening strategy that has been advocated is the performance of CPK estimates on all boys not walking at 18 months. This might enable appropriate genetic counselling to be given with as much effect as with neonatal screening (Gardner-Medwin, 1979).

REFERENCES

Duchenne, G. B. (1868). Recherches sur la paralysie musculaire pseudohypertophique ou paralysie myosclerosique. *Archives of General Medicine*, (6 Ser), **11**, 5–25, 179–209, 305–21, 421–43, 552–88.

Emery A. E. H. and Burt, D. (1980). Intracellular calcium and pathogenesis and antenatal diagnosis of Duchenne muscular dystrophy. *British Medical Journal*, **280**, 355–7.

Firth, M. A. (1983). Diagnosis of Duchenne muscular dystrophy experiences of parents of sufferers. *British Medical Journal*, **286**, 700–1.

Firth, M. A., Gardner-Medwin, D., Hosking, G. and Wilkinson, E. (1983). Interviews with parents of boys suffering from Duchenne muscular dystrophy. *Developmental Medicine and Child Neurology*, **25**, 466–71.

Gardner-Medwin, D. (1979). Controversies about Duchenne muscular dystrophy. 1. Neonatal screening. *Developmental Medicine and Child Neurology*, **21**, 390-3.

Gardner-Medwin, D. (1980). Clinical features and classification of the muscular dystrophies. *British Medical Bulletin*, **36**, 109-15.

Harper, P. (1984). DNA markers and Duchenne muscular dystrophy (annotation). *Archives of Diseases of Childhood*, **59** 195-6.

Hathaway, P. W., Engel, W. K. and Zellweger, H. (1970). Experimental myopathy after micro-anterial embolization - comparison with childhood X-linked pseudohypertrophic muscular dystrophy. *Archives of Neurology* (Chicago), **22**, 365-78.

McComas, A. J., Sica, R. E. P. and Currie, S. (1970). Muscular dystrophy: evidence for a neural defect. *Nature* (London), **226**, 1263-4.

Rowland, L. P. (1976). Pathogenesis of muscular dystrophies. *Archives of Neurology*, **33**, 315-21.

Worden, D. K. and Vignos, P. J. (1962). Intellectual function in childhood progressive muscular dystrophy. *Pediatrics*, **29**, 968-77.

BIBLIOGRAPHY

Dubowitz, V. (1978). *Muscle Disorders in Childhood*. W. B. Saunders Co, London and Philadelphia.

Walton, J. N. and Mastaglia, F. L. (1980). The muscular dystrophies. *British Medical Bulletin*, **36**, 2.

Chapter 27

Muscular Dystrophy – Management

by R. CARTWRIGHT MCSP

Once a diagnosis of muscular dystrophy has been made it is essential for the physiotherapist, occupational therapist and social worker (hospital or patch) to be involved in the team, with the doctor, so as to support and guide the parents through the various stages of the condition. There are many decisions for the family to make, and each needs to have all the facts put to them enough times so that the right conclusions can be made for that particular family. When a friendly relationship has been established it is easier to gain full co-operation and maximum help from the family for the suggested treatment plan. It must be remembered that parents are first and foremost mother and father, and that they will need help and support to achieve the right relationship with their child during treatment sessions.

The treatment of the child with muscular dystrophy is impossible without the parents' co-operation as it needs to be daily, and the majority of it will be carried out and organised by the parents. The physiotherapist needs to assess the agreed treatment at regular intervals to ensure that everything is progressing correctly and be able to plan ahead for the next stage.

EXERCISES

There has been much discussion over the years about the advisability of strong resisted exercises for the patient with muscular dystrophy. It was thought at one time that exercises to the affected muscles would accelerate the condition, but it has been found that resisted exercises (proprioceptive neuromuscular facilitation (PNF)) to those muscles can be beneficial, along with as much normal activity as the child can achieve during the day.

This, of course, will decline, and so exercises using balancing and strengthening techniques in standing, sitting, kneeling and lying can be used. All daily living activities such as feeding, dressing and toileting must be watched so that the parents can be encouraged to let the child do as much for himself at each stage, and for as long as possible. It may be necessary to raise the height of the bed, chair and toilet so that movement from one place to another is easier. Rising from the floor is achieved by the child walking his hands up his legs (Fig. 26/1, p. 581) and this should be encouraged.

STRETCHING AND SPLINTING

Alongside the exercises, the parents need to be taught how to stretch the hips, knees and tendo calcanei; later shoulders, elbows and wrists will need to be stretched also to prevent or delay development of contractures. This must be done daily and must be forceful if full range is to be maintained, and walking continued for as long as possible. Usually, as the condition progresses, flexion at the hips and forward tilting of the pelvis occurs, and the feet take on an equinus position. At first the range of movement in the ankles can be maintained by passive stretching and splinting. The splinting may take the form of:

serial plasters to increase the range gradually,

plaster of Paris night splints, or

by polypropylene ankle-foot orthoses (AFOs) for day or night wear.

Over-correction of the foot can cause the child to reject the splints due to the discomfort.

Another means of helping to obviate hip flexion is through prone lying for 20–30 minutes a day in a good position over a wedge with the feet dorsiflexed. This could be done during a play period or while watching television so that it does not become too tedious or encroach into schooltime.

RECREATION

Advice needs to be given on suitable leisure activities so that they can be continued when the child becomes chairbound, and where possible they should be a means of exercise as well, including swimming and riding. At a later stage the latter may be difficult due to lack of balance and poor chest expansion, but as with all recreational activities they need to be optional. Other suitable activities include fishing, TV games, photography, stamp collecting, chess, bird watching and CB radio.

HOME ADAPTATIONS

Home adaptations need to be considered *before* problems occur and walking is abandoned. The height of the bed, chairs and toilet are critical for independence, and in the later stages for parents when lifting, so must be continually checked. A board with a firm mattress under it can make movement and handling easier. For some of the larger modifications to the home it is necessary for the therapists, social services and local housing authority to be involved in the planning with the family. The width of doorways, the obstruction caused by steps and stairs, the accessibility to living room, kitchen, bedroom, bathroom and toilet all need to be considered. Discussion should take place over the provision of hoists, ramps, lifts, rails, bath inserts, support bars around the toilet, and, possibly in the later stages, some form of moulded seat. There are special sectional bead mattresses available that will relieve pressure areas and minimise the number of times the parents will be called to turn their son during the night. The provision of an alarm can also make night care easier.

Parents need to be aware of what is available to help them, and discussion should take place frequently as they are only able to absorb so much at a time.

SCHOOL

During the ambulatory phase there can be problems in school, and the staff are usually grateful for support from parents and therapists over the amount of help required, the child's capabilities in a PE class and for recreational periods. If the right kind of relationship can be built up with the teaching staff, and contact maintained regularly, this can help when there are problems to be solved, by the teaching staff contacting the therapists, yet always keeping the parents involved. While the child is on his feet the local school can usually manage, but as the weakness increases the child may become vulnerable; failing physically he withdraws into himself and education suffers. At this early stage of education and at the comprehensive stage when most schools are just not geared for a wheelchair, special schools may need to be investigated.

LIFTING

Parents, school staff and school helpers need to be taught how to lift the child. Often it is quicker to lift than wait for the child to perform the movement, but this should be discouraged for as long as possible. The principles of lifting should be explained and holds demonstrated so that from the early stages there is an awareness of the problems of lifting and the damage that can be caused by using the wrong movements. Showing how the child can roll into a bed, and the use of sliding boards and hoists, can also help lessen possible damage to the handler's back.

PROLONGATION OF AMBULATION

The age at which walking becomes impossible varies from as young as 7 years or as old as 13. Walking should be encouraged for as long as possible bearing in mind the child's emotional state and the family's views. The longer the child is on his feet the less is the likelihood of contractures and spinal deformity occurring. Prolongation of walking may be obtained by releasing the tendo calcanei which allows the feet to be maintained at right angles in orthoses which support the lower limbs. Careful assessment is required if orthoses are to be used as there needs to be sufficient power round the hips to maintain the standing/walking position, and the degree of hip and knee contracture will also influence this. Discussion with the family is essential, explaining the purpose of the orthoses and the extent of walking likely to be achieved, so that by the time the child reaches the point of coming off his feet the decision should have already been made to try the use of surgery and orthoses. Delay at this stage waiting for surgery with the child wheelchair bound for a month or two may mean that he will not become ambulant again.

SURGERY AND ORTHOSES

Surgery consists of a percutaneous tenotomy. Long-leg ischial-bearing walking plasters are applied to the legs while on the

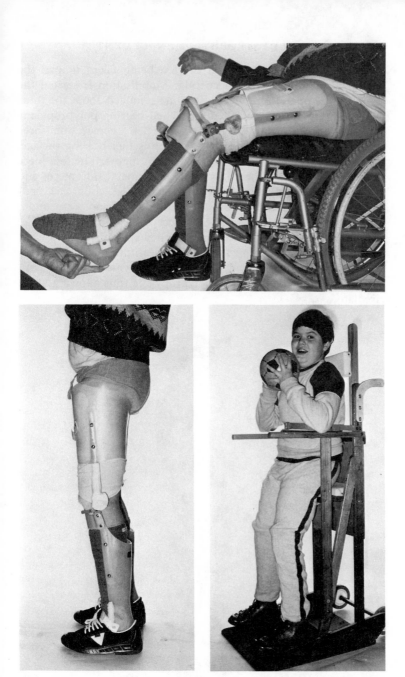

FIG. 27/1 (a) Lateral view of polypropylene knee-ankle-foot orthosis (KAFO); (b) Ischial bearing in KAFOs; (c) Cosmetic appearance and use of standing chair

operating table – a great deal of care being taken to pad the heel area to prevent sores occurring. Mobilisation is started the day after the operation. The plasters are removed about the third or fourth day and a cast taken for ischial-bearing polypropylene knee-angle-foot orthoses (KAFOs). These consist of three polypropylene sections: the thigh with an ischial-bearing surface, the foot piece, and a patellar-bearing knee support. The foot piece and knee support are joined by lightweight metal side-pieces and include a knee-locking mechanism which the child can control himself. The KAFOs are fitting into shoes and worn under trousers making them cosmetically acceptable to the child (Fig. 27/1). The KAFOs are fitted and supplied approximately a week after casting, by which time the child has learnt to walk proficiently in his plasters and the change-over to orthoses causes no problems. Holes may be drilled into the polypropylene thus allowing air to circulate.

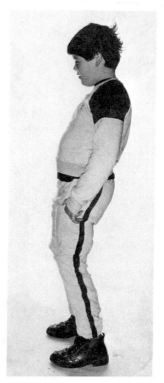

FIG. 27/2 Lordotic position of walking, thumbs holding the rims of the thigh pieces of the KAFO

The child must learn to balance and walk in a lordotic position, without using sticks or a walker as these encourage a forward pattern of movement and balance cannot be maintained. It is quite usual for the child to stabilise his position by tucking his thumbs into the top piece of the moulded thigh sections (Fig. 27/2). Walking is achieved by a rocking motion, the orthoses acting as rigid stabilisers. The length of time ambulation is increased is variable from a few months to three or four years. It is dependent on a number of factors:

1. The child's and the family's desire for ambulation.
2. The encouragement from school.
3. The distances that need to be covered.
4. The availability of equipment, which may need frequent adjustment.
5. The physical barriers that are encountered.

If prolonged ambulation is achieved, it can improve the child's well-being, enable easier handling and help control obesity.

If the feet are at right angles it is sometimes possible to prolong ambulation without surgery by using lightweight ischial-bearing polypropylene KAFOs as described above, but boots are needed to hold the feet in place. As the tendo calcanei tighten, the heels become painful and the orthoses will be rejected, but ambulation can be increased for up to two years in this way.

If there is a tendency to obesity, pinching can take place at the upper end of the thigh pieces. This may be helped by using a covering of ribbed stockinette underneath the polypropylene. Linings need to be washed daily and changed twice a day in hot weather. Due to the hardness of the polypropylene and the length of the KAFOs, and often a sagging chair canvas, changing position from sitting to standing and vice versa can cause pinching; a cushion with a firm base can alleviate this, also padding over the ischial area of the splint. The strength in the child's arms and trunk will determine whether he is able to stand up and sit down independently. The height of the furniture is also critical for this to be achieved, and more often than not help is required when changing from one position to another. A standing chair (Fig. 27/1c) is also beneficial in preventing contractures, allowing supported standing for part of each day. If schoolwork is to be continued in this position the correct height of the desk must be found as the child is unable to lean forward and maintain a standing position. It is essential that parents and school staff are aware of what the child is capable of doing as support from everyone is needed to keep the child mobile. It is important to recognise that when a wheelchair existence eventually becomes necessary there may be a period of depression.

SCOLIOSIS

The spine must be kept under continual review as a progressive scoliosis can cause problems, such as excess pressure under one ischial tuberosity, disturbance of balance, the inability to use one arm as it is acting as a prop and, eventually, as the scoliosis increases there is more likelihood of chest complications occurring. In the terminal stages, sitting for any length of time may be a great problem. Seating needs to be continually reviewed so that the best possible position is achieved as the child's condition changes.

A lightweight polypropylene thoraco-lumbar-sacral orthosis (TLSO), made from a plaster cast with the lumbar spine in a lordotic position, is worn as soon as the child is wheelchair bound and can prevent in some cases, and delay in others, the onset of the scoliosis. It is thought that the lordotic position locks the posterior articular facets preventing the forces causing scoliosis. The TLSO needs to be reviewed every 3 months, and, when re-made, radiographs should be taken in and out of the orthosis to monitor any changes in the spine (Fig. 27/3). If a scoliosis is developing, a pad can sometimes be introduced to correct the position of the spine by placing it on the inside of the TLSO at the apex of the curve and cutting out a hole on the opposite side (Fig. 27/3e). The orthosis must be worn all day. A well-fitting garment with minimal seams, longer than the TLSO – or a vest of ribbed stockinette, should be worn under the orthosis. In hot weather this can be changed during the day as the polypropylene causes excess sweating. The orthosis can also be ventilated by cut-out air holes. When head control becomes difficult a simple head-piece can be fitted to the TLSO (see Fig. 27/6) which can be slotted out and in as necessary to give support, particularly for car journeys where whip-lash injuries may occur on sudden stops. Scoliosis may also be treated surgically by means of the Lucque procedure.

FRACTURES

When walking in orthoses the child may trip and fall, and because of weakness in the arms may be unable to save himself. An arm

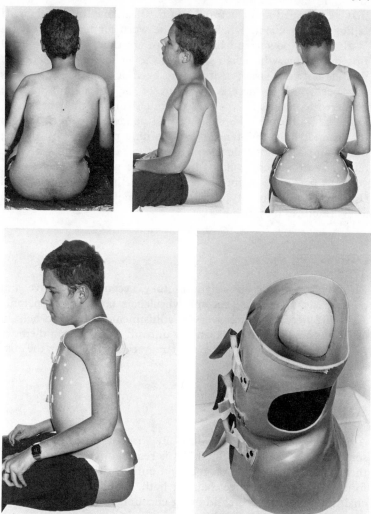

FIG. 27/3 (a) Posterior view of spine showing a scoliosis; (b) Lateral view showing disappearance of lumbar curve; (c) Posterior view in TLSO; (d) Lateral view in TLSO; (e) TLSO showing how further correction is obtained by adding a pad at the apex of the curve, and cutting a hole on the opposite side

may get trapped and fractured and the head may hit the floor. If falling is a problem, a helmet can be worn for head protection. With lack of power and balance there are times when the child tips out of his wheelchair or off the toilet/shower seat because there is no waist strap, or it has not been done up, and fractures may occur. When there is a fracture of the lower limb, and the plastered leg needs to be elevated while sitting in the wheelchair, individual adjustable leg-rests can be padded to cope with legs that cannot be straightened. In the sitting position with the leg raised and a scoliosis developing, pressure can be thrown on to one bony prominence, and if maintained a pressure sore can develop. A personalised cut-out chip-foam cushion can alleviate this (Fig. 27/4). As mobility decreases the bones become brittle and stress fractures may occur.

OBESITY

Most children put on weight as they become less active and particularly when they become wheelchair bound. The parents and child need guidance over the adjustment in diet and help in carrying this through. It is usually difficult when the child enjoys his food as both child and parent may compensate for the disability by over-feeding.

WHEELCHAIRS

As walking becomes more difficult, without or with orthoses, some alternative means of mobility is required for distances when the family are shopping or going on outings. This can be in the form of a buggy or wheelchair, or both. A self-propelled wheelchair may be used, the child being encouraged to do as much for himself as he can, thus helping to maintain chest expansion and muscle power for as long as possible. If the child is still on his feet he should not spend too much time during the day in the sitting position, as contractures can develop. When self-propelling the wheelchair becomes too difficult, a powered wheelchair can be investigated. Powered wheelchairs for use indoors are supplied by the local Artificial Limb and Appliance Centre (ALAC) on prescription from the consultant; for outdoor use there is a range of powered wheelchairs which are supplied by private firms.

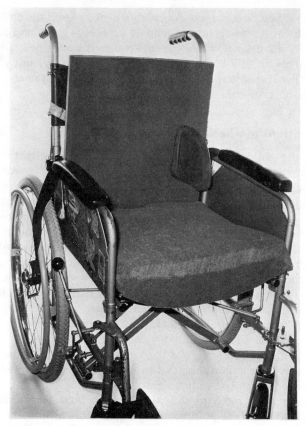

FIG. 27/4 Chip-foam cushion; the base has been curved to accommodate the sag on the seat canvas, and lateral support added to the back rest

It is essential that the correct fitting wheelchair is ordered so that a good sitting position may be maintained, with minimal room on either side of the chair to prevent the child sitting more to one side than the other. The feet should be supported at right angles (90°) so as to discourage the equinus position for as long as possible. The seat sides of the chair should be such that the elbows can be rested comfortably on them with the shoulders in a relaxed position to discourage side flexion of the spine and a slumped position. A safety waist strap should be fitted. Encouragement to the child to do as much for himself as possible overlaps into wheelchair management; propelling the wheelchair, and transferring need to be sustained. It is often easier and quicker for parents/school friends to help when it is not necessary and this should be discouraged. As independence lessens the child can still help with transferring as long as support is given and he can maintain his balance while the movement is performed. Rolling movements on to a bed are also useful to encourage, and sliding boards may be of help. The heights to be transferred to and from must be checked constantly.

Adaptations to wheelchairs

When the child is using his wheelchair continuously the seat cushion should be fitted with a firm base. This may be achieved by placing a board underneath the cushion and encourages a better posture by eliminating the sagging effect of the seat canvas. If this proves uncomfortable it can be replaced by a chip-foam cushion, the base of which has been curved to accommodate the sag on the seat canvas (Fig. 27/4). This cushion should be covered in a semi-permeable plastic Platilon which absorbs sweat but not urine and a loose-fitting stretch cover which maintains the contours. (Platilon is a registered trade mark of Platte Bonne G.mbH. – an elastic polyurethane film which is water vapour permeable.) To enable easier use of a urinal, a seat cushion can be provided with a cut-away in the front.

When the width of the seat is too wide for the child, the sides of the wheelchair should be padded to give hip support and help keep the pelvis central and straight.

A wide strap fitted to the wheelchair behind the calves can discourage the child pulling his feet back and behind the footplates into an equinus position. If this does not control the position, moulded footplates and straps can be added to the wheelchair footplates. Domestic seat sides, that is with the front half cut away, enable the wheelchair to be pushed closer to the table or desk. The back canvas should be high enough to support the shoulders and the angle between it and the seat should be close to a right angle (90°) to encourage a better sitting posture. When the child is wearing a TLSO, pressure may be caused by the lower edge of it pressing on the top of the thighs. This can be helped by keeping the back of the wheelchair as vertical as possible and fitting a wedged seat cushion higher at the back than the front, thus opening out the angle at the hip joints.

When the child uses a powered chair it is important that the position of the controller does not encourage a scoliosis or side flexion. If this is a problem, the chair can be fitted with a central control, usually a bar across the front of the chair which is regu-

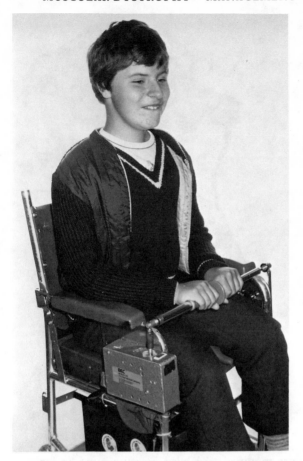

FIG. 27/5 Central control for powered wheelchair

lated by both hands (Fig. 27/5). If this type of control becomes too heavy to operate, a proportional box can be used with a remote controller positioned correctly for that child. Sometimes these controllers are attached to the wheelchair tray, but this can cause problems at mealtimes or when the child wants to sit with the family at table.

When the muscle power becomes poor and the child is unable to maintain his position in the wheelchair, lateral support may be added. This can be discreet, consisting of a padded curved metal plate, which conforms to the shape of the rib cage and is fitted to a curved back rest. Head support can be given by adding a simple extension head rest to the wheelchair or jacket (Fig. 27/6). When

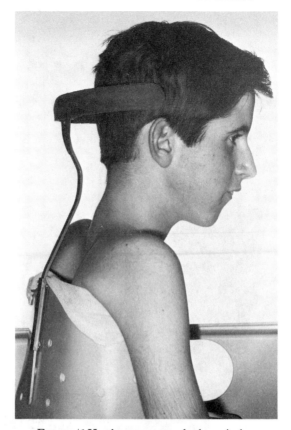

FIG. 27/6 Head support attached to a jacket

seating is modified, the head position must be looked at as the smallest variation can effect the head balance.

As arm power diminishes, hand and arm function can be assisted by arm supports or by the addition of a tray attached to the wheelchair. These need to be easy to connect so that they can be used as and when the problem occurs. If left to himself the child will find his own way around the problem – not always the best – but at least he will feel he does not look any different from his friends in wheelchairs and has overcome the fact that he is gradually getting weaker. Ball-bearing arm supports, supplied by ALAC, or the system of clamps, adaptors, poles and arm pieces (the Orange Aid System developed by Steepers), can be used and must be ordered *before* they are needed.

For the child/young adult who develops a severe scoliosis, the

TLSO will eventually cause problems and have to be discarded. At this stage various forms of cushioning, e.g. contoured or Temper-Foam (a visco-elastic foam) and wheelchair padding must be tried. (Temper-Foam or T-Foam is the trade name for a unique visco-elastic foam.) If this does not overcome the problems, a moulded wheelchair insert plus individual cushioning can be tried. A moulded 'breast plate' of flexible plastic sheet lined with Evazote (B. and L. Ltd.) can prove helpful attached to the moulded seat by adjustable straps. Sheepskin is another means of 'spreading the load' and may prove of use. It may well be that there is no one way of achieving a comfortable position, and it is possible that the child/young adult will need to spend periods of each day in the lying position.

CHEST COMPLICATIONS

As the condition progresses it becomes more and more difficult for the child to clear any chest secretions on his own, so breathing exercises, postural drainage and percussion of the chest and assisted coughing need to be taught to the parents, with backup from the physiotherapy department when it becomes necessary.

CLOTHING

Clothing needs to be loose, light and warm with a minimum amount of fastenings. Ponchos, or anoraks made into ponchos, the sleeves being set into the sides of the anorak, make useful outdoor wear. Lightweight waterproof capes and lap coverings are available. If the lower limbs are very cold, quilted leg bags and sheepskin muffs can be used for warmth. Footwear can cause problems when the feet are in an equinovarus position, but Plastazote boots made from a cast and covered with leather may overcome this problem.

AIDS TO DAILY LIVING

Bedding should be lightweight, duvet covers being ideal; a bed cradle can help in keeping the bedclothes away from the child and make movement in the bed easier. Mattresses have been mentioned on page 591.

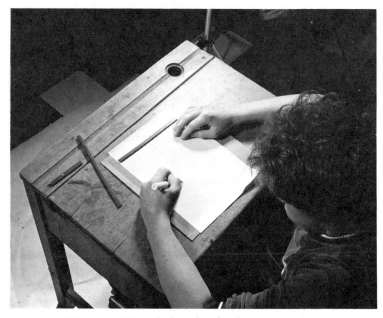

FIG. 27/7 Magnetic board and strip to secure paper

With increasing weakness the problems of function in school need to be thought about. Spring-loaded scissors make cutting easier. Magnets and metal sheets secure the paper while the child is writing, magnets attached to a ruler prevent the ruler from sliding (Fig. 27/7). Eventually electric typewriters, microwriters or computers with customised microswitches need to be investigated. While there is enough power, lazy tongs and croupier sticks may help with reach. Feeding is aided by lightweight cutlery and crockery and plastic straws for drinking.

Travelling in the car when balance is precarious is aided by the use of harness or moulded seating. Transferring into the car can be achieved with the use of a rotating seat which fits into some makes of car, or by hoists.

The Muscular Dystrophy Group of Great Britain, Nattrass House, 35 Macaulay Road, London, SW4 0QP (01-720 8055) is a very active and caring association made up mostly of parents and friends of those suffering with muscular dystrophy, with local groups for parents and the children. The group produces a series of books called *With a Little Help* which look at all aspects of the child with muscular dystrophy, and also publish pamphlets giving a description of the condition.

The Disabled Living Foundation (DLF), 380-384 Harrow Road, London W9 2HU (01-289 6111) runs a comprehensive aids centre where various aids can be demonstrated to parents and the handicapped youngster. They also have numerous publications about all the various aids available.

It is essential to be aware of the changes continually taking place in treatments and the research that is going on so that the best possible regime is found for each individual child.

BIBLIOGRAPHY

Dubowitz, V. (1978). *Muscle Disorders in Childhood*, Chapter 2. W. B. Saunders Co., Philadelphia.

Fowler, W. M. (1982). Rehabilitation management of muscular dystrophy and related disorders. II. Comprehensive care. *Archives of Physical Medicine and Rehabilitation*, **63**, 322-6.

Heckmatt, J. Z., Dubowitz, V., Hyde, S. A., Gabain, A. C., Thompson, N. and Florence, J. (1985). Prolongation of walking in Duchenne muscular dystrophy with lightweight orthoses. *Developmental Medicine and Child Neurology*, **27**, 149-54.

Hyde, S. A., Goddard, C. M., Scott, O. M. and Dubowitz, V. (1982). Prolongation of ambulation in Duchenne muscular dystrophy by appropriate orthoses. *Physiotherapy*, **68**, 4, 105-8.

Hyde, S. A., Goddard, C. M. and Scott, O. M. (1983). The myometer: the development of a clinical tool. *Physiotherapy*, **69**, 12, 424-7.

Hyde, S. A. (1984). Aspects of management of neuromuscular diseases of childhood. Association of Paediatric Chartered Physiotherapists, November Newsletter, 8-14.

Hyde, S. A. (1984). In *Paediatric Developmental Therapy*, pp. 180-94, (ed. Levitt, S.). Blackwell Scientific Publications Limited, Oxford.

Read, L. (1984). The management of scoliosis in Duchenne muscular dystrophy. Association of Paediatric Chartered Physiotherapists, November Newsletter, 2-7.

Robinson, R. O., Cartwright, R., Rockey, J. and Russell, P. (1984). Neuromuscular disorders and muscular dystrophy. In *The Physically Handicapped Child*, pp. 163-74, (ed. McCarthy, G. T.). Faber and Faber, Limited.

Scott, O. M., Hyde, S. A., Goddard, C. M. and Dubowitz, V. (1981a). Prevention of deformity in Duchenne muscular dystrophy. *Physiotherapy*, **67**, 6, 177-80.

Scott, O. M., Hyde, S. A., Goddard, C. M., Jones, R. and Dubowitz, V. (1981b). Effect of exercise in Duchenne muscular dystrophy. *Physiotherapy*, **67**, 6, 174-6.

Scott, O. M. (1984). The effect of increased activity in normal and diseased human muscle. Association of Paediatric Chartered Physiotherapists, November Newsletter, 15–17.

ACKNOWLEDGEMENTS

The author thanks the staff at Chailey Heritage Hospital for all their help in preparing this chapter, and the Department of Medical Photography and Illustration at the Royal Sussex County Hospital, Brighton for taking and developing the photographs. Thanks are also due to the parents and children for allowing the use of the photographs, and to the children for their patience while these were taken.

Chapter 28

Applied Psychology for Physiotherapists

by D. A. HILL BSc, MCSP, DipTP

During the last 15 years the subject of psychology has become increasingly more acceptable to those concerned with education of physiotherapists. The current debate is no longer whether or not we need psychology, but centres on how much psychology, at what stage in training, and in which areas the emphasis should exist.

The arguments have been lengthy, and sometimes heated. They have provided opportunities for educators with interests in discrete areas of psychology to press forward their own specialisms. Fortunately, in psychology, as in other subjects, the foundations of the subject do not change very much, only the refinements developed in the applications of psychology to specific contexts.

DEFINITION

Psychology may be defined as the study of behaviour and experience. Consideration of this definition reveals that there are few, if any, areas of human activity without a psychological component. The scope of the subject necessitates division into areas, and some of these areas are now listed.

Physiological psychology deals with the relationship between physiological processes and behaviour. Activity within the nervous system is closely related to behaviour, and neuropsychology is an important area of physiological psychology.

Comparative psychology compares behaviour between different animal species, and frequently correlates structural differences with differences in behaviour.

Social psychology studies the way in which members of a species, especially man, interact with each other.

Developmental psychology considers the changing processes in organisms as they mature, and whether such changes are due to inherited genetic factors or acquired environmental factors.

Educational psychology deals with those areas of study which have significant parts to play in the learning process, with some emphasis on children of school age.

Clinical psychology is concerned with the study and treatment of those members of society whose behaviour is abnormally undesirable, whether due to inherited or environmental factors.

Occupational psychology is the study of man in relation to his working environment, and deals with organisations in industry, hospitals, offices and the armed forces.

Human behaviour has attracted the attention of experts from many academic disciplines. Biologists, medical practitioners, philosophers, engineers, sociologists, physical scientists and mathematicians have all contributed to the fund of knowledge. It is not surprising, therefore, that various schools of thought have arisen in attempts to explain and ultimately predict human behaviour (Woodworth, 1970). The hard scientific approach of the behaviourist school attempts to explain behaviour in strictly definable and measurable terms and is not much concerned by notions of mind and consciousness which are difficult to define and measure. At the other extreme are the analytical schools which are mainly centred on Freudian psychology. Although at first the conflicting schools appear irreconcilable, deeper study frequently shows that they are looking at similar problems from different viewpoints, and it is unwise to accept blindly the teachings of any one school to the exclusion of all others.

DEVELOPMENTAL PSYCHOLOGY

Literature dealing with anatomical and physiological development reveals that the differences between child and adult are more than differences in body dimensions. Differences in body proportions and composition also exist. Likewise, differences in the quantity and quality of behaviour and mental experience are extensive. The physiotherapist working with children should be aware of these differences, and the approximate ages of transition of development from one stage to another, so that she can tell whether the child's failure to understand the world in adult terms is due to lack of maturity appropriate to the child's age, or due to genuine mental retardation.

A most valuable contribution to developmental psychology has come from Jean Piaget of Geneva (Beard, 1969). His work deals with the development of a child's understanding of the events which occur in the world around him. A brief description of the observed stages follows.

THE SENSORY MOTOR STAGE

This lasts from birth to 2 years. Early behaviour is mainly reflex-ive, and this implies that certain nerve pathways are innate, and the child arrives in the world with certain abilities (see Chapter 3). These innate reflexes combine to give more complex, purpo-sive movements during the first few months of life. The term 'sensory motor' is self-explanatory. The child responds to sensory stimuli with fairly specific motor responses. Towards the end of this stage the use of language and the development of play and imitation reveals that the child is developing real understanding, and not just responding reflexly.

THE PRE-OPERATIONAL STAGE

This lasts from 2 to 7 years. During this stage the child becomes increasingly skilled at handling objects in the material world, but his perception of these objects is still at a very different level from that of the mature adult. For example, if fluid from a container is poured into a container of a different shape, the child will state that the amount of fluid is either more than previously, or less than previously, but not the same. The conservation of volume with change of shape is not appreciated. Similarly it can be de-monstrated that there is lack of appreciation of conservation of mass and number. The rules of simple arithmetic as we know them are just not accepted. Evidence to date suggests that practice and training have little if any effect in speeding up a child's progress through this stage. Presumably one has to wait for appropriate neurological maturation.

THE CONCRETE OPERATIONAL STAGE

This follows and extends to the age of 11. The child now realises that properties such as weight, volume, number, mass, and area are conserved, even though dimensions of objects may be changed. In this stage the child also learns to classify groups of objects according to colour, size, shape and other properties.

THE FORMAL OPERATIONAL STAGE

This starts at 11 years. The child learns to transfer his knowledge and skill from concrete objects to ideas and concepts of a more abstract nature. For example, practical experience with weights and volumes gives rise to the concept of density or specific gravity. Generalisation of the properties of objects enables the child to appreciate scientific laws concerning such phenomena as buoyancy, the laws of reflection of light, and other laws of physics and chemistry.

The above stages demonstrate a progressive understanding of the properties of the physical world.

The development of moral and ethical values has also been studied by Piaget. He simply read stories to children in order to determine a child's sense of right and wrong (Brown, 1966). Children under 7 judge naughtiness by the consequences of an act while older children and adults tend to make moral judgements based on the intentions leading to the act. Thus a child who accidentally broke 15 cups was judged by young children to be naughtier than a child who broke 1 cup while stealing some jam. It is unlikely that a child possesses a conscience, or knowledge of right and wrong as understood by adults. He knows that certain acts will result in punishment if discovered. Distinguishing between different types of naughtiness is difficult for young children. They classify both swearing and the telling of untruths as lying. Both are undesirable forms of verbal behaviour, and therefore go together. As the child matures, the idea of reciprocity develops, in which the level of punishment is equated with the severity of the crime. By the time adolescence is reached ethical values are frequently well developed. Whole complexes of abstract ideas and concepts may be fervently advocated, and may be of a religious, political or social nature. Not only can the adolescent appreciate abstract concepts and laws concerning the material world, but he also feels strongly about how this material world should be manipulated for moral reasons in order to provide, for example, a socialist or a capitalist society.

Learning

Learning is the adaptive change in an organism as a result of experience. It is a change which is inferred because of changes in behaviour. The physiotherapist should be familiar with certain aspects of learning theory, since the majority of patients are required to learn at some stage in their treatment, whether it be breathing exercises, muscle strengthening, or re-education of walking. Some types of learning are more relevant to physiotherapy, and appropriate consideration of these types follows.

CLASSICAL CONDITIONING

This was studied in great detail by Pavlov. His best known experiment involved a bell repeatedly rung in the presence of a dog. Food was presented to the dog shortly after each bell ring. After several such episodes the dog salivated to the sound of the bell in anticipation of the food. Humans show evidence of classical conditioning. We may salivate at the sound of a dinner gong, or experience an increased pulse rate when we hear a police siren. We, in common with Pavlov's dogs, have learned to associate or pair stimuli and events, and the autonomic nervous system responds in a manner appropriate to the anticipated event. Many psychologists believe that classical conditioning plays an important part in attitude formation, and in this respect has some relevance to physiotherapy. Many patients are apprehensive, and a few are possibly terrified on their first visit to the department. The signs of stress will be demonstrated by the activity of the sympathetic nervous system. It is up to the physiotherapist to ensure that favourable attitudes are developed towards therapy. A friendly approach and a comfortable, effective treatment are essential in the early stages. Attitudes are rapidly formed and slow to decay. Imagine the attitude of Pavlov's dog if the bell had been followed by painful stimuli. Further sounds from the bell would have resulted in stress and anxiety.

OPERANT CONDITIONING

This has been investigated by B. Skinner. In this type of learning the organism works for a reward. A rat may learn to press a lever and be rewarded by a pellet of food. A child may run an errand and receive a tip. An adult will work for a month to receive a pay cheque. Operant conditioning involves the use of the voluntary skeletal muscle to create the conditions in which a reward is earned. The therapist can train the patient by operant conditioning to improve his skill level when voluntary movements are involved (O'Gorman, 1975). The most effective rewards will probably be praise and encouragement from the therapist and a realisation of improvement in the patient's condition.

AVOIDANCE CONDITIONING

This is a sophisticated term for punishment, and has little part to play in physiotherapy. The function of punishment is to suppress undesired behaviour, and although the therapist does not usually physically attack an unco-operative patient, it must be remembered that words and facial expressions of disapproval may act as avoidance conditioners, especially to sensitive patients. Punishment is unreliable as an avoidance conditioner, whereas operant conditioning by rewarding a correct response is usually highly successful (Wright and Taylor, 1972).

The three types of conditioning described are all examples of associative learning, in which specific stimuli are paired with specific responses. The timing of reward or punishment is critical. If presented long after the paired behaviour, the links may not be forged and learning will not occur. Consideration of conditioning processes in isolation gives the impression of man as a machine, responding when the appropriate button is pushed, but much evidence exists to suggest that man also learns with conscious understanding. Latent learning takes place when no apparent reward or punishment is involved. You probably know the make of your neighbour's car, the name of the pub at the bottom of your road, and the colour of the walls of the department in which you work. Such learning has gone in as an impression received and retained, simply by existing as part of your environment.

INSIGHT LEARNING

This occurs when the learner receives a flash of inspiration, which results in the solution of a problem. We all know the feeling when 'the pieces all fall into place'. Evidence exists to suggest that many higher mammals enjoy insight learning (Atkinson et al, 1981). Creativity is probably the most advanced form of mental activity, in which a series of mental processes result in a completely new solution to a particular problem in science, or a new form of expression in art, literature or music (Vernon, 1970). Because man is capable of the cognitive processes, the physiotherapist should explain in suitable terms the relevant details of the patient's pathology and the aims and objectives in treatment, in order to harness greater co-operation and higher motivation from the patient.

HABITUATION

This is a form of learning in which a repeated stimulus eventually produces a reduced response. For example, a doctor may take a patient's blood pressure two or three times, and the successive reductions in recorded pressures indicates habituation to the process of taking blood pressure. Patients will habituate to successive physiotherapy treatments and will co-operate more fully and perform at a higher level as their anxiety is reduced.

To return briefly to the theme of child development, we can now consider some of the learning processes involved during the process of socialisation, when the child acquires the accepted values, traditions, and behaviour norms of the culture in which he is reared, and acquires what we loosely refer to as a conscience.

The American sociologist, Talcott Parsons, has called the birth of new generations a recurrent barbarian invasion (Brown, 1966). Behaviourists claim that these barbarians become civilised by conditioning processes applied during maturation of the nervous system. Behaviour is shaped by various mixtures of rewards and punishment until culturally desirable behaviour is elicited. Love-oriented techniques, using the social rewards of praise and affection, and the withdrawing of these rewards for undesired behaviour, produce superior results to object-oriented techniques of tangible rewards and physical punishment. Superior, in that the children have fewer feeding and toilet training problems, and possess a stronger conscience, whereas physical punishment produces individuals low in self-esteem, aggressive and unfriendly (Atkinson et al, 1981). Innate tendencies to certain forms of behaviour do exist, but they can be profoundly modified by conditioning processes.

Biofeedback

During recent years psychologists have developed an interesting area of study known as biofeedback. Originally the term referred to studies in which it was demonstrated that it was possible to exercise voluntary control over certain bodily functions that had previously been described as involuntary. N. E. Miller and others demonstrated that animals could learn to control at will such functions as heart rate, blood pressure, diameter of arterioles, and contractions of the musculature of the digestive tract. Even EEG rhythms could be altered voluntarily.

Much research has now been conducted on human subjects, demonstrating that man can also learn to control these same physiological variables. All this is possible provided that, in the learning stage, rapid feedback of information concerning the physiological parameter under investigation is provided to the subject. These findings have obvious application in the control of some circulatory and neurological disorders such as hypertension, migraine and epilepsy (Harvey, 1978).

The realm of biofeedback has now been extended to include techniques which increase the level of control over voluntary muscles. Here the applications for physiotherapists include training in local and general relaxation, and in rehabilitation of patients suffering from conditions such as hemiplegia, spasmodic torticollis and peripheral nerve injuries (Hurrell, 1980; Skelly and Kenedi, 1982).

Many volumes have now been written on biofeedback, but one particularly useful introductory text, eminently suitable for physiotherapists, is that by Danskin and Crow (1981) (see p. 626).

It must be emphasised that feedback is information. Treatments involving biofeedback therefore increase the amount of information available to the patient, usually by means of sophisticated electronic apparatus. This additional information facilitates voluntary control by the patient.

Intelligence

It is a matter of common observation that some people are more clever than others. But when we attempt to define intelligence a hard-and-fast definition seems impossible. This is because intelligence is an abstract idea which is assumed to exist, and yet remains intangible. Such intangibles are known as constructs. We assess intelligence by observing intelligent behaviour. Hence the rather cynical definition that 'intelligence is what intelligence tests measure'. An intelligence test samples behaviour of individuals. Heim defines intelligence as 'grasping the essentials in a given situation and responding appropriately to them' (Child, 1977). The grasping cannot be assumed until the responding has been observed. Detailed consideration of intelligence testing and measuring is not appropriate in this chapter, and the interested reader should consult standard references (Vernon, 1964). One name which stands out in the history of intelligence testing is Binet, a Frenchman who devised test items which, with slight modifications, are still included in some current tests. Briefly, he identified abilities of average children of all age groups. He then measured the abilities of individual children, and described their mental ages according to the level of test items they could pass. Thus a child of chronological age 12 years who performed at the level of an average 9 year old would be said to have a mental age of 9. From this data the intelligence quotient could be calculated as

$$\frac{\text{Mental Age}}{\text{Chronological Age}} \times \frac{100}{1} = \frac{9}{12} \times \frac{100}{1} = 75$$

After the age of 16 years intelligence does not increase in the same manner as during maturation, but the idea of a spread of ability among the population persists. The precise ranges of scores in a population varies with the type of test, but as a broad generalisation two-thirds of the population have IQs between 85 and 115, the population mean being, by definition, 100. There is strong evidence indicating that intelligence is due to genetic, inherited factors to a much greater extent than environmental factors. For example, genetically identical twins reared apart have closer IQ scores than genetically different twins reared together (Mittler, 1971).

Spearmen identified a general (g) factor (Wiseman, 1967). This g factor contributes to all areas of intellectual activity. The result is that the more intelligent the individual is, the more likely he is to be above average in all areas of ability. In addition to the g factor, possession of specific abilities raises one's performance to higher levels in some areas than in others, so that some excel in maths, others in history or art.

The trained physiotherapist should remember that her proven ability in passing the pre-entry requirements for physiotherapy training, plus her ability to pass the qualifying examinations indicate that, together with other professional people, she is of above average intelligence. Her colleagues at school, work, and in social contexts are also probably of above average intelligence. But if the patients she treats form a typical cross-section of the community, half of them must by definition be of below-average intelligence. They will less easily understand the pathology of their condition and the principles of treatment. It is easy to interpret this inability as stubbornness or lack of co-operation.

Personality

Personality is that area of psychology most concerned with individual differences. When an acquaintance is described as generous, aggressive, kind, greedy or sulky, he is being compared with some mythical averages of these qualities, or behaviour tendencies, which exist in varying degrees in all individuals. Not only do individuals differ from each other in the strength of these tendencies, but the strength varies from time to time within the same individual. The behaviour tendencies are referred to as traits, and one of the aims of students of personality is to identify and measure such traits. Each trait adjective has an opposite, so that a person's score for kindness would exist on a dimension between kindness and cruelty.

Eysenck (1970a) has developed tests which identify two important traits on the dimensions of extroversion-introversion and stability-neuroticism. He describes extroverts and introverts as follows:

> The typical extrovert is sociable, likes parties, has many friends, needs to have people to talk to, and does not like reading or studying by himself. He craves excitement, takes chances, often sticks his neck out, acts on the spur of the moment, and is generally an impulsive individual. He is fond of practical jokes, always has a ready answer, and generally likes changes; he is carefree, optimistic, and likes to 'laugh and be merry'. He prefers to keep moving and doing things, tends to be aggressive, and loses his temper quickly. Altogether, his feelings are not kept under tight control, and he is not always a reliable person.

> The typical introvert, on the other hand, is a quiet, retiring sort of person, introspective, fond of books rather than people; he is reserved and distant except with intimate friends. He tends to plan ahead, 'looks before he leaps' and distrusts the impulse of the moment. He does not like excitement, takes matters of everyday life with proper seriousness and likes a well-ordered mode of life. He keeps his feelings under close control, seldom behaves in an aggressive manner, and does not lose his temper easily. He is reliable, somewhat pessimistic, and places great value on ethical standards.

The behaviour patterns of these two groups may be broadly summarised by saying that the extrovert seeks continuous stimulation, variety, and change, while the introvert avoids these. Eysenck proposes a neurological explanation of these behaviour patterns which should appeal to physiotherapists with their background of neurophysiology. Briefly, the extrovert has an underactive ascending reticular activating system, and he is, therefore, continually seeking stimuli to arouse and alert the cerebral cortex to optimum efficiency. The introvert has an overactive reticular system, and surplus stimuli result in over-arousal of the cortex, with consequent discomfort and loss of efficiency.

A strong case can also be presented for an organic basis of the stability-neuroticism dimension, with manifestations demonstrated via the autonomic nervous system.

These two independent dimensions can interact to give four extreme types. Thus there are neurotic introverts, stable introverts, neurotic extroverts and stable extroverts. Before the reader tries to force himself into one of these categories, it is important to stress that these groups are extreme, and the majority of the population are near to the centre of the dimensions. When large specific groups are studied certain tendencies can be observed. Physiotherapists tend to be slightly extroverted and slightly neurotic when compared with the population mean (Child, 1977). Such a person prefers contact with people and is anxious to do a good job. Physical educationalists, on the other hand, tend to be stable extroverts, which equips them for the stressful conditions of competitive performance (Kane, 1968 personal communication). Other professional groups also display typical personality profiles.

The neurotic extrovert displays hysterical symptoms of a physical nature when under stress. Examples are functional aphasia, hysterical paralysis, and asthma of psychosomatic origin. Such symptoms provide the individual with an escape route away from the stress-producing situation. Thus a man who is required to talk in his job can escape by precipitating aphasia, while a clerk would develop hysterical paralysis of his writing arm.

The neurotic introvert under stress is more likely to develop obsessional neuroses, which consists of unnecessarily repetitive behaviour which is time-absorbing and takes his thoughts away from the stress-or anxiety-producing circumstances. It will be appreciated that a neurosis is not so much an illness as an individual's personal solution to a problem. Furthermore, cure of the symptoms without removal of the stressful cause may result in substitution by an even more severely handicapping set of symptoms. Much tact must, therefore, be employed when treating neurotic patients. When the stress is removed spontaneous recovery frequently follows, but the symptoms may persist as habits, in which case they may be cured without risk of substitution.

Sometimes whole clusters of personality traits appear together to form a personality type. Combinations or clusters of traits can be detected by special tests designed to measure personality types. For example the authoritarian type demonstrates a clustering of patriotism, conservatism, prejudice, tough-mindedness and rigid thinking (Brown, 1966; Eysenck, 1970b).

The importance of early influences on the way in which adults behave is emphasised in an area of development in psychology known as Transactional Analysis. Advocates of this approach point out that our responses to verbal comments from others demonstrate three possible states within us, and that changes from one state to another are apparent in manner, appearance, words and gestures. The three states are known as Child, Parent and Adult and it is assumed that all three states exist in us, waiting to be elicited by appropriate stimuli.

The child is demonstrated by the type of reactions expected from a small child, such reactions being emotional in nature (Berne, 1970; Harris, 1973).

The parent is represented by beliefs and values which were received from parental figures, and internalised without being subjected to logical analysis.

The adult grows in us as a result of our ability to find out for ourselves, taking in data from the real world and submitting it to our own analytical processes.

When interacting with others, an individual's response may be that of the child, the parent, or the adult in him.

Psychotherapy based on transactional analysis usually aims at bringing out the adult in the patient. This does not mean that child and parent responses are always undesirable. Indeed, they provide much of the variety and richness in the quality of life. Treatment is only needed when they exhibit themselves so frequently and emphatically that they impair an individual's relationships and coping abilities.

If a therapist talks to a patient in the manner of parent to child, the patient may accept this relationship as appropriate, or he may resent it, thus erecting a barrier to further communication.

Motivation

Without a motivating or driving force the human organism is totally inactive. Something has motivated the reader to cast his eyes across this page! Motivations or drives may be regarded as inner forces compelling us to action. The hunger and thirst drives compel us to eat and drink. Without such drives we would soon die from malnutrition or dehydration. Such physiological drives ensure our continued survival. The sex drive ensures the perpetuation of the species. Once the biological drives are satisfied we have time for drives ensuring safety and comfort, such as seeking a warm, safe place to live and suitable clothes to wear. Social drives compel us to seek companionship, to obtain a sense of belonging, and to exchange love and affection with other people, and be respected by them. If the physiological and social drives are satisfied man can rise to higher drives in creative spheres and find satisfaction in art, music or other aesthetic or philosophical activities.

This brief description of drives suggests a hierarchical structure, and has been proposed by Maslow (1969). The higher drives are unlikely to receive attention unless the lower ones are satisfied. A man dying from starvation is unlikely to be appreciative of fine art or music. Similarly a patient deprived of the social satisfaction obtained from family and friends, and restricted to a ward bed, may show a regression in behaviour because his motivations have changed. If he is in pain his motivations may appear selfish, but will be concerned with escape from pain. When he is well on the way to recovery he may be more concerned with escape from hospital and the medical team can capitalise on the driving force. Most patients want to be breadwinners and homemakers, but the occasional patient finds life rather pleasant when the physiological drives of hunger and thirst are satisfied by the tender loving care of attentive young nurses. It is the task of the hospital team to shift his motivations higher up the hierarchical list. He should be encouraged to help in routine ward activities or sent to a convalescent or rehabilitation centre where a more independent lifestyle is possible and the circle of interests may be enlarged. It is imperative that during this stage the patient should experience feelings of success and achievement whenever progress is made towards greater independence. Praise should be meted out generously for each step forward, whether the patient is a young motorcyclist with a fractured femur, a middle-aged amputee or an aged hemiplegic. In many ways motivation is the core of psychology. Without it man is virtually lifeless. When present its nature determines our choice of behaviour.

THE ACQUISITION OF MOTOR SKILL

Definitions of skill are many and varied, some experts regarding almost every activity of any living creature as an act of skill. For the purposes of this chapter Guthrie's definition is the most suitable. Skill is defined as 'the learned ability to bring about predetermined results with maximum certainty, often with the minimum outlay of time or energy or both'.

If car driving is taken as an example of a skill, the highly skilled driver is more likely to complete the journey (predetermined result) in a relaxed manner (minimum energy) and shorter time than the learner driver.

Not all skills are 'learned' abilities in some senses of the word. A baby crawls and walks as a result of neurological maturation rather than learning but continued effort increases the ability level. We may, therefore, use the term maturational skill to describe crawling, walking or running as distinct from learned skills such as driving, cycling, swimming or using mechanical apparatus such as a camera or a piano.

The majority of students and practitioners of physiotherapy are more concerned with skill acquisition than with any other area of psychology. The student is required to learn to handle apparatus and equipment which is very unlike anything she has ever used before. In addition she must develop the skill of manipulating the body tissues of the patients in her care. The practitioner of physiotherapy is, in the vast majority of cases, concerned with encouraging the development of new skills, or reviving lost skills in her patient. The majority of treatment sessions include some form of exercise, and for this the co-operation and motivation of the patient are essential. But even with optimum motivation, much of the energy put into skill acquisition may be wasted if the therapist does not follow certain principles.

The first of the principles is guidance during the practice of the skill. Practice may be undertaken for one of three reasons – to acquire a new skill, to improve an existing skill, or to maintain an existing high level of skill. The student is concerned with the first two, the qualified therapist will be fulfilling the second throughout her daily routine, and may become involved with the first when new treatment techniques are introduced. The third reason concerns individuals at peak levels of performance of a skill, such as professional sportsmen or musicians. The patient may be concerned with the first two. Some patients may never have used the diaphragm correctly, and will, therefore, be concerned with a new skill, whereas other patients will be concerned with relearning (re-education) of existing skills such as walking.

Guidance of the learner is most important. Proper guidance results in quicker and more effective skill acquisition. Lack of guidance may mean that the skill learner will never realise his otherwise potential skill level (Knapp, 1967). Usually the initial guidance is verbal, that is an explanation of the nature and requirements of the skill. This should usually be followed by visual guidance, or demonstration, which will assist the learner by providing the opportunity of imitation. Finally, manual or mechanical guidance may be used, as when the teacher places her hands on the student's hands when teaching massage manipulations. Spring or weight-assisted exercises, and plaster slabs to enable patients to use their limbs, are all examples of mechanical guidance. Learning without guidance is learning by trial and error, and this is seldom satisfactory. The learning is slower and less effective, and the maximum possible skill level is seldom achieved. There is little to recommend 'being thrown in at the deep end'. Motivation will certainly be high, but the end result may be fatal!

Having got the learner practising with appropriate guidance, the teacher should provide a continuous feedback of information to the learner concerning progress. To modify a truism, 'practice with feedback makes perfect'. The patient learning to walk with crutches will require continual corrections in the early stages. Length of pace, timing of pace, position of head, general posture, weight on wrists, and many other points will need frequent attention. If the patient is sent to the far end of the gymnasium to practise on his own, the faults will become ingrained and may prove difficult to eliminate. The best feedback is praise for good performance whenever possible. Blame and criticism, if too frequent, are demotivating, and can cause the sensitive learner to give up completely.

The next considerations are spacing, duration, and timing of practice sessions. The optimum duration and frequency for maximum skill level may conflict with administrative desirability. If a new skill is practised for 10 minutes without a break the total gain in learning will probably be less than if the skill is practised for two sessions of 5 minutes. Learning by massed practice results in what is known as reactive inhibition, which reduces total learning (Eysenck, 1970a). Briefer periods of spaced practice suffer less in this way. Two 5-minute sessions of diaphragmatic breathing, or quadriceps exercises, although inconvenient because of time spent travelling by the therapist to and from the ward, will result in more total learning than one 10-minute session. Perhaps a compromise could be reached by going round the patients in a ward twice during one visit, spending less time during each treatment.

Transfer of skill must be considered in most learning situations. Transfer is concerned with what happens when a skill is practised in a different context. Strictly speaking it is impossible to repeat a movement. Even a simple repetitive task, such as throwing darts at a board results in different scores with successive throws. The goal may be the same on each occasion, but success at approximating to the goal varies due to minor modifications in the interpretation of perceptual cues, and variations in muscle action. In skill learning the aim is to achieve maximum positive transfer.

This will mean that skill will be performed at a high level even though the environment or stimulus situation is different. Many skill-training situations necessitate transfer. Air pilots are required to make their initial mistakes in a dummy cockpit before being trusted with a planeload of passengers. The extent to which the skills learned in the simulator can be utilised when placed in the real situation is a measure of the degree of positive transfer. Students practise massage and other therapeutic techniques on each other before they are allowed to treat patients. The greater the similarity between the practice environment and the treatment environment, the larger will be the amount of positive transfer. A student who has only practised a certain treatment technique on the left arm of a healthy, thin, young fellow student sitting on a chair will not enjoy much positive transfer when faced with treating the right arm of a sick, obese, elderly bedridden patient.

Transfer is also important from the patient's point of view. He may have learnt to walk up and down the gymnasium steps, which have a rise of 5 inches and a tread of 10 inches, and a handrail on the right. Confident that he can manage stairs, he is discharged. He then realises that his own stairs have a 7-inch rise, a 9-inch tread, a hand rail on the left and a spiral at the top. The importance of students and patients practising skills in different contexts is obvious, but this aspect of skill acquisition is frequently neglected.

Social skills

Social skills refer to communication abilities and are obviously of considerable importance to professionals who deal with patients in face to face relationships. The whole area of social skill training has been divided for purposes of description into separate subskills. These include skills which operate in interviewing situations, communication to groups and telephone skills.

The aims of such training are to enable the learner to identify and analyse specific social skills, to develop a critical awareness of the behaviours of self and others in interpersonal encounters, and raise the level of performance of such skills.

The range of skills covers non-verbal communication, such as eye contact, facial expressions, bodily gestures. Techniques of questioning, explanation, demonstration, reinforcement, listening and closure of communication are studied and practised. Practise may take the form of role-play in front of video cameras, which are then used to provide rapid feedback of performance standard. Two suitable texts for further information in this area are those by Hargie, Saunders, and Dickson (1981) and Ellis and Whittington (1981) (see p. 626).

Perception

Perception is sometimes considered to be synonymous with vision, but this is a rather limited view of what is really a wide-ranging and complex area of study.

The author chooses to define perception as the organism's interpretation of the environmental stimuli impinging on its sensory receptors. Much laboratory work in perceptual research has been performed on animals and the word organism embraces them. The environment includes internal and external environments. One fascinating area of perception deals with determination of innate perceptual abilities and acquired perceptual abilities. The nature-nurture controversy ranges throughout most areas of psychology. The philosophers Locke and James assumed that the neonate's perceptual awareness was analogous with a blank slate, waiting for impressions to be made by experience. 'A big, booming, buzzing confusion' was how James described the infant's consciousness (Vernon, 1970). Confusion was assumed to decrease as perceptual learning occurred. More recent work by skilled psychologists has demonstrated that the newborn infant possesses many perceptual abilities which earlier workers had been unable to detect. Recognition of human faces, distances, and other perceptual abilities either exist at birth or develop very rapidly (Gregory, 1977). Such abilities are rapidly lost if visual stimuli are absent or distorted, so an interaction between the organism and a normally stimulating environment is essential. There is also much evidence that cultural factors affect perception profoundly. Tribesmen reared in visually restricted jungle environments interpret small retinal images as being necessarily produced by small objects, instead of large distant objects. They are less susceptible to illusions involving straight lines typical of the Westerner's 'carpentered' environment.

The internal environment can also play perceptual tricks. Hungry subjects perceive pictures of food as brighter than other equally illuminated pictures. This is known as perceptual set, and similar forms of set affect us all far more than we normally realise. Southerners have a stereotyped picture of northerners and vice versa. Each will tend to perceive in the other that which they expect to perceive. A special form of set is perceptual defence. This occurs when we raise the threshold of perception to stimuli that we do not wish to be aware of, because we find them embarrassing or annoying. We turn a convenient subconscious blind eye if it suits us.

Pain

Pain is a topic which merits consideration in this chapter, for it is frequently the symptom which first motivates a patient to seek treatment. Relief of pain is often one of the primary aims in physiotherapy treatments. A proper understanding of the psycho-physiology of pain is therefore important.

It has been known for many years that pain impulses travel to the higher centres of the central nervous system via the lateral spinothalmic tracts. Melzack (1973) suggested the existence of a 'pain-gate' in the substantia gelatinosa region of the dorsal horn of the spinal cord. Activity in this area is responsible for suppression, amplification, or variation in the quantity and quality of pain experienced. Such activity is profoundly influenced by the psychological state of the patient.

The therapist should bear in mind that fear, stress, apprehension and ignorance concerning his condition can all increase the amount of pain actually experienced by the patient.

Emotion

Human emotions have interested man throughout history. The supposed anatomical sites of the origin of emotions have varied through the ages from the womb, heart, guts and spleen until present-day theories developed by electrical stimulation techniques point to the brain as the seat of emotion. The mid-brain and hypothalamus are the pleasure centres, while stimulation of discrete regions of the temporal lobe gives rise to feelings of anger and rage.

Brain damaged patients frequently appear in the physiotherapy department and emotional disorders are sometimes present in a subtle form, and may even be wrongly attributed to distress concerning the accompanying physical symptoms such as those of hemiplegia or Parkinson's disease. But depending on the specific areas of brain involvement, signs of depression, anger, distress and weeping, euphoria and rapid swings of mood can be directly due to brain damage. To complicate the issue even further, the displayed behaviour may not even match the mood experienced. Some hemiplegics display uncontrolled weeping even though they report feeling quite cheerful. Close relatives will sometimes report changed moral values in the patient. He may have started telling lies or stealing. The therapist will tend to assume that the patient has always been so inclined unless informed to the contrary.

The physiotherapist is not concerned with treatment of the psychologically abnormal unless she is employed in a hospital unit which specially caters for such patients, in which case she would be well advised to attend courses and refer to books dealing with the psychologically abnormal. For those readers who are interested some suitable textbooks are recommended. Much controversy exists even between experts in the complex area of abnormal psychology. Analytic techniques aim at probing the mental life of the patient and restructuring the personality brick by brick, while behaviourists consider many behaviour disorders as consequences of faulty learning, and the treatment consists of eradication of such learning by avoidance conditioning and substituting correct learning by operant conditioning. The efficiency of treatment frequently seems to be more related to a satisfactory relationship between the patient and clinician than to any particular treatment technique!

Stress

Few people are unaware of the increasing attention paid to stress by psychologists and the medical world generally. We all experience periods of stress from time to time, and stress is blamed for much of the unhappiness in today's technological society. Yet to define stress poses certain problems. Definitions vary depending on the angle from which stress is being considered.

Some definitions are stimulus based. For example, stress can result from extremes of temperature, pain, hunger, or noise. Varying the level of stimulus is therefore equated with varying the level of stress. Other definitions are response based, and variations in responses such as heart rate and blood pressure are taken as indications of changes in stress levels. A more complex but more useful model is one in which stress is regarded as an imbalance between the perceived demands being made on an individual, and the perceived coping ability of the individual (Cox, 1978). According to the model, if a man does not realise that he cannot cope, he will not be stressed. On the other hand, if he is capable of coping, but thinks he cannot cope, he will be stressed.

The conscious state and perceptions of the individual are therefore most important.

Cox continues by describing some of the many pathologies which can arise from continued uncontrolled stress, such as cardiac disease, disorders of the digestive tract, and other psychosomatic disorders. Management of stress may include the following: reduction in the demands being made on the individual, increasing the individuals coping ability, counselling, and the use of certain drugs.

Relaxation techniques have also played a major role in stress management (Mitchell, 1984).

With progress in neurology and biochemistry more and more mental disorders are being recognised as physiological in origin, and the controversy over cause and appropriate treatment recedes.

The day may come when it will be possible to explain all psychology in terms of physiology, but it may not prove to be the most useful and productive way of explaining behaviour. A multidisciplinary approach to the study of man results in a balanced rounded view of homo sapiens, the organism at the top of the evolutionary tree.

REFERENCES

Atkinson, R. C., Atkinson, R. L. and Hilgard, E. R. (1981). *Introduction to Psychology*, 8th edition. Harcourt Brace Jovanovitch, New York.

Beard, R. M. (1969). *An Outline of Piaget's Developmental Psychology*. Routledge and Kegan Paul Limited, London.

Berne, E. (1970). *Games People Play: Psychology of Human Relationships*. Penguin Books, Harmondsworth.

Brown, R. (1966). *Social Psychology*. (Free Press, US). Collier Macmillan, West Drayton.

Child, D. (1977). *Psychology and the Teacher*, 2nd edition. Holt-Saunders, Eastbourne.

Cox, T. (1978). *Stress*. Macmillan Press, London.

Danskin, D. G. and Crow, M.A. (1981). *Biofeedback: An Introduction and Guide*. Mayfield Publishing Company, USA.

Ellis, R. and Whittington, D. (1981). *A Guide to Social Skill Learning*. Croom Helm, London.

Eysenck, H. J. (1970a). *Fact and Fiction in Psychology*. Penguin Books, Harmondsworth.

Eysenck, H. J. (1970b). *Uses and Abuses of Psychology*. Penguin Books, Harmondsworth.

Gregory, R. L. (1971). *Eye and Brain: The Psychology of Seeing*, 3rd edition. Weidenfeld and Nicholson, London.

Hargie, O., Saunders, C. and Dickson, D. (1981). *Social Skills in Interpersonal Communication*. Croom Helm, London.

Harris, T. A. (1973). *I'm O.K. - You're O.K.* Pan Books, London.

Harvey, P. G. (1978). Biofeedback - trick or treatment? *Physiotherapy*, **64**, 333.

Hurrell, M. (1980). Electromyographic feedback in rehabilitation. *Physiotherapy*, **66**, 293.

Knapp, B. (1967). *Skill in Sport*. Routledge and Kegan Paul Limited, London.

Maslow, A. H. (1969). *Toward a Psychology of Being*. Van Nostrand Reinhold Co Limited, Wokingham.

Melzack, R. (1973). *The Puzzle of Pain*. Penguin Books, Harmondsworth.

Mitchell, L. (1984). Relaxation and stress. In *Cash's Textbook of General Medical and Surgical Conditions for Physiotherapists*, pp. 115-30, (ed. Downie, P. A.). Faber and Faber, London.

Mittler, P. J. (1971). *The Study of Twins*. Penguin Books, Harmondsworth.

O'Gorman, G. (1975). Anti-motivation. *Physiotherapy*, **61**, 6, 176-9.

Skelly, A. M. and Kenedi, R. M. (1982). EMG biofeedback therapy in the re-education of the hemiplegic shoulder in patients with sensory loss. *Physiotherapy*, **68**, 2, 34.

Vernon, M. D. (1970). *Psychology of Perception*. Penguin Books, Harmondsworth.

Vernon, P. E. (1964). *Intelligence and Attainment Tests*. University of London Press.

Vernon, P. E. (1970). *Creativity*. Penguin Books, Harmondsworth.

Wiseman, S. (1967). *Intelligence and Ability*. Penguin Books, Harmondsworth.

Woodworth, R. S. (1970). *Contemporary Schools of Psychology*. Methuen and Co Limited, London.

Wright, D. S. and Taylor, A. (1972). *Introducing Psychology: An Experimental Approach*. Penguin Books, Harmondsworth.

BIBLIOGRAPHY

Brearley, G. and Birchley, P. (1986). *Introducing Counselling Skills and Techniques. With Particular Application for the Paramedical Professions*. Faber and Faber, London.

Dunkin, E. N. (1981). *Psychology for Physiotherapists*, The British Psychological Society and Macmillan Publishers Limited, London.

Gillis, L. (1980). *Human Behaviour in Illness: Psychology and Interpersonal Relationships*. Faber and Faber, London.

Rachman, S. J. and Phillips, C. (1975). *Psychology and Medicine*. M. T. Smith, Hounslow, Middlesex.

Shakespeare, R. (1975). *The Psychology of Handicap*. Methuen and Company Limited, London.

Spielberger, C. (1979). *Understanding Stress and Anxiety*. Harper and Row, London.

Williams, M. (1979). *Brain Damage, Behaviour and the Mind*. John Wiley and Sons Limited, Chichester.

ACKNOWLEDGEMENT

The author thanks Mrs G. Dick of the University of Ulster for her secretarial assistance.

Glossary of Neurological Terms

agnosia   inability to recognise a perceived object
akinesia   difficulty in initiating movement (common in Parkinson's disease)
Alzheimer's disease   a frequently occurring degenerative brain disease of later life, producing dementia
amyotrophic lateral sclerosis   motor neurone disease, *q.v.*
amyotrophy   muscle wasting
aneurysm   an expanded segment of an artery. In the brain, its rupture causes subarachnoid haemorrhage
aqueduct stenosis   congenital blockage of the pathway for cerebrospinal fluid in the brainstem: an important cause of hydrocephalus
arachnoiditis   inflammation of the leptomeninges; a cause of spinal and nerve root disorders
astereognosis   inability to perceive shape by touch
astrocytoma   the most important primary brain tumour of adults; a glioma, *q.v.*
basal ganglia disorders   movement disorders due to disease of basal ganglia, e.g. parkinsonism, athetosis, chorea, dystonia
brachial neuritis   pain in an arm due to irritation of a cervical nerve root
Brown-Séquard syndrome   weakness on one side, loss of pain and temperature sensation on the other, due to damage to one side of the spinal cord
bradykinesia   slowed voluntary movement, as in Parkinson's disease
catatonia   freezing of movement. Occurs in Parkinson's disease
Charcot joints   severely damaged joints resulting from loss of pain sensation

Charcot-Marie-Tooth disease peroneal muscular atrophy

chorea fidgety involuntary movements due to basal ganglia disease. Huntington's chorea is an inherited degenerative brain disorder with chorea and dementia

clonus rhythmic rapid repetitive muscle contraction, associated with increased tone

Creutzfeldt-Jakob disease a dementing disease of adults due to a transmissible agent

Déjèrine-Sottas disease a form of hypertrophic peripheral neuropathy

dementia loss of mental function

demyelinating disease disorders – like multiple sclerosis – in which the white matter of brain and spinal cord is damaged

dermatomyositis inflammatory disease of muscle, with skin involvement

diplegia, congenital weakness and spasticity, present from birth, affecting all limbs but legs more than arms

Down's syndrome mongolism. A chromosomal abnormality and most important cause of mental retardation

dysmetria incorrect placing of limbs in testing of cerebellar function, due to cerebellar disorder

dysphagia difficulty in swallowing

dystrophia myotonica slowly progressive muscular dystrophy in which myotonia, q.v., may be prominent

embolism, cerebral a blood clot from elsewhere in the circulation blocking an artery in the brain; one of the causes of a stroke

encephalopathy disorder of the brain substance, producing coma and fits, with many causes

ependymoma tumour of brain and spinal cord, often benign

extrapyramidal disorders synonym for basal ganglia disorders

facio-scapular-humeral dystrophy mild variety of muscular dystrophy mainly affecting face and shoulder muscles

fasciculation visible involuntary contraction of bundles of muscle fibres; may be a prominent feature of motor neurone disease

fibrillation involuntary contraction of individual muscle fibres; visible in tongue

general paresis of the insane meningo-encephalitis occurring in the late stages of syphilis, and producing dementia

glioma the most important group of brain tumours, derived from the connective tissue (glia) of the brain

Guillain-Barré syndrome an acute form of polyneuritis, from which recovery usually occurs

haematoma, intracerebral blood clot in the brain

haematoma, subdural or extradural blood clot inside the skull, compressing the brain

haemorrhage, cerebral bleeding into the brain, causing a stroke. Subarachnoid haemorrhage is bleeding into the coverings of the brain

hemianopia loss of half of the field of vision

hemiballismus violent involuntary movements of a limb

hemiparesis weakness of one side of the body

hypertonia increased muscle tone

hypertrophy increased size (e.g. of muscle, nerve)

hypotonia decreased muscle tone

infarction, cerebral death of brain tissue following blockage of the artery supplying it with blood; one cause of stroke

Kugelberg-Welander disease late onset, relatively benign form of spinal muscular atrophy, *q.v.*

Landry's paralysis old term, often regarded as synonymous with Guillain-Barré syndrome

leuko- (as in leukoencephalitis) affecting the white matter of brain

limb girdle dystrophy moderately severe variety of muscular dystrophy, affecting shoulder and pelvic-girdle muscles

medulloblastoma important malignant cerebellar tumour of children

Ménière's disease disease of the inner ear in middle life, causing giddiness and deafness

meningioma tumour of coverings of brain and spinal cord, usually benign

meningo-encephalitis inflammation of the brain and its coverings

monoparesis weakness of one limb

motor neurone disease fatal, progressively paralysing disease of adults due to degeneration of motor nerve cells

myasthenia gravis muscle disease in which weakness results from blockage of transmission of nerve impulses to muscle

myelitis inflammation of the spinal cord

myoclonus brief shock-like involuntary muscular contraction

myopathy disorder of muscle, producing weakness, and resulting from many causes

myotonia state of persistence of muscle contraction and slowed relaxation after a voluntary movement

neuralgic amyotrophy pain, weakness and wasting in shoulder muscles due to inflammation of cervical nerves

neurofibroma benign tumour of nerve

neurofibromatosis (von Recklinghausen's disease) congenital disorder with skin pigmentation, multiple neurofibromas and other abnormalities

neuromyelitis optica demyelinating disease affecting optic nerves and spinal cord

nystagmus jerky movement of eyes caused by inco-ordination of eye muscles

ocular myopathy variety of muscular dystrophy in which eye movements are affected

oligodendroglioma slow-growing form of glioma, *q.v.*

ophthalmoplegia paralysis of eye movements

optic neuritis inflammation of optic nerves

paraparesis weakness of both legs

polio- (as in poliomyelitis) referring to grey matter of brain and spinal cord

polymyositis inflammatory disorder of muscle

progressive muscular atrophy variety of motor neurone disease, *q.v.*

psychosis severe mental disorder affecting thought processes, e.g. schizophrenia

quadriparesis weakness of all four limbs

radiculitis inflammation of nerve roots

Refsum's disease inherited form of polyneuropathy due to defective lipid metabolism; a cause of hypertrophic neuropathy

retrobulbar neuritis inflammation of optic nerves

Schilder's disease white matter disease of various causes, producing brain damage in children

schwannoma benign nerve sheath tumour, similar to neurofibroma, *q.v.*

scotoma area of defective vision

spinal muscular atrophy group of inherited disorders of motor nerve cells producing wasting and paralysis of muscle

stereognosis tactile perception of shape

striatal disorders basal ganglia disorders, *q.v.*

subacute combined degeneration of cord demyelinating disorder of spinal cord, affecting mainly legs, due to vitamin B_{12} deficiency

subacute sclerosing panencephalitis slowly progressive, usually fatal encephalitis due to persistent measles virus infection

syringomyelia   cavitation of spinal cord producing loss of function in limbs

tabes dorsalis   inflammation of nerve roots occurring in late stages of syphilis, affecting function of limbs, eyes and bladder

tetraparesis   quadriparesis, *q.v.*

torticollis   contraction of neck muscles, sustained or spasmodic, resulting in tilt of head

vertebrobasilar insufficiency   impairment of blood supply to the brainstem, often due to cervical spondylosis

Werdnig-Hoffmann disease   fatal form of spinal muscular atrophy, *q.v.*, in infants

Wernicke's encephalopathy   damage to central areas of grey matter in brain, due to vitamin B_1 deficiency, affecting eye and limb movement

Wilson's disease   inherited disorder affecting copper metabolism, producing basal ganglia disease and dementia

Select Bibliography

In addition to the references and bibliography at the end of most of the chapters, the following is a select list of titles which could be used for further background reading. The current editions are listed, but most textbooks are regularly updated and the reader should check whether there has been a new edition. This can be ascertained by asking the librarian at the hospital or postgraduate centre library, or by checking in Whittaker's *Books in Print* which is to be found in the reference section of all public libraries.

Aids to the Examination of the Peripheral Nervous System (1976). HMSO, London.

Aids to the Investigation of Peripheral Nerve Injuries, 2nd edition revised. HMSO, London.

Bobath, B. and Bobath, K. (1975). *Motor Development in the Different Types of Cerebral Palsy*. William Heinemann Medical Books Limited, London.

Draper, I. T. (1980). *Lecture Notes on Neurology*, 5th edition. Blackwell Scientific Publications Limited, Oxford.

Gloag, S. (1985). Needs and opportunities in rehabilitation. *British Medical Journal*, **290**, 43–6; 132–6; 220–3; 301–3; 368–72; 455–7; 542–4; 699–701; 768–71; 834–7; 913–15; 981–3; 1059–62; 1135–8; 1201–3; 1333–6.

Graham, J. (1981). *Multiple Sclerosis: Self-help Guide to its Management*. Thorsons, Wellingborough.

Greer, R. (1982). *Diets to Help Multiple Sclerosis*. Thorsons, Wellingborough.

Guyton, A. C. (1981). *Basic Human Neurophysiology*. W. B. Saunders Co, Philadelphia.

Holt, K. (1977). *Developmental Paediatrics*. Butterworths, London.

Hosking, G. P. (1982). *An Introduction to Paediatric Neurology*. Faber and Faber, London.

Illis, L. S., Sedgewick, E. M. and Glanville, H. J. (eds.) (1982). *Rehabilitation of the Neurological Patient*. Blackwell Scientific Publications Limited, Oxford.

Jay, P. (1984). *Coping with Disability*, 2nd edition. Disabled Living Foundation, London.

McCarthy, G. T. (ed.) (1984). *The Physically Handicapped Child. An Interdisciplinary Approach to Management*. Faber and Faber, London.

McKeran, R. O. (1986). *Diagnosis and Management of Nervous Disorders*. Blackwell Scientific Publications Limited, Oxford.

Marshall, J. (1976). *The Management of Cerebrovascular Disease*, 3rd edition. Blackwell Scientific Publications Limited, Oxford.

Matthews, W. B. and Miller, H. (1979). *Diseases of the Nervous System*, 3rd edition. Blackwell Scientific Publications Limited, Oxford.

Pact, V., Sirotkin-Roses, M. and Beatus, J. (1984). *The Muscle Testing Handbook*. Little Brown, Boston: Quest, London.

Robinson, G. (1980). *Multiple Sclerosis: Simple Exercises*. Multiple Sclerosis Society, London.

Rose, F. C. (ed.) (1984). *Progress in Motor Neurone Disease*. Pitman, London.

Walton, J. N. (ed.) (1981). *Disorders of Voluntary Muscle*, 4th edition. Churchill Livingstone, Edinburgh.

There is a useful series of books on equipment, aids, wheelchairs and other items for disabled persons. They can be obtained from: Equipment for the Disabled, c/o Mary Marlborough Lodge, Nuffield Orthopaedic Centre, Headington, Oxford OX3 7LD.

A full list of titles is available from this address – a stamped addressed envelope should be enclosed for a reply.

Useful Organisations

Of necessity this is only a select list of organisations and agencies which can offer help, advice and counselling. Mostly they relate to the conditions mentioned in this book. A useful guide book for extensive information about many organisations is the *Directory for the Disabled* edited by A. Darnbrough and D. Kinrade and published by Woodhead-Faulkner, Cambridge CB2 3PF. It is regularly updated. The reference departments of many public libraries now contain much information relating to the disabled; similarly post offices and Citizens Advice Bureaux carry lists of local and national organisations and self-help groups.

Disabled Living Foundation
380–384 Harrow Road
London W9 2HU   01-289 6111

Royal Association for Disability and
Rehabilitation (RADAR)
25 Mortimer Street
London W1N 8AB   01-637 5400

Consultant Assessment Service for
the Disabled
c/o R. Jefcoate Esq
Willowbrook, Swanbourne Road
Mursley, Bucks MK17 0JA   029672 533

Physically Handicapped and Able
Bodied (PHAB)
42 Devonshire Street
London W1N 1LN   01-637 7475

Association to Aid Sexual and
Personal Relationships of Disabled
People (SPOD)
286 Camden Road
London N7 0BJ   01-607 8851

Riding for the Disabled Association
Avenue R, National Agricultural Centre
Kenilworth
Warwickshire CV8 2LY   (Coventry) 0203 56107

British Sports Association for the Disabled
Stoke Mandeville Stadium
Harvey Road, Aylesbury
Bucks HP21 8PP   (Aylesbury) 0296 27889

Leonard Cheshire Foundation
26–29 Maunsel Street
London SW1P 2QN   01-828 1822

ACTIVE (with the Toy Libraries
Association)
68 Churchway
London NW1 1LT   01-387 6592

Possum Controls Limited
Middlegreen Road, Langley
Slough, Bucks SL3 6DF   Slough 79234

SEQUAL (Formerly Possum Users
Association)
The Bungalow, 31A Northfield Close
South Cave, N. Humberside
HU15 2EW

Chest, Heart and Stroke Association
Tavistock House North, Tavistock Square
London WC1H 9JE   01-387 3012

Multiple Sclerosis Society of Great
Britain and Northern Ireland
25 Effie Road
London SW6 1EE   01-736 6267

Action for Research into Multiple
Sclerosis (ARMS)
71 Gray's Inn Road
London WC1X 8TR   01-568 2255

Parkinson's Disease Society
36 Portland Place
London W1N 3DG   01-323 1174

Spinal Injuries Association (SIA)
76 St James' Lane
London N10 3DF   01-444 2121

Motor Neurone Disease Association
38 Hazelwood Road
Northampton NN1 1LN   0604 22269

Spastics Society
12 Park Crescent
London W1N 4EQ   01-636 5020

Bobath Centre
5 Netherall Gardens
London NW3 5RN   01-794 6084

Association for Spina Bifida and
Hydrocephalus (ASH)
Tavistock House North, Tavistock
Square
London WC1H 9HJ   01-388 1382

Muscular Dystrophy Group of Great
Britain
35 Macaulay Road
London SW4 0QP   01-720 8055

The International Cerebral Palsy
Society
5a Netherall Gardens
London NW3 5RN   01-794 9761

Scottish Council on Disability
Princes House, 5 Shandwick Place
Edinburgh EH2 4RG   031-229 8632

Scottish Spinal Cord Injury Association
3 Cargill Terrace
Edinburgh EH5 3ND   031-552 8459

Scottish Spina Bifida Association
190 Queensferry Road
Edinburgh EH4 2BN   031-332 0743

Scottish Council for Spastics
22 Corstophine Road
Edinburgh EH12 6HP   031-337 9876

Multiple Sclerosis Society in
Scotland
27 Castle Street
Edinburgh EH2 3DN   031-225 3600

Chest Heart and Stroke Association
(Scotland)
65 North Castle Street
Edinburgh EH2 3LT   031-225 6527

Northern Ireland Council for the
Handicapped
Information Service for Disabled
People   *Information Service*
NI Council of Social Service   Belfast 649555
2 Annadale Avenue
Belfast BT7 3JH   Belfast 640011

Demonstration and Aids Centres

DHSS Demonstration Centres
DHSS, Alexander Fleming House
London SE1 6BY

Joint Aids Centres Committee
c/o Medical Aids Department
British Red Cross Society
76 Clarendon Park Road
Leicester LE2 3AD   0533 700747

Professional groups

The following are Specific Interest Groups of the Chartered
Society of Physiotherapy. Anyone interested should write to the
secretary of the relevant group, c/o the Chartered Society of
Physiotherapy, 14 Bedford Row, London WC1R 4ED.

Association of Chartered Physiotherapists with a Special Interest
  in Neurology

Association of Paediatric Chartered Physiotherapists

Association of Community Physiotherapists

Riding for the Disabled

Index